The Bud Tender

The Bud Tender

by
Linda Broadway

The Bud Tender is a comprehensive reference guide that sheds light on how herbal alternatives are helping people cope with various conditions. *The Bud Tender* explains illnesses and ways to relieve the symptoms. The International Classification of Diseases, Tenth Revision (lCD), is an excellent reference for the profiling of medical conditions, and is useful to medical doctors, recreational, medical dispensaries and caregivers. Herbal alternatives can play a significant role in coping with the symptoms of many medical conditions that interfere with the normal function of everyday life.

Copyright © 2018 by Linda Broadway.

Library of Congress Control Number:		2018902600
ISBN:	Hardcover	978-1-9845-1170-6
	Softcover	978-1-9845-1171-3
	eBook	978-1-9845-1172-0

All rights reserved. No part of this book may be reproduced or transmitted in any form or by any means, electronic or mechanical, including photocopying, recording, or by any information storage and retrieval system, without permission in writing from the copyright owner.

Any people depicted in stock imagery provided by Getty Images are models, and such images are being used for illustrative purposes only. Certain stock imagery © Getty Images.

Print information available on the last page.

Rev. date: 11/23/2018

To order additional copies of this book, contact:
Xlibris
1-888-795-4274
www.Xlibris.com
Orders@Xlibris.com
763152

Enjoy reading the history of herbal medicine and the healing property.

This book is dedicated to my creative husband, Robert B. Taylor, whom I share my life with and my loving family.

Indica strains

These are sedatives relaxants are useful for treating the symptoms of medical conditions such as anxiety, chronic pain, insomnia, muscle and tremors. Indica has a higher level of cannabinoids than saliva, which results in a sedated-body-type stone. Because indica strains may cause a feeling of sleepiness and heaviness, many consumers prefer to medicate with this type of cannabis at night.

Sativa strains

Sativa is more of a stimulant and are useful in appetite stimulation also, relieving depression, migraines, chronic pain, and nausea. Sativa has an antrorse level of tetrahydrocannabinol (THC) than indica, which results in a psychoactive and energetic mind—high. Because saliva may cause feelings of alertness and optimism many consumers prefer to medicate with this type of cannabis during the day.

Tetrahydrocannabinol (THC)

Tetrahydrocannabinol (THC) is the first compound responsible for the psychoactive effects of cannabis. The mixture is a mild analgesic, and cellular research has shown that the compound has an antioxidant breakdown. THC is believed to obtrude with parts of the brain typical controllers by the endogenous cannabinoid neurotransmitter and anandamide. Anandamide is thought to play a role in pain sensation, memory and sleep.

Caryophyllene

Caryophyllene are part of the mechanism by which medical/recreational cannabis has been shown to reduce tissue inflammation is via the compound B-caryophyllene. A cannabinoid receptor called CB2 plays a vital part in reducing inflammation in humans and other animals. B-caryophyllene has been shown to be a selective activator of the CB2 receptor. B-caryophyllene is primarily concentrated in cannabis essential oil. This CB2 and B-caryophyllene contains about 12-35 percent caryophyllene.

Three main classification types are Hybrid, Indica, and Sativa cannabis.

Cannabis has three primary categories:

1. Hybrid cannabis (50/50) strains give a balance of head and body calmness.
2. Indica-dominant hybrid cannabis provides a full-body pain relief and a relaxing high.
3. Sativa-dominant hybrid, cerebral high with a relaxing body effect, provides physical and mental relief.

Hybrid cannabis strains are perfect for people who suffer from autoimmune diseases, insomnia and depression.

Cannabis ruderalis, another type of cannabis, grows wild in parts of eastern Europe and Russia. Cannabis ruderalis grows better in colder weather. Ruderalis plants have lower percentages of THC.

These hybrids are auto-flowering strains. Because of the short flowering period of Cannabis ruderalis, growing period is two to three weeks with highest level Cannabidiol (CBD).

Cannabis sativa is a strain originated in the tropical countries of Columbia, Mexico, Thailand and Southeast Asia and thrive in warmer weather. Sativa leaves are much narrower and are typically a lighter shade of green.

Sativa plants can grow to a height of up to twenty feet when raised outside, for a longer more extended (flowering) it can take ten to sixteen weeks to mature. Because the growing time is so long sativa plants produce much higher yield, about three ounces to one pound per plant but has a lower THC percentage around 12-16 percent.

Sativa plants have an incredibly strong aromas of sweet and fruity to peppery to earthy smell of diesel fuel.

Cannabis sativa is suitable for mental and behavioral stress anxiety, depression and Attention Deficit Hyperactivity Disorder (AFHD). Cannabis sativa is known for uplifting, cerebral high, energizing, stimulating, laughing and engaging in deep conversations and being very analytical and creative.

Butane hash oil is also known as BHO or butane honey oil. This concentrated form of cannabis split up the essential oils of the cannabis plant from the plant. The result is tremendously strong resembling beer and steep liquor plant.

A portion of butane hash oil should be the size of a grain of rice. For first-time users, use half a pellet. If you accidentally take too much, you are going to have a bad day if you don't recognizable the concentrates of(butane hash oil (BHO).

Vape Oil (concentrates) are essentially concentrated cannabis oil. Carbon dioxide (CO_2) extracted cannabis oil that's refined with organic ethanol which means no chemicals, lipids, waxes or impurities.

The Bud Tender overview includes a detailed explanation of each stage of the plant production and supply chain process, including

- breeding
- cloning
- cultivating
- vegetation
- flowering
- harvesting and drying
- trimming
- curing
- packaging
- distribution.

Quality control and testing are included in our outcome safety plan and monopolizing plant matter for manufacturing edibles.

The Bud Tender cultivation plan describes a hydroponic drip ground plan. This technique gives a plant literally what, when and the amount it needs to be as healthy as possible while meeting sustainability. The plant has to be as hardy as is genetically possible while also meeting sustainability target.

Dab are concentrated butane hash oil, wax honey oil, dangerous Tetrahydrocannabinol (THC) nights is often compared to hard alcohol of the cannabis universe. Dabs come in many forms. Dabs are extracted and concentrated into potent wax forms that are essential oils and waxes of the cannabis plant.

Dabs are known for their high concentration of Tetrahydrocannabinol (THC). Smoking a dab is much stronger than burning bud. You must be a regular cannabis consumer with high tolerance. Proceed with extreme caution.

Some extracts that have not been purged correctly can contain small amounts of butane. Carbon Extracts (CO_2) oil is often noted as the safest oil because critical extraction machines use Carbon Dioxide Extracts (CO_2) as the only water extract in it.

Marijuana that's accepted in some states has been opened to the extensive range of cannabis both medicinal and recreational.

The Bud Tender inform the patient and the public of the different psychoactive effects of cannabis and how it affects you.

INDICA

Indica is short and stout in composure and will grow two to four feet tall and yield smaller crops (1.5 to 2.5 ounces) per plant and higher quality plants (18 percent) Tetrahydrocannabinol (THC) than sativa.

Cannabis indica is believed to have originated in the Middle East (Pakistan and Afghanistan) and thrive in colder weather.

Cannabis indica strains are typically darker green leaves. The buds are thick and dense. Flowering takes about anywhere from eight to twelve weeks to grow.

The flavors and smell of cannabis indica is pine, pungent skunk, earth, hash or a sweet and sugary fruit flavor.

Cannabis indica has been known to relieve stress, full body pain, muscle spasms, anxiety, and nausea. To induce relaxation to stimulate appetite and to combat sleep deprivation.

Diseases like fibromyalgia, lupus, multiple sclerosis, and insomnia tend to benefit from the effects of indica.

Quality control and testing are included in our outcome safety plan and monopolizing plant matter for manufacturing edibles.

The Bud Tender cultivation plan describes the technology and facility designs to simplify and streamline the hydroponic growing process. The hydroponic design content represents today's advanced indoor growing systems for sustainable plant production. There are many different ways to grow the primary cultivation method is outdoors or greenhouse.

The hydroponic section includes topics on

- hydroponic facility setup
- innovative growing systems
- advanced lighting setups
- organic nutrients and additives
- organic growing medium
- nonharmful pest and disease control
- environmental controls
- irrigation systems and controls
- propagation and cloning
- postharvest
- cannabis indica strains

Acquired Hypothyroidism: Hashimoto Thyroiditis is a disruption that does not let the Thyroid Gland make sufficient Thyroid hormone. The Thyroid Gland is found in the neck and shaped like a butterfly.

Acute Gastritis: sudden swelling or inflammation of the covering of the stomach. It causes severe and nagging pain.

Adrenal Cortical Cancer (ACC): Cortical Carcinoma is a rare disease. It is caused by a cancerous growth in the adrenal cortex which is the outer layer of the Adrenal Glands.

Agoraphobia: fear of being outside or various things one cannot escape or from which escaping would be awkward or humiliating.

AIDS-Related Illness: people with Acquired Immune Deficiency Syndrome (AIDS) have weakened immune systems. People with AIDS are more prone to infections called opportunistic infections. These organisms attack when there's an opportunity to infect.

Alcohol Abuse: previous psychiatric diagnosis in which there is a recurring harmful use of ethanol despite its negative consequences.

Alcoholism: also known as Alcohol Use Disorder (AUD). Alcohol dependence syndrome is a broad term for any drinking of alcohol that results in problems.

Alzheimer Disease: mental destruction that can occur in midlife or advancing years. Because of a general deterioration of the brain most common cause of premature senility.

Amphetamine Dependency: because of the frequent and long-term use of this drug some people become dependent faster than others.

Amyloidosis: is a rare disease that results from an accumulation of inappropriately folded proteins. These misfiled proteins are called amyloids.

Amyotrophic Lateral Sclerosis (ALS): also known as Lou Gehrig disease and charcot disease. A particular disorder that involves the death of neurons.

Angina Pectoris: also known as stable angina the medical term for chest pain or discomfort because of coronary heart disease.

Ankylosis: Immobility and consolidation of a joint because of disease, injury and surgical procedure. Ankylosis may be caused by the destruction of the membranes that line the joint or by a weak bone structure that can be a result of chronic rheumatoid arthritis.

Anorexia: eating disorder characterized by low weight fear of gaining weight and a strong desire to be thin and food restriction.

Anorexia Nervosa: has physical and emotional components that require the attention of different health care providers such as primary care physicians, mental health counselors, psychologists and psychiatrists.

Arteriosclerotic Health Disease: thickening and hardening of the walls of the coronary arteries as a result of invasion and accumulation of white blood cells.

Arthritis: joint pain will occur if there is damage because of disease or trauma. The illness or injury will interfere with normal movement of the joint and produce pain.

Arthritis Rheumatoid: chronic inflammatory disorder that typically affects the small joints in your hands and feet. Rheumatoid arthritis can affect the lining of your joints that cause a painful swelling that can eventually result in bone and joint erosion. Rheumatoid arthritis occurs when your immune system inadvertently attacks your own body's tissues. Rheumatoid arthritis sometimes can affect other organs of the body such as the skin, eyes, lungs and blood vessels.

Arthropathy: gout is a form of arthropathy that involves inflammation of one or more joints.

Asthma: is a common chronic inflammatory disease of the airways characterized by variable and recurring symptoms reversible airflow obstruction and bronchospasm.

Attention-Deficit hyperactivity disorder (ADD/ADHD): similar to a hyperkinetic disorder which is a neurodevelopment psychiatric disorder in which there are significant problems.

Autism/Asperger: Brain Disorder is when communication and interaction with others is involved.

Autoimmune Disease: develops when your immune system attacks healthy cells in the system that defends your body against disease.

Back Pain: pain in the back that usually originates from the bones, muscles, nerves, joints and the spine. Also, Gallbladder and Pancreas may also refer pain to the back. Most back pain is felt on the lower end to other areas.

Back Sprain: injury to either a muscle or a tendon. The tight fibrous bands of tissue that connect muscle to bone. With back pressure, the muscles and tendons that support the spine are twisted, pulled or torn.

Bells' Palsy: a form of facial paralysis resulting from a dysfunction of the cranial nerve VII (the facial nerve) causing an inability to control facial muscles. Most often the eye on the affected side cannot be closed. The eye should be protected from drying up, or the cornea may be permanently damaged resulting in impaired vision. This condition is a rapid onset of partial or complete paralysis that often occurs overnight. Bell's palsy is defined as a unilateral facial nerve paralysis of unknown cause. Several other conditions can also cause facial paralysis brain tumor, stroke, myasthenia gravis, and Lyme Disease.

HYBRID

HYBRID

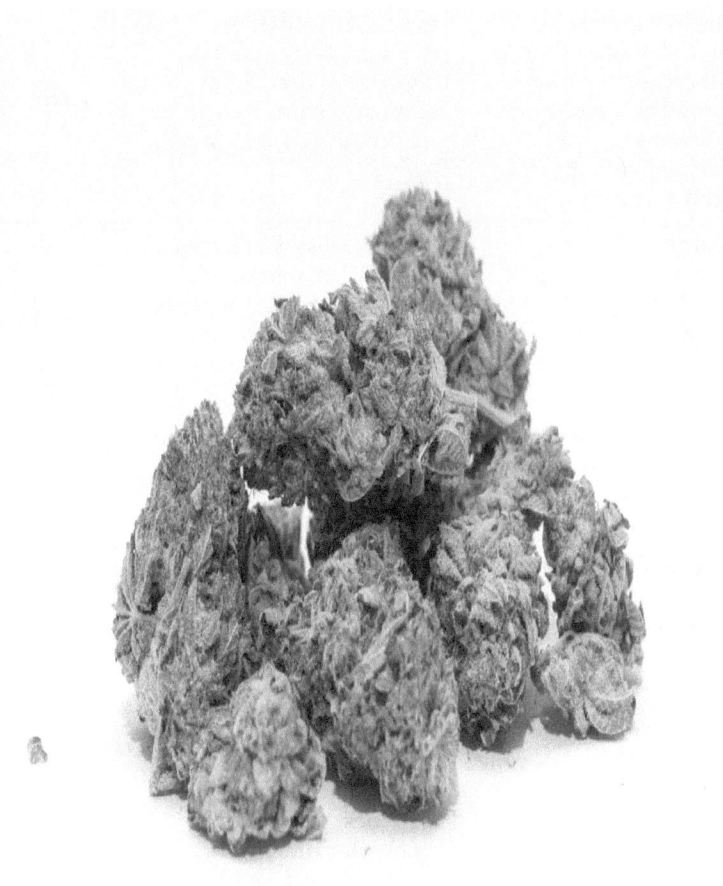

HYBRID

Medical Conditions	Symptoms	Desired Effects	Flavored Scents
Acquired Hypothyroidism: conditions in which your thyroid gland doesn't produce enough of certain hormones. Hypothyroidism cause many health problems such as infertility, joint pain, heart disease and obesity.	Fatigue, increased sensitivity to cold, constipation, dry skin, feeling sad or depressed, tired, joint or muscle pain, muscle weakness and weight gain.	Arousal	Dank
Acute Gastritis: abrupt inflammation or swelling of the stomach lining, can cause nagging and severe pain.	Appetite loss, black stools, indigestion, nausea and bloody vomiting that looks like used coffee grounds. Pain in the upper part of the abdomen.	Creativity	Earthy
Adrenal Cortical cancer/ Carcinoma (ACC): rare disease.	Increased facial, body and hair, particularly in females. Will deepened voice in women	Energy	Fruity
Agoraphobia: is a phobia of unrelenting fear of a situation, activity or thing that one cannot escape or avoid.	Enclosed spaces like bus, bridges, elevator, movie theaters, train and airplane. Leaving home along and crowds or waiting in line.	Euphoria	Hash
Alcohol Abuse: recurring harmful use of ethanol despite its adverse consequences	Tolerance withdrawal, loss of control, desire to stop but can't, neglecting other activities, alcohol takes up greater time, energy and focus and continued use despite negative consequences.	Happiness	Pink
Alcohol Use Disorder: (AUD) and alcohol dependence syndrome	Can't go a day or even two days without drinking alcohol.	Happiness	Minty
Alzheimer Disease: the progressive mental decline that can occur in middle- aged or geriatrics because of widespread decaying of the brain.	Constant questions or conversations, misplacing personal belongings, forgetting events, appointments and getting lost on a familiar route.	Serenity	Skunks

Amphetamine Dependency: a potent stimulant that is used medically to keep a person alert as in narcolepsy. Health problem for people that fall asleep at times.	Decreased appetite, breathing, dry mouth, dilated pupils, euphoria, fatigue increased energy, alertness and increased blood pressure.	Sleepiness	Spicy
Amyloidosis: is a rare disease with no cure. Amyloidosis occur with a substance called amyloid build up in an organ. Amyloid is a protein that is produced in your bone marrow and can deposit in any tissue or organ that will affects the digestive tract, heart, kidneys, liver nervous system and spleen.	Patients with amyloidosis can result from abnormal functioning of the bowels, hear, kidneys, liver, nerves, skin and lungs.	Upliftedness	Woody
Angina Pectoris: is known as stable angina, chest pain or discomfort due to coronary artery disease.	Chest pain, squeezing, burning or fullness, dizziness, fatigue, shortness of breath, sweating and nausea. Pain in your arms, neck, jaw, shoulder or back accompanying chest pain.	Serenity	Skunks
Ankylosing: is an inflammatory disease of the vertebrae of the spine. Fusing makes the boneless moveable and can cause hunched - forward posture, affecting the ribs and making it difficult to breathe deeply.	Can affect the cartilage between the breastbone, hips, pelvis (sacroiliac), lower back (vertebrae), shoulder joints, spine, ligaments and tendons attach to bones (entheses).	Sleepiness	Spicy
Anorexia: a eating disorder characterized by low weight, fear of gaining weight fear of increasing heaviness a strong desire to be thin.	Fearful of the slightest weight gain and takes all precautionary measures to avoid weight gain and becoming overweight.	Upliftedness	Woody
Anorexia Nervosa: can be a physical and emotional illness that requires the attention of primary care physicians, mental health counselors, psychologists and psychiatrists.	Individuals with anorexia display varying symptoms. Mostly obviously associated with malnutrition such as abnormally low body weight, exhibit depression and solitude.	Happiness	Minty

Any Chronic Medical condition: is referred to a mental health condition that last 6 months to years.	Recognizing health problem and unusual pattern in your day to day living.	Serenity	Skunks
Arteriosclerotic Health Disease: is a narrowing of the arteries due to plaque buildup on the artery walls.	There is no symptoms only when a plaque ruptures or the blood flow is very restricted. Over the course of years for this to occur, causing chest pain, coughing, difficulty breathing, extreme anxiety, facial numbness, feeling faint, paralysis, renal arteries and vomiting.	Sleepiness	Spicy
Arthritis: joints are associates of the bones that allow flexibility and movement. Joint pain will occur if there is damage because of disease or trauma. The illness or injury will interfere with normal movement of the joint and produce pain.	Inflammation in the hands, feet, knees and ankles	Upliftedness	Woody
Arthritis Rheumatoid: is a chronic inflammatory disorder that typically affects the small joints in your hands and feet. Eventually results in bone erosion.	Tender, warm, swollen joints, morning stiffness that may last for hours. Firm bumps of tissue under the skin on your arms (rheumatoid nodules), fatigue, fever and weight loss	Happiness	Minty
Arthropathy: gout arthritis is a form of arthropathy that involves inflammation of one or more joints.	Gout can affect the joints of the feet, ankles, knees, wrists, fingers and elbows. Gout can be confused with other forms of arthritis.	Hunger	Pink
Autism/Asperger: is a brain disorder in which communication and interaction with others are involved.	Autism may fluctuate from total lack of communication with others to difficulty in understanding others' feelings.	Sleepiness	Spicy

Autoimmune Disease: develops when your immune system which defends your body against infection, decides your healthy cells are foreign. As a result your immune system attacks healthy cells.	Autoimmune diseases usually go between periods of remission (little or no symptoms) and flare-ups (worsening symptoms).	Upliftedness	Woody
Back Pain: in the back that usually originates from the muscles, nerves, bones, joints or other structures in the spine.	Back pain can be a sharp piercing or burning feeling. The pain may travel into the arms and hands as well as the legs or feet.	Upliftedness	Minty
Back Sprain: injury to either a muscle or a tendon. With back strain the muscles and tendons that support the spine are twisted and pulled or torn.	Pain that worsens with movement, muscle cramping or spasms (suddenly uncontrollable muscle contractions). Decreased function and range of motion of the joint.	Hunger	Pink
Bell's Palsy: a form of facial paralysis resulting from a dysfunction of the cranial nerve. Sometimes the affected side will not be closed. Permanent damage resulting in an impaired vision of this condition is a rapid onset of partial or complete paralysis. That often occurs overnight.	The facial nerve controls some functions, such as taste sensations, blinking and closing the eyes, smiling, frowning, lacrimation, salivation, flaring nostrils and raising eyebrows and two-thirds of the tongue chords.	Serenity	Skunks
Bipolar Disorder: also known as a bipolar affective disorder and manic-depressive illness with periods of elevated mood swings and periods of depression.	Mania is the defining presence of bipolar disorder and can occur with different levels of grimness.	Sleepiness	Spicy
Brain Tumor cancer: disease of the brain in which cancer cells occur in the tissue of the brain.	Difficulty walking, dizziness, seizures, weakness and headaches	Minty	Woody
Bruxism: chewing, grinding of the teeth because of clenching of the teeth other than eating.	Dehydration, anxiety, gum disease, tongue problems and headache	Happiness	Minty

Bulimia Nervosa: This mental illness is characterized by episodes of bingeing and somehow purging the food and weight loss.	Uncontrollable overeating, inability to stop eating, eating until a person has physical discomfort and pain.	Hunger	Minty
Cachexia (cancer): marked weight loss, muscular loss, resistant to natural therapies. Difficulties in performing routine activities and fatigue.	Fatigue, physical disability along with a loss of skeletal muscle mass. The sudden or gradual appearance of weight loss in any individual is highly unusual.	Serenity	Skunks
Cancer: types include breast, lung, colon, skin, prostate and ovarian cancer.	Has no symptoms, signs and symptoms only appear as the mass continues to grow or ulcerates.	Sleepiness	Spicy
Carpal Tunnel Syndrome: (pinched nerve) known as the arm and hand condition that causes numbness, tingling and other symptoms.	Carpal tunnel syndrome is a pinched nerve.	Upliftedness	Woody
Cerebral Palsy: is the inability of movement of the muscle tone and posture that is caused by damage that occurs in the immature developing brain often before birth.	Signs of cerebral palsy can be during infancy or preschool years. Noticing the impaired abnormal reflexes, floppiness, a rigidity of the limbs, trunks, posture with unsteady walking, eating, speaking and picking up a crayon or spoon can be difficult.	Happiness	Minty
Cervical Disc Disease: degeneration common cause of neck pain most frequently felt like a stiff neck.	Cervical disc pain that is usually related to activity and will flare up at times or the pain will go away entirely.	Hunger	Pink
Cervicobrachial Syndrome: common cause of neck pain most frequently felt like a stiff neck. Cervical degenerative disc disease is far less common than disc degeneration in the lumbar spine.	As we mature the cervicobrachial changes occur in the body which becomes weaker, fragile and has thin cartilage.	Serenity	Skunks

Chemotherapy: often abbreviated to chemo, a category of cancer treatment that uses chemical substances especially one or more anticancer drugs.	Some of the most common side effects of chemotherapy involve the digestive tract, mouth sores and dry mouth can make it difficult to chew and swallow.	Sleepiness	Spicy
Chronic Fatigue Syndrome: significant fatigue that can't be explained by any initial medical specification. The fatigue may decline with physical or mental activity but doesn't improve with rest.	Loss of memory or concentration, feeling unrepressed after sleep, muscle pain, headaches, multijoint pain, persistent sore throat without redness or swelling and tender lymph in your neck and armpits.	Minty	Woody
Chronic Pain: often pain lasting more than twelve weeks. Whereas, acute pain is a normal feeling.	Pain that won't go away as expected after an illness or injury, pain that may be described as aching, burning, shooting or electrical.	Happiness	Minty
Chronic Renal (kidney) failure: the gradual loss of kidney function. Kidneys filter wastes and excess fluids from your blood and then excreted in your urine. When chronic kidney disease reaches a progressive stage dangerous levels of fluid, electrolytes and wastes can build up in your body.	Natural bruising, muscle twitching or cramps, breath odor, blood in the stool and excessive thirst.	Hunger	Pink
Cluster Headaches: can awaken you in the middle of the night causing penetrating pain around one eye on one side of your head.	Agonizing pain generally located in or around the eye but may radiate to other areas of your face, head, neck and shoulders (one-sided pain).	Serenity	Skunks

Cocaine Dependence: also called coke or blow is a dangerous stimulant that is in both powdered and crack rock (hard) appearance. Powdered cocaine can be snorted by melting the power and injecting it. Crack cocaine is consumed by heating the stone in a pipe and inhaling the smoke. The high resulting from cocaine varies depending on the method used.	Anxiety, irritability, paranoia, restlessness, loss of sense of smell, nosebleeds, difficulty swallowing, hoarseness and chronically runny nose.	Happiness	Fruity
Colitis: inflammation that affects the large intestine and symptoms may recur. After a period of remission of months or even years you could experience what's commonly known as a flare.	Constant urge to have a bowel movement. Tenesmus may exist with abdominal pain, may come in waves, building diarrhea and continuous pain.	Upliftedness	Woody
Conjunctivitis: pink eye can be highly contagious and level of inflammation or infection of the membrane of the lining of the eyelid that covers the white part of the eye.	Pink eye is commonly caused by a bacterial or viral infection or an allergic in one or both eyes. Also redness, itchiness and discharge.	Focus	Hash
Constipation: when stools are hard and hard to pass.	hard stools	Happiness	Minty
Cystic fibrosis (CF): is a common inherited disease in which the exocrine (secretory) glands that produce abnormally thick mucus that causes a problem with digestion, breathing and body cooling.	CF mainly affects the lungs, pancreas, liver, intestines, sinuses and sex organs.	Serenity	Skunks
Damage Spinal Cord injury: to the spinal cord or nerves at the end of the spinal canal (cauda equina), can cause permanent changes in sensation and other body functions.	Effects your injury mentally, emotionally and socially. Bladder or bowel control, back pain or pressure in your back, head, neck, numbness, tingling weakness or paralysis balance, walking and impaired breathing.	Sleepiness	Spicy

Darier Disease: dark crusty patches on the skin sometimes containing pus. The crusty pieces are also known as keratotic papules.	Darier's disease, bleeding under the skin, wart-like blemishes on arms, back, chest, elbows and behind the ears and scalp.	Focus	Hash
Degenerative Arthritis: can cause local pain in the affected area. All areas of the spine can be affected by disc decaying.	Degenerative arthritis, ages, inflammation joints and increases swelling.	Hunger	Pink
Delirium Tremens: also known as alcohol withdrawal delirium (AWD) the most severe form of alcohol withdrawal. It causes sudden and severe problems in your brain and nervous system.	Delirium Tremens anxiety, chest pain, delusion, fatigue, increased breathing or heart rate, sweating, restlessness and mood swings.	Sleepiness	Spicy
Dermatomyositis: an uncommon incendiary disease often occurs when muscles become inflamed (inflammatory myopathy). It is one of only three known inflammatories.	Weakness in the muscles, tenderness, problems swallowing, lung problems and hard calcium deposits underneath the skin.	Happiness	Minty
Diabetes Adult onset Metabolic Disorder: that can be characterized by hyperglycemia (high blood sugar), with the lack of insulin resistance and relative lack of insulin. Diabetes is in contrast to diabetes mellitus type 1.	Excess thirst, frequent urination. Type 2 diabetes makes up about 90 percent of cases.	Hunger	Pink
Diabetes Adult onset type 2 Diabetes: once known as adult-onset noninsulin-dependent diabetes. Type 2 diabetes is a chronic condition that affects the way the body metabolizes sugar.	Areas of darkened skin, blurred vision, fatigue, frequent urination, increased thirst, slow-healing sores or frequent infections and weight loss.	Happiness	Minty
Diabetes Peripheral Arterial Disease: called (PAD). Occurs when blood vessels in the legs are narrowed or blocked by fatty deposits and blood flow to your feet and legs decreases.	Leg pain can occur especially when walking or exercising, numbness, tingling or coldness in the lower legs.	Sleepiness	Spicy

Diarrhea: caused by an increased flow of water into the intestine. Reduce absorption of fluid from the organ or rapid passage of stool through the body.	Bowel movements are frequent and watery.	Upliftedness	Woody
Diverticulitis: is a bulging pouch or sac that can form on internal organs. Diverticula can occur anywhere in the colon but most commonly develop near the end of the colon on the left side (sigmoid colon).	Diverticulitis can go unnoticeable for quite a while before complications start to occur. Most people live their whole lives without the knowledge that they have diverticulitis until a doctor orders tests for an unrelated condition.	Happiness	Minty
Dysthymic Disorder: materializes as depression can last at least two years or longer.	Loss of interest in activities, sadness or feeling down, hopelessness, tiredness and lack of energy, low self-esteem, self-criticism or feeling incapable, trouble concentrating and making decisions, irritability or excessive anger.	Hunger	Pink
Eczema (atopic dermatitis): condition that can make your skin red and itchy. With flare up periodically and then subside most common in children but can occur at any age with symptoms of hay fever and asthma.	Severe itching red to brownish-gray patches on ankles, eyelids, feet, hands, wrists, neck, upper chest, inside the bend of the elbows and knees. Also in infants the face and scalp.	Serenity	Skunks
Emphysema: can gradually damage the air sacs (alveoli) in your lungs, making you progressively more short of breath. Emphysema is one of the several diseases known collectively as the chronic obstructive pulmonary disease (COPD).	Some people have emphysema for many years without symptoms. The primary symptom of emphysema is shortness of breath which begins gradually.	Sleepiness	Spicy

Endometrial Cancer: began in the uterus (a hollow, pear-shaped pelvic organ) where fetal development occurs. Endometrial cancer is sometimes called uterine sarcoma. Endometriosis is the materialization of uterine-lining tissue outside the uterus.	An abnormal watery or blood-tinged discharge from your vagina, pelvic pain, pain during intercourse, painful periods (dysmenorrhea). Pelvic pain and cramping may begin several days before and into your period with lower back and abdominal pain.	Focus	Hash
Epidermolysis Bullosa: accumulation of rare diseases that cause the skin to blister. The blisters appear in response to minor injury, heat or friction.	A swollen scrotum, testicle pain and tenderness, usually on one side, painful urination, enlarged lymph nodes in the groin.	Hunger	Pink
Epididymitis: red swollen or warm scrotum with testicle pain or tenderness usually on one side. Painful urination and frequent urinate discharge from the penis, painful intercourse or ejaculation a lump on the penis. Also, discomfort in the lower abdomen or pelvic area and blood in the semen.	Warmth in the scrotum area with low-grade fever, chills, pain, pressure, enlarged lymph nodes, urination, bowel movements, pain in the pelvic area during intercourse and ejaculation.	Serenity	Skunks
Epilepsy: uncontrollable jerking movements tend to begin and end suddenly and last for about five to 10 seconds. Although they can last longer and occur several times a day.	Triggers can be bright lights, flashing lights or patterns, caffeine, alcohol, medicines or drugs, illness or fever, lack of sleep and stress. Skipping meals, overeating or specific food ingredients.	Sleepiness	Spicy
Felty Syndrome: long-standing rheumatoid arthritis. Felty syndrome is defined by three conditions, rheumatoid arthritis, an enlarged spleen (splenomegaly) and an abnormally low white blood cell count. Felty syndrome is uncommon. It affects less than 1 percent of patients with rheumatoid arthritis.	Sleep difficulties, pain all over, brain fog, morning stiffness, digestive disorders, muscle knots and cramping.	Focus	Hash

Fibromyalgia: is a disorder of the musculoskeletal system with painful body aches with fatigue, sleep, memory and mood disorders that amplifies unpleasant sensations by affecting the way the brain process pain.	Irritable bowel, interstitial cystitis or painful syndrome. Migraine headaches and temporomandibular joint disorders.	Happiness	Fruity
Friedreich Ataxia (FRDA): is a rare inherited disease of the nervous system. It usually begins in childhood and leads to impaired muscle coordination (ataxia) that worsens over time.	Aggressive scoliosis (of the spine), diabetes mellitus (insulin - dependent, fatigue, loss of coordination in arms and legs, energy deprivation and muscle loss.	Hunger	Hash
Gastritis: inflammation of the lining of the stomach. The swelling of gastritis is most often the result of infection with the same bacterium that causes most stomach ulcers. Injury and drinking too much alcohol also can contribute to gastritis.	Nausea or recurrent upset stomach, abdominal bloating, abdominal pain, vomiting, indigestion, burning or gnawing feeling in the stomach between meals or at a night, hiccups and loss of appetite.	Serenity	Minty
Herpes Simplex virus type 1 (HSV-1): is often the cause of cold sores or fever blisters and genital herpes.	A burning sensation when having intercourse or urinating. Numbness, tingling or burning in the genital area with watery blisters.	Sleepiness	Spicy
Glaucoma: causes damage to your optic nerve and gets worse over time. It is often associated with a buildup of pressure inside the eye. Glaucoma may be inherited and may not show up until later in life.	Seizure, nausea, vomiting, headache, memory loss, and hemiparesis. The single most prevalent is a progressive memory.	Focus	Earthy
Glioblastoma Multiforme (GBM): classification name is glioblastoma also known as grade IV astrocytoma, the most common and most aggressive.	Drowsiness, headaches, nausea and vomiting, difficulty with memory speech, weakness on one side of the body and changes in vision.	Happiness	Fruity

Graves Disease: also known as toxic diffuse goiter and Flajani-Basedow-Graves disease. Autoimmune disease that affects the thyroid.	Increased appetite, diarrhea, excessive sweating, hair loss, hand tremor, heat intolerance, hyperactivity, itching, muscle weakness, moistness, muscle weakness, palpitations and skin warmth.	Hunger	Hash
Hemophilia A: is when your body doesn't have enough protein called factor VIII that the body needs to make clots and stop bleeding.	Blood in the stool or urine, nosebleed. Suffering from a small injury start and stop bleeding and massive bruising.	Happiness	Minty
Henoch-Schonlein purpura: a disorder that causes inflammation and bleeding in the small blood vessels in your skin, joints, intestines and kidney.	A disease of the skin mucous membranes and sometimes other organs that most commonly affects children.	Sleepiness	Spicy
Hepatitis C: is an infection that causes by liver inflammation with severe liver damage. Hepatitis C is spread through contaminated blood.	Bleeding, bruising easily, dark-colored urine, confusion, drowsiness, slurred speech, fatigue, fluid buildup in abdomen, itchy skin. Poor appetite, swelling in your legs, weight loss and spider-like blood vessels on your surface (spider angiomas).	Focus	Earthy
HIV/AIDS (human immuno-deficiency virus): condition caused by infection. Stages of HIV are complicated by a disease of the lung known as pneumocystis pneumonia severe weight loss. A type of cancer known as Kaposi sarcoma, or other AIDS-defining conditions.	Fever, headache, large tender lymph nodes, sores of the mouth and genitals and throat inflammation.	Woody	Earthy
Hospice Patient Care: that focuses on the palliation of a chronically ill, terminally ill seriously ill patients. Attending to their emotional and spiritual needs for the sick, wounded or dying as well.	Hospice is for a terminally ill person who's expected to have six months or less to live.	Hunger	Happiness

Huntington Disease: an inherited disease that causes the progressive breakdown (degeneration) of nerve in the brain cells. Huntington disease has a substantial impact on a person's functional abilities and usually results in movement, thinking (cognitive) and psychiatric disorders.	An inherited disorder that results in the death of brain cells. Earliest symptoms are a subtle problem with mood or mental abilities, lack of coordination, unsteady, jerky body movements, physical skills gradually worsen. Awkward and unable to talk with the decline into dementia.	Hunger	Hash
Hypertension High Blood pressure: a common condition in which there is long-term force of the blood against your artery walls such as heart disease.	Weakness, fainting, dizziness, confusion, agitation, a feeling of being outside yourself	Sleepiness	Spicy
Hyperventilation Syndrome: more accurate and relates to an overbreathing pattern that happens under certain conditions. This overbreathing results in a group of symptoms.	For some people, hyperventilation is rare can be the occasional panicked response to fear, stress, or a phobia, for some people, emotional states such as depression, anxiety or anger.	Upliftedness	Woody
Hypoglycemia: also known as low blood glucose or low blood sugar, occurs when blood glucose drops below normal levels. Glucose a vital source of energy for the body. Carbohydrates are the primary dietary source of glucose. Rice, potatoes, bread, tortillas, cereal, milk, fruit and sweets are all carbohydrate-rich foods.	Clamminess, drowsiness, dizziness, includes hunger, irritability, low blood sugar, paleness, rapid heartbeat, shakiness, sweating and weakness.	Woody	Earthy
Impotence: is a problem among men with the inability to achieve an erection or ejaculation.	Anxiety, chest pain, depression, heart disease, high blood pressure, cholesterol, obesity, metabolic and substance abuse.	Happiness	Fruity
Inflammatory Bowel Disease (IBD): combination of gut-brain axis problems gut motility disorders, pain sensitivity, infections including small intestinal bacterial overgrowth.	Abdominal pain and cramping. Blood in your stool, diarrhea, fever, fatigue, reduced appetite and unintended weight loss.	Sleepiness	Spicy

Intermittent Explosive Disorder (IED): behavioral disorder repeated, sudden episodes of impulsive, aggressive, violent behavior or angry verbal outbursts. Overreacting grossly out of proportion to the situation, road rage, domestic abuse, throwing or breaking objects or other temper tantrums.	Energy changes, mood changes and tension.	Upliftedness	Woody
Intractable Vomiting: repeated vomiting with nausea that resists. People can develop this symptom for some reasons and therapy is focused on providing supportive care.	Migraine, seizure disorders, chronic intestinal pseudo-obstruction, gastroparesis, irritable bowel syndrome, bacteria, bacterial toxins, food-borne toxins and pneumonia.	Focus	Earthy
Lipomatosis: believed to be an autosomal dominant condition in which multiple lipomas are present on the body (fatty tumors). Disease is benign. Many discrete encapsulated lipomas form on the trunk and extremities. This is most commonly found mutations in solitary lipomatous tumors. But lipomas often have multiple variations. Reciprocal translocations involved have been observed.	Abdominal pain containing the mass decreased function (range of motion) enlargement of varicose veins, fatigue, numbness, painful swelling and weight loss	Happiness	Fruity
Lou Gehrig Disease: or amyotrophic lateral sclerosis (ALS). Rapidly progressive uniformly fatal neurodegenerative disease, the loss of motor neurons in the brainstem, spinal cord and cerebral cortex leading to a decline in muscular function. It eventually results in weakness, speech deficits and difficulty swallowing. ALS is almost always fatal in two to three years.	Cramps, chewing, difficulty with writing or buttoning a shirt, leg or arm weakness causing an awkward gait or stumbling Twitching, stiff muscles, difficulty swallowing and slurred speech.	Hunger	Hash

Lyme Disease (Borrelia burgdorferi): caused by the most common tick-borne illness (tick bite) in North America and Europe. Lyme disease is transmitted by the bite of an infected black-legged tick.	Eye inflammation, liver inflammation (hepatitis), rashes, severe fatigue, nausea and vomiting.	Serenity	Minty
Lymphoma Hodgkin: is cancer that originates in your lymphatic system. Causing tumors develop from lymphocytes that will spread throughout the body.	Abdominal pain, chest pain, coughing or trouble breathing, fever, painless, swollen lymph nodes in your neck, armpits or groin or swelling, night sweats, persistent fatigue and unexplained weight loss.	Sleepiness	Spicy
Major Depression: feeling sad or weak at some point in their lives. Clinical depression is a depressed mood most of the day.	Angry outbursts, anxiety, agitation, concentrating, back pain, feelings of worthlessness or guilt. Fixating on past failures, frustration over small matters, lack of energy, loss of interest, loss of appetite, insomnia or sleeping too much, tiredness and suicide.	Upliftedness	Woody
Malignant Melanoma: a kind of cancer. That can develop from the pigment-containing cells known as melanocytes.	Melanomas usually occur in the skin but may rarely occur in the mouth, intestines or eye, sometimes develop from a mole.	Focus	Earthy
Mania: abnormally elevated mood arousal energy level. A state of heightened overall activation with enhanced practical expression together with a liability of effect.	Disconnected and speedy (racing) thoughts, grandiose beliefs, inappropriate happiness or euphoria. Inappropriate irritability markedly increased energy, inappropriate social behavior, increased talking speed or volume and increased sexual desire.	Happiness	Fruity

Melorheostosis: also known as Leri disease unusual mesenchymal dysplasia manifesting as regions of sclerosing bone with the unique dripping wax appearance or flowing candle appearance that began in childhood.	Absent or abnormal muscles, irregular bone growth, dripping candle wax appearance on x-ray imaging, cortical thickening unequal length of limbs, joint swelling, soft tissue abnormalities, subcutaneous calcification, tendon and ligament shortening	Hunger	Hash
Meniere Disease: is a disarrange of the inner ear that causes spontaneous episodes of vertigo a sensation of a spinning motion.	Feeling of fullness in the ear, hearing loss, ringing in the ear (tinnitus) and recurring episodes of vertigo.	Serenity	Minty
Migraine Headaches: neurological disease characterized by recurrent moderate to severe headaches.	Constipation, food cravings, frequent yawning, increased thirst, mood changes from depression to euphoria, neck stiffness and urination.	Minty	Spicy
Motion Sickness or Ketosis: also known as travel sickness. Condition in which a disagreement exists between visually perceived movement and the vestibule's sense of movement. Depending on the cause it can also be referred to as seasickness, car sickness, simulation sickness and airsickness.	Motion sickness can strike suddenly feeling of uneasiness to cold sweat, dizziness and vomiting. Any form of transportation (car, ship, plane and train) can cause motion sickness.	Spicy	Woody
Mucopolysaccharidosis: is a disorder that divided into three separate syndromes 1. Hurler syndrome (MPS I-H) 2. Hurler-Scheie syndrome (MPS I-H/S) 3 Scheie syndrome (MPS I-S) these are metabolic disorders caused by the malfunctioning of the liposomal enzymes, needed to break down molecules called glycosaminoglycans.	Enlarged cheeks, head, lips, tongue and nose. Vocal cords, deep voice and sleep apnea, carpal tunnel syndrome, heart (valve) disease and upper respiratory infections.	Focus	Earthy

Multiple Sclerosis (MS) disease: that attacks the protective sheath (myelin) that covers your nerves in your immune system. Myelin can disrupt communication between your brain and the rest of your body.	Bowel and bladder dysfunction partial or complete loss of vision. Usually in one eye at a time dizziness, fatigue, electric shock that occurs with specific neck movements especially bending the neck forward, weakness in one or more limbs that occurs on one side of your body, slurred speech, tingling in parts of your body, tremor and lack of coordination or unsteady gait.	Happiness	Fruity
Muscle Esophageal spasms: are painful muscle contractions that affect your esophagus. The hollow tube between your throat and your stomach. Sudden have severe chest pain that may last for few minutes to an hour.	Difficulty swallowing liquids such as red wine or extremely hot or cold liquids. The feeling that an object is stuck in your throat and the return of food and fluids back up your esophagus (regurgitation).	Hunger	Hash
Muscular Dystrophy disease: that causes increasing weakness with loss of muscle mass. Irregular muscular dystrophy. Progressive genes (mutations) interfere with the production of proteins needed to form healthy tissue.	Hard to get up from a lying or sitting position. Frequent falls, large calf muscles, learning disabilities, muscle pain, stiffness. Trouble running, jumping, waddling gait and walking on the toes.	Serenity	Minty
Myeloid Leukemia or acute myelogenous leukemia (AML): Cancer of the blood and bone marrow tissue inside bones where blood cells are made.	Early stages of acute leukemia may mimic the flu or other common diseases. Fever, bone pain, lethargy, fatigue, shortness of breath, pale skin, frequent infection, easy bruising and unusual bleeding.	Sleepiness	Spicy

Nail-Patella Syndrome: also known as HOOD syndrome. Genetic disorder that results in small poorly developed nails and kneecaps, elbows, chest, and hips. The name nail-patella can be misleading because the syndrome often affects other areas of the body including the production of specific proteins.	Fingernail and toenail absence (aplasia). Abnormally increased fluid pressure in eyes (glaucoma). The toenail is less often affected. Kneecap abnormalities are the second most common signs associated with this disorder.	Upliftedness	Woody
Nightmares: troubling dreams associated with negative feelings such as anxiety or fear.	The dream may seem vivid real and very upsetting. Often becoming disturbing as the dream unfolds. Leaving you feeling anxious, angry, scared, sad and disgusted. With pounding heartbeats and sweaty. Upon awakening you can recall details of your dream.	Focus	Focus
Obesity: complicated disorder involving an excessive amount of body fat. Obesity isn't just a cosmetic concern. BMI is calculated by dividing your weight in kilograms (kg) by your height in meters squared (m^2).	Obesity can be a concern with overweight-related health problem.	Focus	Fruity
Obsessive-Compulsive Disorder (OCD): with irrational thought and anxieties (compulsions) that will lead you to be repetitive. Compulsions or behavior problems. A person can have just one obsession or compulsions and still have OCD.	Fear of uncleanness or dirt needing things methodical and symmetrical. Aggressive or horrific thoughts about harming yourself or others useless reflections including aggression, sexual or religious subjects.	Serenity	Minty

Opiate Dependence: on morphine injection is used to relieve direct to severe pain. It may also be used before or during surgery with an anesthetic.	Opiates development of tolerance (meaning the need to use more significant amounts). Withdrawal symptoms after reducing or stopping. Use can cause depression, upset stomach, insomnia, muscle aches and difficulty meeting social or work obligations	Sleepiness	Spicy
Osteoarthritis: occurs when the protective cartilage on the ends of your bones wears down over time.	Joint pain and stiffness. Treatment of affected joint including the hand, wrist, neck, back, knee and hip involves medication and exercise.	Upliftedness	Woody
Panic Disorder: with sudden episode of severe fear with severe physical feelings with no real danger or apparent cause. You feel like you are losing control having a heart attack or dying.	Palpitations, pounding heart or accelerated heart rate, sweating, trembling, shaking, sensations, shortness of breath, smothering or feeling of choking.	Focus	Hash
Parkinson Disease: is a chronic and progressive disorder of the central nervous system. It affects how your body moves and can also change the way you think. Parkinson's belongs to a group of diseases known as movement disorders.	Resting tremors, slow movement (bradykinesia), stiff muscles, lack of balance or falling, being stuck in place while walking. Reduced arm swings on one side of your body. Dragging foot, small voice, loss of automatic movements like blinking, swallowing, speech, writing, smell and taste	Happiness	Fruity
Peripheral Neuropathy: is a result of damage to your peripheral nerves. Often causes weakness, numbness and pain usually in your feet, hands and other areas of your body.	Gradual feeling of numbness, prickling or tingling in your feet, hands that spreads upward into your legs and arms. Sharp jabbing, throbbing, freezing or burning pain, sensitivity to touch, lack of coordination, falling muscle weakness or paralysis.	Hunger	Hash

Peritoneal Pain: associated with peritoneal dialysis. Caused by germs around the catheter after receiving peritoneal dialysis.	Results of damage to your peripheral nerves. Often causes weakness, numbness, and pain usually in your feet, hands and other areas of your body.	Serenity	Minty
Persistent Insomnia: is a inability to sleep that persists for several nights. Lasting for months depending on the gravity of the problem.	Anxiety, depression and stress are some of the most common causes of chronic insomnia.	Sleepiness	Spicy
Porphyria: is a collection of disorders that can cause nerve or skin problems.	Abdominal pain often severe chest pain with increased heart rate, blood pressure, back pain, limb muscle weakness, tingling, loss of sensation, cramping. Vomiting and constipation, personality changes or mental disorders, agitation, confusion and seizures.	Upliftedness	Spicy
Post-polio Syndrome (PPS): affects some people who have had polio (poliomyelitis) for many years typically from age ten to forty after recovery from infections.	Muscle weakness, extreme fatigue, joint pain, skeletal deformities such as scoliosis. PPS symptoms copy those of the disorder known as Lou Gehrig disease.	Arousal	Dank
Post-Traumatic Arthritis: is inflammation of a joint. Common cause is wearing out joint surface cartilage (osteoarthritis) that has had a physical injury. The injury could be a sport fall, vehicle accident or any source of physical trauma.	Joint pain, with fluid accumulation in the joint, causes swelling, decreased tolerance for walking, sports, stairs and other activities that stress the joint.	Creativity	Earthy

Post-Traumatic Stress Disorder (PTSD): is an anxiety disorder that can develop after a person is exposed to one or more traumatic events. Such as significant stress, sexual assault, warfare or other threats on the person's life.	Flashback, nightmares, avoid crowds, because they feel dangerous. You may have a hard time sleeping. Trouble concentrating, startled by a loud noise or surprise. Have back to a wall in a restaurant or waiting room.	Energy	Fruity
Premenstrual Syndrome (PMS): is changes that happen before a woman's monthly period.	Moodiness, depression, abdominal cramping, bloating, food cravings, headaches, muscle aches, breast tenderness and fatigue and acne.	Happiness	Minty
Prostate Cancer: in a man's prostate gland. Prostate is the small walnut-shaped gland that produces the seminal fluid that nourishes and transports to the male reproductive system. The cancer cells spread mainly to the bones and lymph nodes.	Blood in semen, trouble urinating, decreased force in the stream of urine. Discomfort in the pelvic area bone pain and erectile dysfunction.	Hunger	Pink
Prostatitis: is inflammation and swelling of the prostate gland located below the bladder in men. The prostate gland produces fluid (semen) that nourishes and transports sperm.	Prostatitis often causes painful or difficult urination. Other symptoms include pain in the groin, pelvic area or genitals and sometimes flu-like symptoms.	Upliftedness	Skunks
Psoriasis: is a chronic disease that comes and goes. The primary goal is to stop the skin cells from proliferating.	Red patches of skin seen in children covered with thick silvery scales or spots. Dry skin that may bleed, burning or itching with pitted nails that are swollen and stiff joints.	Sleepiness	Spicy
Pulmonary Fibrosis: is thickens and scar tissue around and between the (alveoli) air sacs in the lungs. Causing difficult for oxygen to pass through the bloodstream.	Shortness of breath (dyspnea), fatigue, aching muscles and joints. Shortness of breath, widening rounding the fingertips or toes (clubbing).	Upliftedness	Woody

Radiation Therapy: is used as a high-energy radiation to shrink tumors and kill cancer cells. X-rays and charged particles are types of radiation used for cancer treatment.	Some people who received radiation therapy experience, dryness, blistering, peeling, fatigue head, neck, chest, stomach, abdomen and pelvis pain.	Energy	Fruity
Raynaud Disease (ray-NOHZ): is arteries narrowing your vessels and temporarily limiting blood supply to your fingers and toes. Which go into vasospasm when exposed to cold or stress.	Cold finger or toes can change your skin's response to cold and stress. Causing stinging or numb pain upon warming or stress relief	Focus	Minty
Reiter Syndrome: is a inflammatory reaction to an infection. Somewhere in the body. It usually follows a urogenital or intestinal disease.	Pain and stiffness most commonly occur in your knees, ankles, feet, low back, buttocks, eye inflammation (conjunctivitis), urinary problem, also inflammation of the prostate gland or cervix.	Happiness	Pink
Restless Legs Syndrome (RLS): is not entirely known can be related to genetic factors. Low iron levels in the brain or diseases such as chronic kidney or diabetes.	Aching, crawling, twitching, itching and throbbing in the legs.	Focus	Hash
Rheumatoid Arthritis (RA): is a formed arthritis that causes swelling, stiffness and pain with loss of function in your joints. It can also affect the wrist and fingers.	Stiffness, swelling and pain in the affected joints.	Happiness	Minty
Rosacea: is chronic is potentially life-troublesome disorder mainly of the facial skin. Often characterized by flare-ups and remissions.	Pimples and bumps often develop in severe cases. The nose may grow swollen and bumpy from excess tissue.	Hunger	Pink
Schizoaffective Disorder: is a chronic mental health condition. Characterized mainly by symptoms of delusions, hallucinations, mood disorder such as mania and depression.	Symptoms of schizophrenia may vary but typically include delusions, hallucinations, disorganized thinking, speaking and abnormal motor behavior.	Serenity	Skunks

Schizophrenia: is a mental disorder represented by abnormal social behavior and failure to understand what is real.	False beliefs, confused or unclear thinking, hearing voices that others do not hear. Reduced social engagement, emotional expression and lack of motivation.	Sleepiness	Spicy
Scoliosis: when the spine has a sideways curve usually S- or C-shaped. In some the degree of curvature is stable. While in others it increases over time. Mild scoliosis does not usually cause problems while severe cases can interfere with breathing. Pain is not often present.	Back, shoulders, neck buttock pain. Pain nearest bottom of the back, respiratory and cardiac problems in severe cases. Constipation because of curvature causing "tightening" of the stomach and intestines. Limited mobility secondary to pain or functional limitation in adults and painful menstruation.	Upliftedness	Woody
Sedative Dependence: includes an assortment of drugs depressing the central nervous system. Barbiturates and benzodiazepines are the most common. But other painkillers include chloral hydrate, glutethimide, methaqualone and meprobamate.	Cravings for the drugs, anxiety, insomnia, nervousness, tremors, loss of appetite, nightmares, rapid breathing, fast heartbeat and up and down in blood pressure.	Arousal	Dank
Seizures: is based on the type of behavior and brain activity. Seizures are divided into two broad categories generalized and partial (also called local or focal).	Violent shaking, loss of control, sudden feeling of fear or anxiousness. Feeling sick to your stomach, dizziness, vision change, jerking of the arms, legs that may cause you to drop things. An out-of-body sensation and headache.	Focus	Earthy
Senile Dementia: is a severe mental deterioration in old age. Represented by the loss of memory and control of bodily functions.	The ability to focus, pay attention, communication, language, memory, judgment and visual perception.	Euphoria	Hash

Severe Nausea: is appearing shortly after eating. Nausea or vomiting may be caused by gastritis (inflammation of the stomach lining), bulimia, food poisoning or ulcer.	Headache, fever, diarrhea, gas, vomiting, dizziness, lightheadedness, diarrhea, abdominal pain. General feeling of being sick to one's stomach.	Focus	Minty
Shingles (herpes zoster): is a highly contagious infection usually spread through sex. Occurs soon after a person is infected. Starts as small blisters that ultimately, break open and fertile painful. Raw sores that scab that can heal over few weeks. This disease is usually caused by the herpes simplex virus-2.	Headache, itching, rash, blisters, flu-like symptoms, vision change, fever and swollen lymph nodes.	Happiness	Pink
Sinusitis Inflammation: is swelling of the tissue lining the sinuses. Sometimes sinuses are filled with air. But when sinuses become blocked and filled with fluid, bacteria, fungi, germs viruses can grow and cause an infection.	Facial pain, pressure, nasal stuffiness, nasal discharge, loss of smell, cough and congestion.	Happiness	Minty
Skeletal Muscular somatic nervous system (SoNS: or voluntary nervous system): is the part of the peripheral nervous system associated with skeletal muscular optional control of body movements.	Increased muscle tone, overactive reflexes, involuntary movements which may include spasms brisk or sustained involuntary muscle contraction and clonus.	Hunger	Pink
Spasticity: is a muscle control disorder when the muscles are tight or stiff. Inability to control those muscles. Also reflexes may persist for too long and may be too high (hyperactive reflexes).	Increased muscle tone, overactive reflexes, involuntary movements. Which may include spasms brisk or sustained involuntary muscle contraction and clonus.	Sleepiness	Spicy
Spinal Stenosis: is a narrowing space within the spine which can put pressure on the nerves. Spinal stenosis occurs most often in the lower back and the neck.	Tingling and weakness in the arm, hand, foot, leg and problem balance and walking.	Upliftedness	Woody

Surge-Weber Syndrome (SWS): is a neurological disorder marked by a distinctive port-wine stain around the eyes, forehead and scalp. This stain is a birthmark caused by an overabundance of capillaries near the surface of the skin. Blood vessels on the same side of the brain as the dye may also be affected.	Cognitive impairment, developmental delays, paralysis, seizures and weakness on one side of the body.	Creativity	Earthy
Stuttering: is not uncommon for children between the ages of two and five years old. It may come and go and last a few weeks or a couple of years. Most children outgrow stuttering without professional intervention.	Difficulty starting a word, sentence or phrase, prolonging a word, repetition of a sound, syllable or word, brief silence for certain syllables, words. Pauses within a nutshell and (broken word) addition of extra words like "um".	Energy	Fruity
Tardive Dyskinesia (TD): is a difficult to treat and often incurable form of dyskinesia. A disorder resulting in involuntary body movements. In this type of dyskinesia, the involuntary movements are tardive and have a slow onset.	Arm and leg movements, lip smacking, facial grimacing, finger tapping and rapid eye blinking.	Euphoria	Hash
Temporomandibular Joint (TMJ): disorder is connects your jaw to the temporal bones of your skull which are in front of each ear. Allowing you move your jaw up and down and side to side so you can talk, chew and yawn.	Earaches, dizziness, headaches, hearing problem, toothaches, neck aches, ringing in the ears (tinnitus). Jaw that gets "stuck" or "locked" in the open- or closed-mouth position.	Focus	Minty
Tenosynovitis: is a painful condition affecting the tendons on the thumb side of your wrist.	Difficulty moving your thumb and wrist when you're doing something that involves grasping or pinching. A "sticking" or "stop-and-go" sensation in your thumb when moving it. Pain or swelling near the base of the thumb.	Happiness	Minty

Tension Headache: is the most common type of headache. A tension headache is mild to moderate pain in your head that feels like having a tight band around your head.	Aching head pain with tightness or pressure across or side of your forehead. The side and back of your head, scalp, neck and shoulder with muscle pain	Hunger	Pink
Terminal Illness: is a home-based family-centered care for individuals facing a terminal illness. Hospice addresses these aspects of a terminal disease when appropriate.	A methodical process, denial, listen, accept ask the person what they want.	Serenity	Skunks
Testicular Cancer: testicles that produce male sex hormones and sperm for reproduction. Which occurs in the testicles (testes). Located inside the scrotum a loose bag of skin underneath the penis.	A lump or enlargement in either testicle. A feeling of heaviness in the scrotum. A dull ache in the abdomen or groin. A sudden collection of fluid in the scrotum. Pain or discomfort in a testicle, scrotum enlargement or tenderness of the breasts and back pain.	Sleepiness	Spicy
Thyroiditis: is a swollen thyroid. It primarily affects women from early adulthood to middle age although anyone can get it.	Anxiety, fatigue, insomnia, irritability, rapid heartbeat or palpitations, tremor. Unexplained weight loss and increased sensitivity to heat.	Upliftedness	Woody
Tic Douloureux: also called trigeminal neuralgia. The trigeminal nerve's function is disrupted. Usually the problem is the contact between a typical blood vessel—in this case. An artery or a vein—and the trigeminal nerve at the base of your brain. This communication puts pressure on the nerve and causes it to malfunction.	Episodes of severe shooting or jabbing pain when shaving, touching your face. Eating, drinking, brushing your teeth, talking, putting on makeup, encountering a breeze, smiling and washing your face.	Arousal	Dank

Tietze Syndrome costochondritis: is an inflammation of the cartilage that connects a rib to the breastbone (sternum). Pain caused by costochondritis might mimic that of a heart attack or other heart conditions.	Can occur on the left side of your breastbone with a sharp aching or pressure. Can affect more on a rib. Worsens when you take a deep breath or a cough.	Creativity	Earthy
Tinnitus: is noise or ringing in the ears. Inner ear cell damage. Tiny hairs in your inner ear move about the pressure of sound waves.	Buzzing, clicking, hissing, ringing and roaring.	Energy	Fruity
Tobacco Dependence: is being addicted to tobacco products induced by the drug nicotine.	Can't stop smoking, physical, mood swings, intense cravings, anger, anxiety, difficulty concentrating, constipation, depressed mood, irritability, restlessness, frustration, increased hunger, insomnia and diarrhea.	Euphoria	Happiness
Tourette Syndrome Nervous system (neurological) disorder: that starts in childhood. It involves unusual repetitive movements or unwanted sounds that can't be controlled (tics).	Eye blinking, head jerking, stepping in a particular pattern, touching or smelling objects, repeating observed movements, shoulder shrugging, eye darting, obscene gesturing, nose twitching, bending or twisting, mouth movements and hopping.	Focus	Minty
Trichotillomania (also known as hair pulling disorder): A disorder characterized by the compulsive urge to pull out one's hair.	Many people also pick their skin, bite their nails or chew their lips. Sometimes pulling hairs from pets or dolls or materials.	Happiness	Pink
Uterine Cancer: is a type of cancer that begins in the uterus. The uterus is the hollow pear-shaped pelvic organ in women where fetal development occurs.	Vaginal bleeding after menopause bleeding between periods an abnormal watery or blood-tinged discharge from your vagina and pelvic pain.	Focus	Hash

Viral Hepatitis: is an infection caused by a virus that attacks the liver and leads to inflammation. Most people are infected with the hepatitis C virus (HCV).	Some people have no symptoms. Others may have yellow discoloration of the skin and whites of the eyes. Abdominal diarrhea pain, reduced appetite, vomiting, or tiredness.	Happiness	Minty
Wasting Syndrome (AIDS): patients are said to have it when they have lost at least 10 percent of their body weight. Because of diarrhea for at least a month. Extreme weakness and fever that are not related to an infection especially muscle.	Depression, opportunistic infections, like a painful throat or feeling full and lack of energy. Medication side effects are nausea, changes in taste and or mouth tingling.	Hunger	Pink
Whiplash: occurs when the head and neck are suddenly forced backward and then forward. Allowing the cervical spine to pass through lightning-quick motions and extreme stresses.	Tendons and muscles in the neck stretch and tear, leaving you with a painful, sore, and stiff neck.	Serenity	Skunks
Wittmaack–Ekbom Syndrome also known as restless legs syndrome (RLS) or Willis-Ekbom disease (WED): a neurological disorder. An urge to move one's body to stop uncomfortable or odd sensations. It most commonly affects the legs but can affect the arms, torso and head.	An urge to move legs twitching during sleep and motor restlessness.	Sleepiness	Spicy
Writer's Cramp: also known as (scrivener's palsy) and (mogigraphia) cramps or spasms of specific muscles of the hand and forearm. Writer's cramp happens when performing fine motor tasks such as writing or playing an instrument.	Addition of the finger during writing making the pen difficult to hold. Gripping the pen too hard and unusual postures of the wrist or elbow.	Upliftedness	Woody

INDICA

INDICA

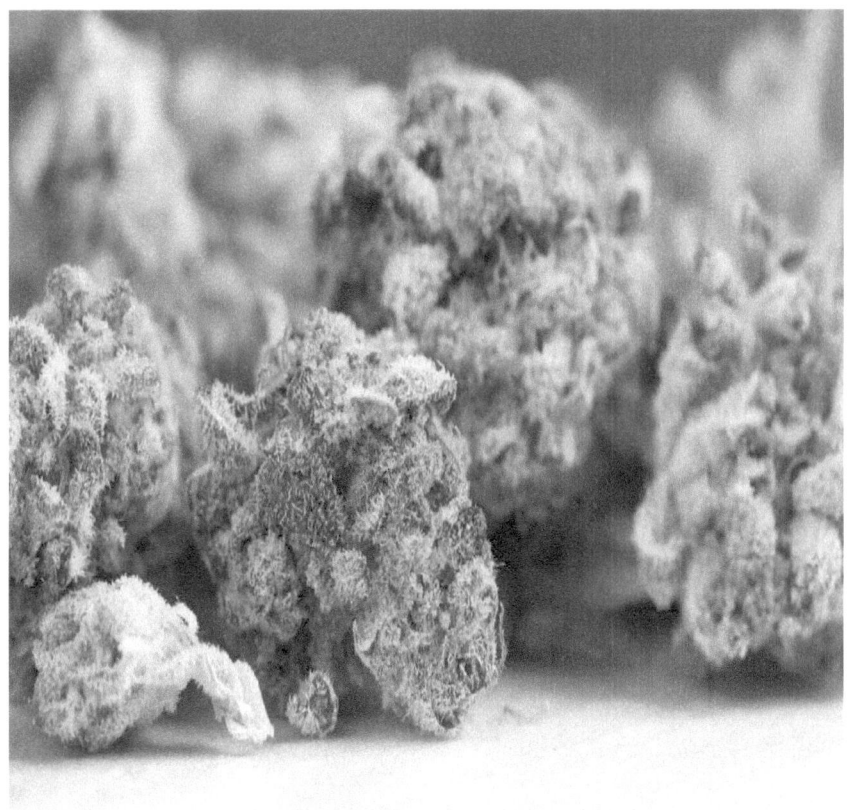

INDICA

Medical Conditions	Symptoms	Desired Effects	Flavored Scents
Acquired Hypothyroidism: is sometimes called "Hashimoto thyroiditis.	Slow growth, not starting puberty, early periods that aren't regular, tired, dry skin, constipation, slow heart rate and weight gain.	Arousal	Dank
Acute Gastritis: is an abrupt inflammation or swelling of the stomach lining. Can cause nagging and severe pain.	Appetite loss, black stools, indigestion, nausea, bloody vomiting that looks like used coffee grounds. Pain in the upper part of the abdomen.	Creativity	Earthy
Adrenal Cortical Cancer: carcinoma (ACC) is a rare disease	Increased facial and body hair particularly in females that deepened voice in women.	Energy	Fruity
Agoraphobia: a phobia is defined as the severe.	Agoraphobia includes anxiety that feel like a panic attack. Situation from one can't escape or not possible or is awkward and embarrassing.	Euphoria	Hash
Aids Related Illness: is an opportunistic infection that is caused by a viruses, bacteris, fungus even parasites. (CANCER)	Coughing and shortness of breath difficult or painful swallowing, extreme fatigue, fever mental symptoms such as confusion and forgetfulness. Nausea, abdominal cramps, vomiting, seizures, lack of coordination, severe, persistent diarrhea, severe headaches, vision loss and weight loss.	Focus	Minty
Alcohol Abuse: is a is a recurring harmful use of ethanol despite its adverse consequences is a psychiatric diagnosis.	Low tolerance, withdrawal, loss of control, desire to stop-but can't, neglecting other activities, alcohol takes up greater time, energy, focus, continued use despite negative consequences.	Happiness	Pink

Alcoholism: people who drink almost everyday. Can't go a day without drinking.	A person that drink almost everyday.	Happiness	Pink
Alcohol (AUD) disorder: alcohol dependence syndrome is a broad term for any drinking of alcohol those results in problems.	Constant questions or conversations misplacing personal belongings, forgetting events or appointments. Getting lost on a familiar route.	Serenity	Skunks
Alzheimer's: is the progressive mental decline that can occur in middle or geriatrics due to widespread decaying of the brain.	Repetitive questions or conversations, misplacing personal belongings, forgetting events, appointments and getting lost.	Sleepiness	Spicy
Amphetamine Dependency: is caused by the frequent and long-term use of the drug. Some people become dependent faster than others.	Decreased appetite, breathing problem, dry mouth, euphoria, fatigue, increased energy and high blood pressure.	Upliftedness	Woody
Amyloidosis: is a rare disease that results from an accumulation of inappropriately folded proteins. These misfolded proteins are called amyloids.	Patient with any amyloidosis can result from abnormal functioning of the bowels, heart, kidneys, liver, nerves, skin and joints.	Upliftedness	Focus
Ankylosing: unresponsiveness and consolidation of a joint due to disease, injury or surgical procedure.	Some people have early symptoms of ankylosing spondylitis include constant pain and stiffness.	Serenity	Skunks
Ankylosing: unresponsiveness and consolidation of a joint due to disease, injury or surgical procedure.	Refusal to maintain a healthy body mass a symptom that occurs after prolonged weight loss.	Sleepiness	Spicy
Anorexia: is an eating disorder characterized by a small weight fear of gaining weight, fear of increasing heaviness and a strong desire to be thin.	Fearful of the slightest weight gain and takes all precautionary measures to avoid weight gain. Noticeable rapid dramatic weight loss 15% under normal body weight.	Upliftedness	Woody

Anorexia Nervosa: can be a physical and emotional Illness. Anorexia Nervosa requires the attention of primary care physicians, mental health, counselors, psychologists and psychiatrists.	Individuals with anorexia display varying symptoms. Mostly obviously associated with malnutrition such as abnormally low body weight. Individuals also exhibit depression and solitude.	Happiness	Minty
Any Chronic Medical Symptom: that limits significant life activities (disability).	Allergy, anxiety, arthritis, asthma, autism symptom, back pain, blood, bronchitis, clinical depression, flu, hernia, night sweats, sleep apnea, stress anxiety and panic attacks.	Serenity	Skunks
Arteriosclerotic Health disease: is a thickening and hardening of the walls of the coronary arteries. As a result of invasion and accumulation of white blood cells.	Symptoms only occur after severe contraction or closure impedes blood flow to different organs enough to induce symptoms.	Hunger	Pink
Arthritis Joints: are the associates of the bones that allow flexibility and movement. Joint pain will occur if there is damage due to disease or trauma. The illness or injury will interfere with normal movement of the joint and produce pain.	Inflammation in the hands, feet, knees and ankles.	Serenity	Skunks
Arthritis Rheumatoid: is a chronic inflammatory disorder that typically affects the small joints in your hands and feet. Eventually result in bone erosion.	Tender, warm, swollen joints, morning stiffness that may last for hours. Firm bumps of tissue under the skin on your arms (rheumatoid nodules) fatigue, fever and weight loss.	Sleepiness	Spicy

Arthropathy Gout Arthritis: is a form of arthropathy that involves inflammation of one or more joints, bone and tissues.	Chronic gout in mature adults may be less painful and can be perplexed with other forms of arthritis. Gout may lead to inflammation in the fluid sacs that cushion tissues of the elbow (olecranon bursitis) and knees (prepatellar bursitis) and other conjuncts.	Upliftedness	Woody
Asthma: is an airway inflammatory disease, characterized by variable and recurring symptoms, reversible airflow obstruction and bronchospasm.	Symptoms include coughing, (SOB) shortness of breath, tightness in the chest and wheezing.	Happiness	Minty
Attention Deficit Hyperactivity Disorder (ADD, ADHD): similar to hyperkinetic disorder is a neurodevelopment psychiatric disorder in which there are significant problems.	These symptoms begin by age six to twelve and continue for more than six months. In school-aged individuals inattention often results in poor school performance. Although it causes impairment many children have a right attention span for tasks they find interesting.	Hunger	Pink
Autism / Asperger's: is a brain disorder in which communication and interaction with others are involved.	Autism may fluctuate from total lack of communication with others to difficulty in understanding others' feelings.	Sleepiness	Spicy
Autoimmune Disease: develops when your immune system defends your body against infection decides your healthy cells are foreign. As a result your immune system attacks healthy cells.	Autoimmune diseases usually go between periods of remission (little or no symptoms) and flare-ups (worsening symptoms).	Upliftedness	Woody
Back Pain: in the back usually originates from the muscles, nerves, bones, joints or other structures in the spine.	Back pain can be a sharp piercing or burning feeling. The pain may travel into the arms and hands as well as the legs or feet.	Happiness	Minty

Condition	Symptoms		
Back Sprain: is an injury to either a muscle or tendon. With a back strain the muscles and tendons that support the spine are twisted, pulled or torn.	Pain that worsens with movement. Muscle cramping or spasms (suddenly uncontrollable muscle contractions). Decreased function and range of motion of the joint.	Hunger	Pink
Bells' Palsy: is a form of facial paralysis resulting from a dysfunction of the cranial nerve Sometimes the affected side will not be closed. Permanently damaged resulting in an impaired vision of this condition is a rapid onset of partial or complete paralysis. That often occurs overnight.	The facial nerve controls some functions such as taste sensations, blinking, closing the eyes, smiling, frowning, lacrimation, salivation, flaring nostrils, raising eyebrows and two - thirds of the tongue chords.	Serenity	Skunks
Bipolar Disorder: also is known as a bipolar affective disorder and manic-depressive illness with periods of elevated mood and periods of depression.	Mania is the defining presence of bipolar disorder and can occur with different levels of grimness.	Sleepiness	Spicy
Brain Tumor: cancer is a disease of the brain in which cancer cells occur in the tissue of the brain.	Brain Tumor symptoms can be difficulty walking, dizziness, seizures, weakness and headaches.	Minty	Woody
Bruxism: can be chewing and grinding of the teeth due to clenching of the teeth other than eating.	Symptoms can be dehydration, anxiety, gum disease, tongue and headache.	Happiness	Minty
Bulimia Nervosa: is one of many eating disorders. This mental illness is a characterized by episodes of bingeing and somehow purging the food with weight loss.	Uncontrollable over eating. Eating until a person has physical discomfort and pain.	Hunger	Minty
Cachexia (CANCER): marked weight loss, muscular loss with resistant to natural therapies difficulties in performing routine activities and fatigue.	Fatigue and physical disability along with a loss of skeletal muscle mass. The sudden or gradual appearance of weight loss in any individual is highly unusual.	Serenity	Skunks
Cancer types: including breast, lung, colon, skin, prostate and ovarian cancer.	Has no symptoms, signs and symptoms only appear as the mass continues to grow or ulcerates.	Sleepiness	Spicy

Carpal Tunnel Syndrome: (pinched nerve) is known as the arm and hand condition that causes numbness, tingling and other symptoms.	Carpal Tunnel Syndrome is a pinched nerve.	Upliftedness	Woody
Cerebral Palsy: is a disrupt of movement with muscle toning or posture that is caused by an insult to the immature developing the brain.	Stiff muscles and exaggerated reflexes, lack of muscles, tremors, slow movements, delay motors skill. Dragging a leg while crawling and seizures.	Happiness	Minty
Cervical Disk Disease: degeneration is a common cause of neck pain most frequently felt like a stiff neck.	Cervical Disk pain that is usually related to activity and will flare up at times. The pain can go away entirely.	Hunger	Pink
Cervicobrachial Syndrome: common cause of neck pain, most frequently felt like a stiff neck. Cervical degenerative disc disease is far less common than disc degeneration in the lumbar spine.	As we mature the cervicobrachial changes the in the body that becomes weaker, more fragile and thin cartilage.	Serenity	Skunks
Chemotherapy (often abbreviated to chemo): and is a category of cancer treatment that uses chemical substances especially one or more anti-cancer drugs.	Some of the most common side effects of chemotherapy involve the digestive tract. Mouth sores and dry mouth can make it difficult to chew and swallow.	Sleepiness	Spicy
Chronic Fatigue Syndrome: is a complicated disorder significant fatigue that can't be explained by any initial medical specification. The fatigue may decline with physical or mental activity but doesn't improve with rest.	Chronic fatigue is the loss of memory or concentration. Feeling unrepressed after sleep, muscle pain, headaches, multi-joint pain, persistent sore throat. Without redness, swelling and tender lymph in your neck and armpits.	Minty	Woody
Chronic: pain is often pain lasting more than 12 weeks. Whereas acute pain is a normal feeling.	Pain that won't go away as expected after an illness or injury. Pain that may be described as aching, burning, shooting or electrical.	Happiness	Minty

Chronic Renal (kidney): Failure is the gradual loss of kidney function. Kidneys filter wastes and excess fluids from your blood then excreted in your urine. When chronic kidney disease reaches a progressive stage dangerous levels of fluid, electrolytes and wastes can build up in your body.	Natural bruising muscle twitching, cramps, breath odor, blood in the stool and excessive thirst.	Hunger	Pink
Cluster Headaches: can awaken you in the middle of the night causing penetrating pain around one eye on one side of your head.	Agonizing pain generally located in or around the eye. May radiate to other areas of your face, head, neck and shoulders. Can be a one-sided pain.	Serenity	Skunks
Cocaine Dependence: also called coke or blow is a dangerous stimulant that is in both powdered and cracks rock (hard) appears. Powdered cocaine can be snorted by melting the power and injecting it. Crack cocaine is consumed by heating the stone in a pipe and inhaling the smoke. The high resulting from cocaine varies depending on the method used.	Anxiety, irritability, paranoia, restlessness. Loss of the sense of smell nosebleeds, difficulty swallowing hoarseness and chronically runny nose.	Happiness	Fruity
Colitis Inflammation: affects the large intestine and symptoms may recur. After a period of remission of months or even years you could experience what's commonly known as a flare.	Constant urge to have a bowel movement. Tenesmus may exist with abdominal pain may come in waves building diarrhea and continuous pain.	Upliftedness	Woody
Conjunctivitis: also called (Pinkeye) is redness and infection of the thin tissues layer with the whites of the eyes and the membranes on the inner part of the eyelids. Pinkeye is most often caused by a virus or by a bacterial infection.	Bacteria and viruses such as gonorrhea or chlamydia can irritant by shampoos, dirt, smoke, dust, pollen, contact leans and pool chlorine.	Focus	Hash

Constipation: occurs when stools are difficult to pass. Some people are overly concerned with the frequency of their bowel.	Hard compacted stools that are difficult or painful to pass. Straining during bowel movements; fewer bowel movements than usual stomachache or cramping that is relieved by bowel movements.	Happiness	Minty
Cohn's Disease: can affect any part of the GI tract from the mouth to the anus. It most commonly affects the end of the small intestine (the ileum) where the joins the beginning of the colon. Crohn's disease may appear in "patches" affecting some areas of the GI tract while leaving other sections completely untouched.	Persistent Diarrhea rectal bleeding urgent need to move bowels, abdominal cramps and pain. Sensation of incomplete evacuation constipation (can lead to bowel obstruction). General symptoms that may also be associated with IBD. Fever, loss of appetite, weight loss, fatigue, night sweats, loss of normal menstrual cycle.	Hunger	Pink
Arteriosclerotic Heath Disease: is a thickening and hardening of the walls of the coronary arteries. As a result of invasion and accumulation of white blood cells.	Other symptoms include sinus infections, growth, fatty, clubbing of the finger and toes. Infertility in males among others. Different people may have different degrees of symptoms.	Serenity	Skunks
Cystic Fibrosis (CF): also known as mucoviscidosis is an inherited disorder that mostly affects the lungs but can affect the pancreas, liver, kidneys and intestine. Long-term issues include difficulty breathing and coughing up sputum as a result of frequent lung infections.	Breathlessness, a cough that produces thick mucus (sputum), exercise intolerance, stuffy nose, lung infections and wheezing	Sleepiness	Spicy
Damage to Spinal Cord: is a collection of nerves that travels from the bottom of the brain down your back.Injuries can cause weakness or complete loss of muscle function.	Damage to spinal cord bladder or bowels. Control, problem moving arms or legs, headache, numbness or tingling in extremities. Pain, pressure or stiffing in the back and neck area also unconsciousness.	Upliftedness	Woody

Condition	Symptoms		
Delirium Tremens: is alcohol withdrawal delirium (AWD) is the most severe form of alcohol withdrawal. It causes sudden and severe problems in your brain and nervous system.	Anxiety, chest pain, delusion, fatigue, increased breathing or heart rate, sweating, restlessness and mood swings.	Sleepiness	Spicy
Dermatomyositis: is an uncommon incendiary disease. Offen occurs when muscles become inflamed, inflammatory myopathy). It is one of only three known inflammatories.	It is one of only three known inflammatories. Is weakness in the muscles, tenderness problems swallowing, lung problems and hard calcium deposits underneath the skin.	Happiness	Minty
Diabetes Adult Onset: is a metabolic disorder that can be characterized by hyperglycemia (high blood sugar) with the lack of insulin resistance and relative lack of insulin. Diabetes is in contrast to diabetes mellitus type 1.	The classic symptoms are excess thirst, frequent urination and constant.	Hunger	Pink
Diabetes Insulin Dependent Mellitus (IDDM): also known as type 1 diabetes, usually starts before 15 years of age but can occur in adults too. Diabetes involves the pancreas gland which is located behind the stomach.	Weight loss or poor weight gain even if eating large amounts of food More thirst than usual Enuresis (bedwetting) Frequent urination, feeling tired all the time. Dry skin and mouth, hard to breathe, sugar and acetone will be positive blood sugar is very high (above 126 mg/dL). Loss of appetite "fruity" odor to the breath and stomach pain.	Happiness	Minty
Diabetes Neuropathy: nerve damages that happen when a person has diabetes, high blood sugar, diabetes neuropathy cause nerves damages in feet and legs.	Balance or coordination, burning or tingling sensation, cramps or pain in the feet and legs and numbness or reflexes in the ankle. Ulcers on foot, infection, deformities to bone and joint pain.	Sleepiness	Spicy

Diabetes Peripheral Arterial Disease: called PAD occurs when blood vessels in the legs are narrowed or blocked by fatty deposits and blood flow to your feet and legs decreases.	Autonomic neuropathy causes symptoms associated with dysfunction of an organ system. Pain, burning, tingling and numbness in the feet and lower legs.	Happiness	Minty
Diarrhea: is caused by an increased flow of water into the intestine reduced absorption of fluid from the organ or rapid passage of stool through the body.	Diarrhea can be the bowel movements are frequent and watery.	Hunger	Pink
Dysthymic Disorder: materializes as depression that can last at least two years or longer.	Loss of interest in actives, sadness or feeling down hopelessness, tiredness and lack of low energy, self-esteem, self-criticism or feeling incapable. Trouble concentrating and making decisions. Irritability or excessive anger.	Serenity	Skunks
Endometrial Cancer: is cancer that began in the uterus (a hollow pear-shaped pelvic organ) where fetal development occurs. Endometrial cancer is sometimes called uterine sarcoma.	An abnormal watery or blood-tinged discharge from your vagina pelvic pain. Pain during intercourse, painful periods (dysmenorrhea). Pelvic pain and cramping may begin several days before and into your period with lower back and abdominal pain.	Sleepiness	Spicy
Endometriosis: is the materialization of uterine-lining tissue outside the uterus.	Painful periods (dysmenorrhea). Pelvic, abdominal pain, heavy periods, infertility and cramping. May begin until several days into your period lower back and abdominal pain with intercourse.	Focus	Hash
Epidermolysis Bullosa: is an accumulation of rare diseases that cause the skin to blister. The blisters appear in response to minor injury, heat or friction.	A swollen scrotum, testicle pain and tenderness usually on one side. Painful urination enlarged lymph nodes in the groin.	Happiness	Serenity

Condition	Symptoms		
Epididymitis: is a red swollen or warm scrotum with testicle pain or tenderness usually on one side. Painful urination and frequent urinate discharge from the penis. Painful intercourse or ejaculation a lump on the penis. Also discomfort in the lower abdomen or pelvic area blood in the semen.	Warmth in the scrotum area with low-grade fever, chills, pain, pressure, enlarged lymph nodes, urination, bowel movements, pain during intercourse and ejaculation in the pelvic area.	Hunger Serenity	Pink Skunks
Epilepsy: is a central nervous system disorder, also know as (neurological disorder) in which nerve cell activity in the brain become disrupted. When that occurs seizures or unusual behavior, sensation or loss of consciousness can happen.	Anxiety, fear, temporary confusion, staring spell, jerking of the arms and legs.	Sleepiness	Spicy
Felty's Syndrome: is of long-standing rheumatoid arthritis. felty's syndrome is defined by three conditions: rheumatoid arthritis, an enlarged spleen (splenomegaly), and an abnormally low white blood cell count. Felty's syndrome is uncommon. It affects less than 1% of patients with rheumatoid arthritis.	Loss of appetite, deformities, eye discharge, fatigue, general discomfort, infections, joint pain, stiffness and swelling.	Focus	Hash
Fibromyalgia: means enormous pain all over the body without signs of inflammation. Fibromyalgia causes many other symptoms.	Anxiety, chronic fatigue, depression, breathing disorder, lack of energy and sleep.	Happiness	Fruity
Frederica's Ataxia (FRDA): is a genetic progressive neurodegenerative movement disorder with a mean age of onset between 10 and 15 years.	The Initial symptom of FRDA is progressive ataxia of the limbs and during walking. Ataxia involves poor muscle coordination that results in an unsteady gait and poor control of subtle movements.	Hunger	Hash

Condition	Symptoms		
Gastritis: is inflammation of the lining of the stomach. The swelling of gastritis is most often the result of infection with the same bacterium that causes most stomach ulcers. Injury and drinking too much alcohol also can contribute to gastritis.	Nausea or recurrent upset stomach, abdominal bloating, abdominal pain, vomiting, indigestion, burning or gnawing feeling in the stomach between meals or at a night. Hiccups and loss of appetite.	Serenity	Minty
Genital Herpes: there's no cure for genital herpes. Genital herpes is a sexually transmitted infection disease called herpes simplex virus (HSV). Genital herpes lies dormant in your body and can reactivate several times a year.	Pain and itching with no visible sores in your genital area. You may have no sign or symptoms.	Sleepiness	Spicy
Glaucoma: will cause damage to your eye's optic nerve and gets worse over time. It's often associated with a buildup of pressure inside the eye. Glaucoma may be inherited and may not show up until later in life.	Glaucoma may be inherited and may not show up until later in life.	Focus	Earthy
Glioblastoma Multiforme(GBM): classification name "glioblastoma" also known as Grade IV astrocytoma is the most common and most aggressive (Brain Cancer).	Glioblastoma includes seizure, nausea and vomiting, headache, memory and speech, weakness on one side of the body and change in vision.	Happiness	Fruity
Graves' Disease: (Toxic Diffuse Goiter) and Flajani-Basedow-Graves' disease is an autoimmune disease that affects the thyroid.	Increased appetite, diarrhea, excessive sweating, hair loss, hand tremor, heat intolerance, hyperactivity, itching, muscle weakness, moistness, muscle weakness, palpitations and skin warmth.	Hunger	Hash
Hemophilia A: is when your body doesn't have enough protein called factor VIII that the body needs to make clots and stop bleeding.	Blood in the stool or urine and nosebleed. Suffering from a small injury start and stop bleeding and massive bruising.	Happiness	Minty

Henoch-Schonlein Purpura: is a disorder that causes bleeding and inflammation in the small blood vessels, skin, joints, intestines and kidneys.	A disease of the skin mucous membranes and sometimes other organs, rash and swollen joints.	Sleepiness	Spicy
Hepatitis C Virus: is a liver disease. The virus causes acute and chronic hepatitis infection. Hepatitis C Virus was ranging from severity to a mild illness from a few weeks to a lifelong disease. Hepatitis C transfusion of unscreened blood and blood products.	Acute liver failure result, decreased appetite, fatigue, joint pains, muscle, nausea and weight loss.	Focus	Earthy
Hereditary Spinal Ataxia: is a lack of muscle control or involuntary movements of the muscle.	Change in speech, difficulty with fine motor tasks, such as eating, writing, swallowing or buttoning a shirt. Involuntary back-and-forth eye movements (nystagmus). Poor coordination and unsteady walking with a tendency to stumble.	Happiness	Fruity
HIV/AIDS (Human immunodeficiency virus) HIV/AIDS: is a condition caused by infection. Stages of HIV complicated by a disease of the lung known as pneumocystis pneumonia. Severe weight loss, a type of cancer known as Kaposi's sarcoma or other AIDS-defining conditions.	Fever, headache, large tender lymph nodes, sores of the mouth, genitals and throat inflammation.	Hunger	Happiness
Huntington's Disease: is an inherited disease causes the (degeneration) progressive breakdown of nerve in the brain Cells. Huntington's disease has a substantial impact on a person's functional abilities and usually results in movement, thinking (cognitive) and psychiatric disorders.	An inherited disorder that results in the death of brain cells. Earliest symptoms are a subtle problem with mood or mental abilities. Lack of coordination, unsteady, jerky body movements, physical skills gradually worsen. Awkward and unable to talk with the decline into dementia.	Hunger	Hash

Hypertension: is high blood pressure is a common condition in which the long-term force of the blood against your artery walls such as heart disease.	Confusion, dizziness, weakness, fainting a feeling of being outside yourself.	Sleepiness	Spicy
Hyperventilation Syndrome: is more accurate and relates to an over breathing pattern that happens under certain conditions. This over breathing results in a group of symptoms.	Some people hyperventilation is rare. Occurs can be the occasional panicked response to fear, stress or a phobia. For some people emotional states such as depression, anxiety or anger.	Woody	Earthy
Hypoglycemia: also known as low blood glucose or low blood sugar occurs when blood glucose drops below normal levels. Glucose a vital source of energy for the body. Carbohydrates are the primary dietary source of glucose. Rice, potatoes, bread, tortillas, cereal, milk, fruit and sweets are all carbohydrate-rich foods.	Clamminess, drowsiness, dizziness, include hunger, irritability, low blood sugar, paleness, rapid heartbeat, shakiness and sweating and weakness.	Happiness	Fruity
Impotence: is a common problem among men consistent inability to sustain an erection. Erectile dysfunction can vary in men.	Anxiety, diabetes, alcoholism, impotence, medical conditions, (alcoholism,) medications, trauma, and outside influences can contribute to impotence.	Sleepiness	Spicy
Inflammatory of the Bowel Disease (IBD): combinations of gut-brain axis problems, gut motility disorders, pain sensitivity, infections including small intestinal bacterial overgrowth.	Abdominal pain and cramping. Blood in your stool, diarrhea, fever, fatigue, reduced appetite and unintended weight loss.	Focus	Woody
Intermittent Explosive Disorder (IED): behavioral disorder repeated sudden episodes of impulsive, aggressive, violent behavior or angry verbal outbursts. Over react grossly out of proportion to the situation. Road rage, domestic abuse, throwing or breaking objects, or other temper tantrums.	Energy changes, mood changes and tension.	Focus	Earthy

Intractable Vomiting: is repeated vomiting with nausea that resists medical treatment. People can develop this symptom for some reasons and therapy is focused on providing supportive care.	A migraine, seizure disorders, chronic intestinal pseudo-obstruction, gastroparesis, irritable bowel syndrome, bacteria, bacterial toxins, food-borne toxins and pneumonia.	Happiness	Fruity
Lou Gehrig's Disease: amyotrophic lateral sclerosis (ALS) is a rapidly progressive uniformly fatal neurodegenerative disease. The loss of motor neurons in the brainstem, spinal cord and cerebral cortex leading to a decline in muscular function. It eventually results in weakness, speech deficits and difficulty swallowing. ALS is almost always fatal in two to three years.	Cramps, chewing, difficulty with writing, buttoning a shirt, leg or arm weakness causing an awkward gait or stumbling. Twitching or stiff muscles, swallowing and Slurred speech.	Hunger	Hash
Lyme Disease (Borrelia burgdorferi): is caused by the most common tick-borne illness (tick bite) in North America and Europe. Lyme disease is transmitted by the bite of an infected black-legged tick.	Lyme disease is often a bite mark that often becomes red swollen and very tender. As the bacteria spread in the body severe headaches and neck stiffness and rash on other parts of the body. Particularly the knees and others large joints of the body. facial palsy	Serenity	Minty
Lymphoma Hodgkin: cancer that affects the immune system. It is a cancer of immune cells called lymphocytes.	Pain in armpits, fatigue, fever, groin, itching, lymph, night sweats and weight loss.	Sleepiness	Spicy
Major Depression: feel sad or weak at some point in their lives. Clinical depression is a depressed mood most of the day.	Major Depression mostly people feel sad or weak at some point in their lives. But clinical depression is marked by a depressed mood most of the day.	Upliftedness	Woody

Malignant Melanoma: is a kind of cancer. That can develop from the pigment-containing cells known as melanocytes. Exposure to the sun such as your arms, back, face and legs.	Melanomas can develop anywhere on your body. A change in an existing mole, new pigmented or unusual looking growth on the skin.	Serenity	Minty
Melorheostosis: also know as Leri Disease is unusual mesenchymal dysplasia manifesting as regions of sclerosing bone. With the unique dripping wax appearance or flowing candle was appearance began in childhood.	Absent or abnormal muscles, irregular bone growth, dripping candle wax" appearance on x-ray imaging, cortical thickening unequal length of limbs, joint swelling, soft tissue abnormalities, subcutaneous calcification, tendon and ligament shortening.	Minty	Spicy
Meniere's Disease: is a disarrange of the inner ear that causes spontaneous episodes of vertigo a sensation of a spinning motion.	Feeling of fullness in the ear, hearing loss, ringing in the ear (tinnitus) and recurring episodes of vertigo.	Focus	Earthy
Mucopolysaccharidosis (MPS): is a collection of metabolic disorders caused by the absence or malfunctioning of lysosomal enzymes, that needed to break down molecules called glycosaminoglycan's. Long chains of sugar carbohydrates in each of our cells.	Enlarged cheeks, head, lips, tongue and nose. Vocal cords, deep voice and sleep apnea, carpal tunnel syndrome, heart (valve) disease and upper respiratory infections.	Happiness	Fruity
Multiple Sclerosis (MS): is a disease where attacks the protective sheath (myelin) that covers your nerves and immune system. Myelin can disrupt communication between your brain and the rest of your body.	Bowel and bladder function, partial or complete loss of vision. Usually in one eye at a time, dizziness, fatigue, electric-shock that occur with specific neck movements, especially bending the neck forward. Weakness in one or more limbs that occurs on one side of your body, slurred speech, tingling in parts of your body, tremor and lack of coordination or unsteady gait.	Serenity	Minty

Muscle Spasm Esophageal spasms: are painful muscle contractions that affect your esophagus. The hollow tube between your throat and your stomach. Sudden severe chest pain that may last for few minutes to an hour.	Chest Pain so intense it's mistaken for a heart attack, feeling sometimes in your chest or throat heart burn, liquid back - up your mouth and trouble swallowing.	Sleepiness	Spicy
Myeloid Leukemia Acute: myelogenous leukemia (AML) is a cancer of the blood and bone marrow tissue inside bones where blood cells are made.	Early stages of acute leukemia may mimic the flu or other common diseases. Fever, bone pain, lethargy, fatigue, short of breath, pale skin, frequent infection, easy bruising and unusual bleeding.	Upliftedness	Woody
Nightmares: is a troubling dream associated with negative feelings such as anxiety or fear.	Nightmares are common. A nightmare is a troubling dream associated with negative feelings such as anxiety or fear.	Focus	Focus
Obesity: is a complicated disorder involving an excessive amount of body fat. Obesity isn't just a cosmetic concern. (BMI) Is calculated by dividing your weight in kilograms (kg). Your height in meters (m^2) squared.	Obesity isn't just a cosmetic concern. Concern with overweight-related health problems.	Happiness	Fruity
Obsessive-Compulsive Disorder (OCD): is an irrational thought and anxieties (compulsions). That will lead you to do repetitive compulsions behaviors. A person can have just one obsession or compulsions and still have OCD.	Obsessive-compulsive disorder (OCD Is an irrational thought and anxieties (compulsions). That will lead you to do repetitive compulsions behaviors. A person can have just one obsession or compulsions and still have OCD.	Serenity	Minty
Opiate Dependence: morphine injection is used to relieve direct to severe pain. It may also be used before or during surgery with an anesthetic.	Opiate Dependence it acts on the central nervous system (CNS) to relieve pain.	Sleepiness	Spicy

Osteoarthritis: is the most common form of arthritis affecting millions of people worldwide. It occurs when the protective cartilage on the ends of your bones wears down over time.	Osteoarthritis. It occurs when the protective cartilage on the ends of your bones wears down over time.	Upliftedness	Woody
Panic Disorder: is a sudden episode of intense fear that triggers severe physical reactions. When there is no real danger or apparent cause. Panic attacks can be very frightening. When a panic attacks occur you might think you're losing control having a heart attack or even dying.	Feeling of choking, accelerated heart, palpitations, pounding of the heart, sweating and trembling.	Focus	Hash
Parkinson's Disease: is a progressive disorder of the nervous system that affects movement. It develops gradually, sometimes starting with a barely noticeable tremor in just one hand. But while a tremor may be the most well-known sign of Parkinson's disease. The disorder also commonly causes stiffness or slowing of movement.	Resting tremors, slow movement (bradykinesia) stiff muscles, balance or falling, being stuck in place while walking, reduced arm swings on one side of your body. Dragging foot, small voice, loss of automatic movements like blinking, swallowing, speech, writing, smell and taste.	Happiness	Fruity
Peripheral Neuropathy: a result of damage to your peripheral nerves often causes weakness, numbness and pain. Usually in your hands and feet. It can also affect other areas of your body.	Gradual feeling of numbness, prickling or tingling in your feet or hands that spread upward into your legs and arms. Sharp, jabbing, throbbing, freezing or burning pain sensitivity to touch lack of coordination, falling muscle weakness or paralysis.	Hunger	Hash
Persistent Insomnia: is a persistent disorder that can make it hard to fall asleep. Hard to stay asleep or both despite the opportunity for adequate sleep.	Anxiety, depression and stress are some of the most common causes of chronic insomnia.	Sleepiness	Spicy

Porphyria: can be a rare hereditary disease in which the blood pigment hemoglobin is abnormally metabolized.	Abdominal pain, often severe chest pain with increased heart rate, blood pressure, back pain, limb muscle weakness, tingling, loss of sensation, cramping with vomiting and constipation. Personality changes or mental disorders agitation, confusion and seizures.	Upliftedness	Woody
Post-Polio Syndrome (PPS): is an infectious viral disease that can strike at any age and affects a person's nervous system.	Can affected muscles weakness, extreme fatigue, joint pain, skeletal deformities such as scoliosis PPS copycat those of the disorder known as Lou Gehrig's.	Arousal	Dank
Post-Traumatic Arthritis: is a common form of osteoarthritis (OA) is the wearing away of cartilage in the joint. This condition can occur in any joint including the shoulder, elbow, wrist, hip, knee and ankle.	Joint pain fluid accumulation in the joint swelling, decreased tolerance for walking, sports, stairs and other activities that stress the joint.	Creativity	Earthy
Post-Traumatic Stress (PTSD): is an anxiety disorder that can develop after a person is exposed to one or more traumatic events. Such as major stress, sexual assault, warfare or other threats on a person's life.	Emotional numbness, difficulty concentrating and sleeping, feeling jumpy, flashbacks, nightmares, avoidance activities, people, places easily being irritated and angered.	Energy	Fruity
Premenstrual Syndrome (PMS): changes that happen before a woman's monthly period. Including symptoms ranging from bloating, weight gain to mood swings and depression.	Moodiness, depression, abdominal cramping, bloating, food cravings, headaches, muscle aches,breast tenderness and fatigue, acne.	Happiness	Minty
Prostate Cancer: in a man's prostate gland a small walnut-shaped gland that produces the seminal fluid that nourishes and transports to the male reproductive system. Cancer cells that spread mainly to the bones and lymph nodes.	Blood in semen trouble urinating, decreased force in the stream of urine. Discomfort in the pelvic area, bone pain and erectile dysfunction.	Hunger	Pink

Prostatitis: is inflammation and swelling and of the prostate gland located below the bladder in men. The prostate gland produces fluid (semen) that nourishes and transports sperm.	Prostatitis often causes painful or difficult urination. Other symptoms include pain in the groin, pelvic area or genitals and sometimes flu-like symptoms.	Serenity	Skunks
Psoriasis: is a chronic disease that comes and goes. The primary goal is to stop the skin cells from proliferating.	Red patches of skin seen in children covered with thick silvery scales spots. Dry skin that may bleed, burning or itching with pitted nails that are swollen and stiff joints.	Sleepiness	Spicy
Pulmonary Fibrosis: is the thickness and scars tissue around and between the (alveoli) air sacs in the lungs. Causing difficult for oxygen to pass into the bloodstream	Shortness of breath (dyspnea) fatigue, aching muscles, joint. Shortness of breath, widening and rounding the finger tips or toes (clubbing).	Upliftedness	Woody
Quadriplegia Paralysis: can be either periodic partial, complete or incomplete. Paralysis of both the arms and legs.	Is a spinal cord injury. Other conditions such as strokes and cerebral palsy can cause a similar appearing paralysis.	Arousal	Dank
Radiation Therapy: is used as a high energy radiation to shrink tumors and kill cancer cells. X- rays and particles are types of radiation used for cancer treatment.	Some people who received radiation therapy experience dryness, blistering, peeling, fatigue, head, neck, chest, stomach, abdomen and pelvis pain.	Energy	Fruity
Reynaud's Disease (ray-NOHZ Arteries: were narrowing your vessels and temporarily limiting blood supply to your fingers and toes go into vasospasm when exposed to cold or stress.	Cold finger or toes can change in your skin in response to cold and stress. Causing stinging or numb pain upon warming or stress relief.	Focus	Minty
Reiter's Syndrome: is an inflammatory reaction to an infection somewhere in the body. It usually follows a urogenital or intestinal disease.	Pain and stiffness most commonly occur in your knees, ankles, feet, low back, buttocks and eye. Inflammation (conjunctivitis) a urinary problem also inflammation of the prostate gland or cervix.	Happiness	Pink

Condition	Symptoms		
Restless Legs Syndrome (RLS): is not entirely known can be related to genetic factors. Low iron levels in the brain or diseases such as chronic kidney or even diabetes.	Include aching, crawling, twitching, itching and throbbing in the legs.	Focus	Hash
Rheumatoid Arthritis (RA): is a form arthritis that causes swelling, stiffness, pain with loss of function in your joints and impact the wrist and fingers.	Stiffness, swelling, pain in the affected joints.	Happiness	Minty
Rosacea: is a chronic and potentially life-troublesome disorder mainly of the facial skin. Often characterized by flare-ups and remissions.	Pimples and bumps often develop in severe cases. The nose may grow swollen and bumpy from excess tissue	Hunger	Pink
Schizoaffective Disorder: is a chronic mental health condition. Characterized mainly by symptoms of delusions, hallucinations and mood disorder such as mania and depression.	Symptoms of schizophrenia may vary but typically include delusions, hallucinations, disorganized thinking or speaking and abnormal motor behavior.	Serenity	Skunks
Schizophrenia: is a mental disorder represented by abnormal social behavior and failure to understand what is real.	Include false beliefs, confused thinking or unclear, hearing voices that others do not hear. Reduced social engagement and emotional expression and a lack of motivation.	Sleepiness	Spicy
Scoliosis: the spine has a sideways curve usually "S"- or "C"-shaped. In some the degree of curvature is stable while in others it increases over time. Mild scoliosis does not usually cause problems while severe cases can interfere with breathing.	Back pain, shoulders, neck, buttock pain nearest bottom of the back, respiratory and cardiac problems in severe cases. Constipation due to curvature causing "tightening" of the stomach, intestines limited mobility.	Upliftedness	Woody

Sedative Dependence : includes an assortment of drugs that depressing the central nervous system. Barbiturates and benzodiazepines are the most common. But other painkillers include chloral hydrate, glutethimide, methaqualone and meprobamate.	Cravings for the drugs, anxiety, insomnia, nervousness, tremors, loss of appetite, nightmares, rapid breathing, fast heartbeat and ups and down in blood pressure.	Arousal	Dank
Seizures: are based on the type of behavior and brain activity. Seizures are divided into two broad categories generalized and partial (also called local or focal).	Violent shaking and a loss of control a sudden feeling of fear or anxiousness. Feeling sick to your stomach, dizziness with vision change. A jerking of the arms and legs that may cause you to drop things an out of body sensation and headache.	Creativity	Earthy
Senile Dementia: is severe mental deterioration in old age. Represented by the loss of memory and control of bodily functions.	Memory, communication and language problem. Unable to focus and pay attention, reasoning, judgment and visual perception.	Euphoria	Hash
Severe Nausea: appearing shortly after eating. Nausea or vomiting may be caused by gastritis (inflammation of the stomach lining), bulimia, food poisoning and ulcer.	A headache, fever, diarrhea, gas, vomiting, dizziness, lightheadedness, diarrhea, abdominal pain and a general feeling of being sick to one's stomach.	Focus	Minty
Shingles (Herpes Zoster): highly contagious infection usually spread through sex. Occur soon after a person is infected. Start as small blisters that ultimately break open and fertile painful raw sores scab that can heal over few weeks. This disease is usually caused by the herpes simplex virus-2.	A headache, itching, rash, blisters, flu-like symptoms, vision change, fever and swollen lymph nodes.	Happiness	Pink

Sinusitis inflammation: or swelling of the tissue lining the sinuses. Usually sinuses are filled with air but when sinuses become blocked and filled with fluid, bacteria, fungi, germs the viruses can grow and cause an infection.	Facial pain, pressure, nasal stuffiness, nasal discharge, loss of smell cough and congestion.	Happiness	Minty
Skeletal Muscular: somatic nervous system (Sons or voluntary nervous system) is the part of the peripheral nervous system associated with skeletal muscle optional control of body movements.	Increased muscle tone with overactive reflexes, involuntary movements. Which may include spasms brisk or sustained involuntary muscle contraction.	Hunger	Pink
Sleep Apnea: means that your breathing is blocked or partly blocked during sleep.	Excessive daytime sleepiness. Waking with an unrepressed feeling after sleep.	Serenity	Skunks
Spasticity: is a muscle control disorder that is characterized by tight or stiff muscles and an inability to control those muscles. Also reflexes may persist for too long and maybe too thick (hyperactive reflexes).	Numbness or weakness most often in the legs, feet, and buttocks. Numbness, weakness, cramping or pain in the legs, feet or buttocks.	Sleepiness	Spicy
Spinal Stenosis: of the lower back also called lumbar area. Is a narrowing of the space within the spine.	Arm, back pain, bladder, foot or leg, tingling in hands and weakness.	Upliftedness	Woody
Stuttering: is not uncommon for children between the ages of 2 and five years old. It may come and go or last a few weeks or a couple of years. Most children outgrow stuttering without professional intervention.	Difficulty starting a word, sentence or phrase. Repetition of a sound syllable or word, brief silence for certain syllables or words or pauses within a nutshell (broken word). Addition extra words like "UM."	Energy	Fruity

Surge- Weber Syndrome (SWS): is a neurological disorder marked by a distinctive port-wine stain around the eye, forehead and scalp. This stain is a birthmark caused by an overabundance of capillaries near the surface of the skin. Blood vessels on the same side of the brain as the dye may also be affected.	Cognitive impairment, developmental delays, paralysis, seizures and weakness on one side of the body.	Creativity	Earthy
Tardive Dyskinesia (TD): is a difficult-to-treat and often incurable form of dyskinesia. A disorder resulting in involuntary body movements. In this type of dyskinesia is the involuntary movements are tardive and have a slow onset.	Arm and leg movements, lip smacking, facial grimacing, finger tapping and rapid eye blinking.	Euphoria	Hash
Temporomandibular Joint Disorder (TMJ): is a joint that connects your jaw to the temporal bones of your skull that is in front of each ear. Allowing you move your jaw up and down and side to side so you can talk, chew and yawn.	Ear aches, dizziness, headaches, hearing problem, toothaches, neck aches, ringing in the ears (tinnitus). Jaw that get "stuck" or "lock" in the open - or closed- mouth position.	Focus	Minty
Tenosynovitis: is a painful condition affecting the tendons on the thumb side of your wrist.	Difficulty moving your thumb and wrist when you're doing something that involves grasping or pinching. A "sticking" or "stop-and-go" sensation in your thumb when moving it with pain or swelling near the base of the thumb.	Happiness	Minty
A Tension Headache: is mild to moderate pain in your head that's as feeling like a tight band around your head.	Aching head pain with tightness or pressure across the side of your forehead or the side and back of your head. Your scalp, neck and shoulder have muscles pain.	Hunger	Pink

Terminal illness: is a home based family care for individuals facing a terminal illness. Hospice addresses these aspects of a terminal disease when appropriate.	A methodical process denial, listen, accept ask the person what they want and grief.	Serenity	Skunks
Testicular Cancer: the testicles produce male sex hormones and sperm for reproduction occurs in the testicles (testes). They are located inside the scrotum a loose bag of skin underneath the penis.	A lump or enlargement in either testicle with a feeling of heaviness in the scrotum. A dull ache in the abdomen or groin. A sudden collection of fluid in the scrotum. Pain or discomfort in a testicle or the scrotum enlargement or tenderness of the breasts and back pain.	Sleepiness	Spicy
Thyroiditis: is swollen thyroid called thyroiditis. It primarily affects women from early adulthood to middle age although anyone can get it.	Anxiety, fatigue, insomnia, irritability, rapid heartbeat or palpitations. Tremor and unexplained weight loss with increased sensitivity to heat.	Upliftedness	Woody
TIC DouloureuxIn Trigeminal neuralgia: is also called tic douloureux the trigeminal nerve's function is disrupted. Usually the problem is contact between a typical blood vessel in this case an artery or a vein. The trigeminal nerve at the base of your brain. This communication puts pressure on the nerve and causes it to malfunction.	Episodes of severe, shooting or jabbing pain, shaving, touching your face, eating, drinking, brushing your teeth, talking, putting on makeup, encountering a breeze, smiling and washing your face.	Arousal	Dank
Tietze's Syndrome: Costochondritis is an inflammation of the cartilage that connects a rib to the breastbone (sternum). Pain caused by costochondritis might mimic that of a heart attack or other heart conditions.	Can occur on the left side of your breastbone with a sharp aching or pressure. Can affect more than the rib worsens when you take a deep breath or a cough.	Creativity	Earthy
Tinnitus: is noise or ringing in the ears. The inner ear cell damage. Tiny hairs in your inner ear move about the pressure of sound waves.	Buzzing, clicking, hissing, ringing and roaring.	Energy	Fruity

Tobacco Dependence Nicotine: is an addiction to tobacco products induced by the drug nicotine.	Can't stop smoking, physical and mood swings, intense cravings, anger, anxiety, difficulty concentrating, constipation depressed mood irritability, restlessness, frustration, increased hunger, insomnia and diarrhea.	Euphoria	Happiness
Tourette's Syndrome: is a nervous system (neurological) disorder that starts in childhood. It involves unusual repetitive movements or unwanted sounds that can't be controlled (tics).	Eye blinking, head jerking, stepping in a particular pattern. Touching or smelling objects, repeating observed movements shoulder shrugging, eye darting, obscene gesturing, nose twitching, bending or twisting, mouth movements and hopping.	Focus	Minty
Trichotillomania: known as hair pulling disorder characterized by the compulsive urge to pull out one's hair.	Many people also pick their skin, bite their nails or chew their lips. Sometimes pulling hairs from pets or dolls or other materials.	Happiness	Pink
Uterine Cancer: is a type of cancer that begins in the uterus. The uterus is the hollow pear-shaped pelvic organ in women where fetal development occurs.	Vaginal bleeding after menopause. Bleeding between periods an abnormal, watery or blood-tinged discharge from your vagina pelvic pain.	Focus	Hash
Viral Hepatitis: an infection caused by a virus that attacks the liver and leads to inflammation. Most people infected with the hepatitis C virus (HCV).	Some people have no symptoms others may have yellow discoloration of the skin and whites of the eyes. Abdominal, diarrhea pain that's reduced appetite, vomiting and tiredness.	Happiness	Minty
Wasting Syndrome: AIDS patients are said to have it when they have lost at least 10% of their body weight due to diarrhea for at least a month. Extreme weakness and fever that not related to an infection especially muscle.	Depression opportunistic infections, like a painful throat or feeling full, lack of energy. Medication side effects like nausea, changes in taste or mouth tingling.	Hunger	Pink

Whiplash: occurs when the head and neck are suddenly forced backward and then forward. Allowing the cervical spine pass thought lightning-quick motions and extreme stresses.	Tendons and muscles in the neck to stretch and tear leaving you with a painful, sore and a stiff neck.	Serenity	Skunks
Wittmaack – EkbomsRestless Legs Syndrome (RLS): also known as Willis-Ekbom disease (WED) or Wittmaack-Ekbom syndrome is a neurological disorder. An urge to move one's body to stop uncomfortable or odd sensations. Commonly affects the legs but can change the arms, torso and head.	An urge to move leg twitching during sleep and motor restlessness.	Sleepiness	Spicy
Writers' Cramp: is also known as scrivener's palsy and mogigraphia is a disorder of cramps or spasms of specific muscles of the hand and forearm. Writers' Cramp happens when performing fine motor tasks such as writing or playing an instrument.	Addition of the finger during writing making the pen difficult to hold hold. Gripping the pen too hard, unusual postures of the wrist or elbow.	Upliftedness	Woody

SATIVA

SATIVA

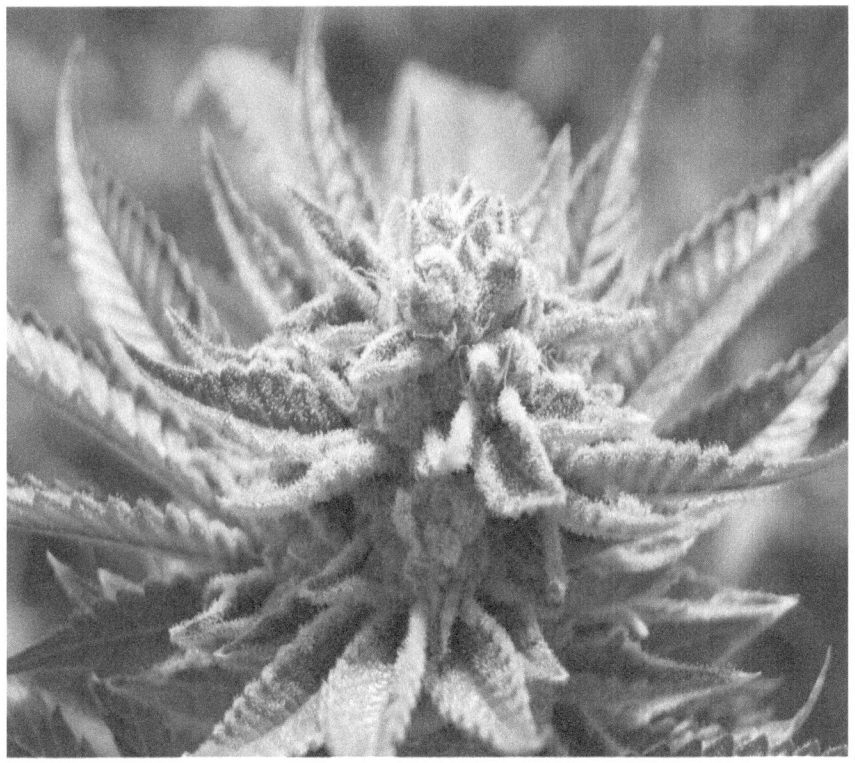

SATIVA

Medical Conditions	Symptoms	Desired Effects	Flavored Scents
Acquired Hypothyroidism: is sometimes called Hashimoto thyroiditis. The thyroid gland is located in the neck and is shaped like a butterfly. Acquired hypothyroidism is a disorder that does not allow the thyroid gland to make enough thyroid hormone.	Slow growth not starting puberty early, periods aren't regular, tiredness, dry skin, constipation, slow heart rate and weight gain	Arousal	Dank
Acute Gastritis: is abrupt inflammation or swelling of the stomach lining can cause nagging and severe pain. Fortunately, the pain usually only lasts for a short period.	Black tarry stools, abdominal bloating, abdominal pain, burning in the stomach. Between meals or at night, hiccups, indigestion, loss of appetite, nausea or recurrent upset stomach, vomiting, vomiting blood or coffee ground-like material.	Creativity	Earthy
Adrenal Cortical Cancer: also known as Adrenal Cortical Carcinoma (ACC) is a rare disease. It is caused by a cancerous growth in the adrenal cortex. Which is the outer layer of the adrenal glands.	Increased facial and body hair particularly in females. The deepened voice in women.	Energy	Fruity
Agoraphobia: is a phobia is defined as the severe unrelenting fear of activity situation or thing that causes one to want to avoid it.	Agoraphobia includes anxiety that feel like a panic attack when in a situation from which escape is not possible or is awkward or embarrassing.	Euphoria	Hash

AIDS-Related Illness: because people with AIDS have weakened immune systems. They're more prone to infections called opportunistic infections. Opportunistic infections are caused by organisms that typically don't cause disease in healthy people but affect people with damaged immune systems.	Coughing and shortness of breath, difficult or painful swallowing, extreme fatigue, fever, mental. Symptoms such as confusion and forgetfulness, nausea, abdominal cramps, vomiting, seizures, lack of coordination. Severe persistent diarrhea, severe headaches, vision loss and weight loss.	Focus	Minty
Alcohol Abuse: is a medical term used as a psychiatric diagnosis in which there is a recurring harmful use of ethanol despite its adverse consequences.	Low tolerance, withdrawal, loss of control, desire to stop but can't. Neglecting of activities, alcohol takes up greater time, energy and focus. Continued use despite negative consequences.	Happiness	Pink
Alcoholism: also known as alcohol use disorder (AUD) and alcohol dependence syndrome. Drinking of alcohol that results in problems.	A person who drinks almost every day may comment that they can't go a day or even two days, without alcohol.	Happiness	Minty
Alzheimer Disease: is a mental deterioration that may occur in old age because of degeneration of the brain. Most common cause of premature senility.	Repetitive questions or conversations, misplacing personal belongings. Forgetting events or appointments, getting lost on a familiar route.	Serenity	Skunks
Amphetamine Dependency: is caused by the frequent and long-term use of the drug. Some people become dependent faster than others.	Patient with amphetamine has violence and mood disturbance, decreased appetite, dry mouth, low energy and high blood pressure.	Sleepiness	Spicy
Amyloidosis: is a rare disease that results from an accumulation of inappropriately folded proteins. These misfolded proteins are called amyloids.	Patients with amyloidosis has abnormal functioning of the bowels, heart, kidneys, liver, nerves, skin, joints and lungs can be affected.	Upliftedness	Woody

Amyotrophic Lateral Sclerosis (ALS): also known as Lou Gehrig disease and Charcot disease. Specific disorder that involves the death of neurons.	ALS is characterized by stiff muscles, muscle twitching and worsening. Also weakness because of muscle wasting, difficulty speaking, swallowing and breathing.	Happiness	Minty
Angina Pectoris: is also known as stable angina. The medical term for chest pain or discomfort because of coronary heart disease.	Common symptoms of angina include chest pain, vertigo, queasiness and sweating. Chest pain because of angina also may be accompanied by pain in the back, neck and shoulders. Individuals with angina also may feel tired and experience shortness of breath.	Serenity	Skunks
Anorexia: is a eating disorder characterized by low weight, fear of gaining weight, a strong desire to be thin and food restrictions.	Fearful of the slightest weight gain and takes all precautionary measures to avoid weight gain. Becoming overweight. noticeable rapid dramatic weight loss, 15 percent under normal body weight, soft beautiful hair growing on the face and body. Obsession with calories and fat content of food.	Upliftedness	Woody
Anorexia Nervosa: has physical and emotional components. That's why it can require the attention of different health care providers such as primary care physicians, mental health counselors, psychologists and psychiatrists.	Individuals with anorexia display varying symptoms. Most obviously associated with malnutrition such as abnormally low body weight. Individuals also exhibit depression and solitude.	Happiness	Minty
Arteriosclerotic Health Disease: is thickening and hardening of the walls of the coronary arteries. As a result of invasion and accumulation of white blood cells.	Symptoms only occur after severe contraction or closure impedes blood flow to different organs enough to induce symptoms.	Hunger	Pink

Arthritis: joints that are associates of the bones that allow flexibility and movement. Joint pain will occur if there is damage because of disease or trauma. The illness or injury will interfere with normal movement of the joint and produce pain.	Inflammation in the hands, feet, knees and ankles.	Serenity	Skunks
Arthritis Rheumatoid: is a chronic inflammatory disorder that typically affects the small joints in your hands and feet. Eventually results in bone erosion.	Tender, warm, swollen joints, morning stiffness that may last for hours. Firm bumps tissue under the skin on your arms (rheumatoid nodules) fatigue, fever and weight loss.	Sleepiness	Spicy
Arthropathy Gout Arthritis: is a form of arthropathy that involves inflammation of one or more joints.	Gout can affect the joints of the feet, ankles, knees, wrists, fingers and elbows. Gout may first appear as nodules on the hands, elbows or ears. Gout can be confused with other forms of arthritis.	Upliftedness	Woody
Asthma: is a common chronic inflammatory disease of the airways characterized by variable and recurring symptoms. Reversible airflow obstruction and bronchospasm.	Wheezing, coughing, chest tightness and shortness of breath.	Happiness	Pink
Attention-Deficit Hyperactivity Disorder (ADHD/ADD): is a neurodevelopment psychiatric disorder.	Symptoms may begin by age six to twelve and persist for six months to make a diagnosis. Although it causes impairment particularly in modern society many children have attention span for tasks they find interesting.	Hunger	Spicy

Autism, Asperger: is a brain disorder is when communication and interaction with others are difficult.	Symptoms of autism spectrum disorder (ASD) may range from lack of communication with others to difficulty in understanding others feelings. Because of the variety of symptoms this condition is now called Autism Spectrum Disorder (ASD).	Sleepiness	Fruity
Autoimmune Disease: that develops when your immune system which defends your body against disease attacks healthy cells. Depending on the type an autoimmune disease can affect one or many different types of body tissue. Autoimmune disease can also cause abnormal organ growth and changes in organ function.	Autoimmune diseases usually fluctuate between periods of remission (little or no symptoms) and flare-ups (worsening symptoms). Currently treatment of autoimmune illnesses focuses on relieving symptoms there is no curative therapy.	Upliftedness	Woody
Back Pain: is felt in the back that can originate from the muscles, nerves, bones, joints or other structures in the spine.	An ache or a sharp or piercing, burning sensation that may radiate to the arm, hands, legs and feet with muscle cramping or spasms. (sudden uncontrollable muscle contractions). Decreased function and range of motion of the various joints difficulty walking, bending forward or sideways or standing straight.	Happiness	Minty
Back Sprain: a sprain is an injury to either a muscle or tendon. Tendons are the tight fibrous bands of tissue that connect muscle to bone. With back pressure. The muscles and tendons that support the spine are twisted, pulled or torn.	Pain with movement, muscle cramping, spasms (sudden uncontrollable muscle contractions). Decreased function and range of motion of the joint difficulty walking, bending forward or sideways or standing straight. In some cases the person may feel pop or tear at the time of injury.	Hunger	Pink

Bells' Palsy: is a form of facial paralysis resulting from a dysfunction of the cranial nerve (the facial nerve) causing an inability to control facial muscles on the affected side. Often the eye on the affected side cannot be closed.	The facial nerve controls some functions such as blinking and closing the eyes, smiling, frowning, lacrimation and salivation.	Serenity	Skunks
Bipolar Disorder: is known as bipolar affective disorder. Manic-depressive illness is a mental disorder with high mood swings and periods of depression.	Bipolar Disorder (manic is the defining feature) can occur with different levels of severity. With milder levels of obsession known as hypomania. Individuals appear energetic, excitable and may be highly productive. As madness worsens a person begins to exhibit erratic and impulsive often making bad decisions with unrealistic ideas and sleep very little.	Sleepiness	Spicy
Brain Tumor: is the illness of the brain in which cancer cells (malignant cells) occur in the brain tissue that affects the brain. Functions such as muscle control, sensation, memory, and other typical body functions.	Difficulty walking, dizziness, seizures, weakness and headaches.	Minty	Woody
Bruxism: is grinding and gnashing of the teeth. Bruxism is because of clenching of the teeth that is associated with dominant lateral or protrusive jaw movements.	Dehydration, anxiety, gum disease, tongue problems, headache and stress.	Happiness	Minty
Bulimia (Bulimia Nervosa): is one of many eating disorders. This mental illness is characterized by episodes of bingeing and somehow purging the food and associated calories in the pursuit of weight loss.	Low blood pressure (hypotension), constipation, abdominal pain, bloating, gas, colitis, endometriosis, food poisoning, GERD, IBS and ovarian dehydration.	Hunger	Minty

Cachexia (Cancer): is marked weight loss, muscular loss, resistant to normal therapies, difficulties in performing routine activities and fatigue	Symptoms associated with cancer therapy fatigue, anorexia-cachexia, mucositis and chronic pain.	Serenity	Skunks
Cancer: is a types include breast, lung, colon, skin, prostate and ovarian cancer.	Sometimes has no symptoms. Signs and symptoms only appear as the mass continues to grow or ulcerates.	Sleepiness	Spicy
Carpal Tunnel Syndrome: is the hand and arm condition that causes numbness, tingling and other symptoms. Carpal tunnel syndrome is because of a pinched nerve.	Carpal Tunnel Syndrome is a pinched nerve.	Upliftedness	Woody
Cerebral Palsy: is the disruption of movement in the muscle toning or posture that is caused by an injury to the immature develop brain.	Stiff muscles and exaggerated reflexes, lack of muscles tremors, slow movements, delay motors skill, dragging a leg while crawling and seizures.	Happiness	Minty
Cervical Disc Disease: is a degeneration disease. Common cause of neck pain most frequently felt like a stiff neck.	Cervical disc pain that is usually related to activity and will flare up at times or the pain will go away entirely.	Serenity	Skunks
Chemotherapy (often abbreviated to chemo): is a category of cancer treatment that uses chemical substances. Especially one or more anticancer drugs.	Some of the most common side effects of chemotherapy involve the digestive tract. Mouth sores and dry mouth can make it difficult to chew and swallow.	Sleepiness	Spicy
Chronic Fatigue Syndrome: is a is a complicated disorder characterized by significant fatigue that can't be explained by any initial medical specification. The fatigue may decline with physical or mental activity but doesn't improve with rest.	Chronic fatigue can be the loss of memory or concentration. Feeling unrepressed after sleep, muscle pain, headaches, multijoint pain, persistent sore throat, without redness or swelling. Tende lymph in your neck and armpits.	Minty	Woody

Chronic Pain: that is often pain lasting more than twelve weeks. Whereas acute pain is a normal feeling.	Pain that won't go away as expected after an illness or injury. Pain that may be described as aching, burning, shooting or electrical.	Happiness	Minty
Chronic Renal (kidney) Failure Disease (CKD): is a renal disease that occurs when the kidneys don't work as well to filter waste, toxins and excess fluid from your body.	Breath odor, drowsiness, blood in stool, easy bruising, excessive thirst, hard time concentrating, fatigue, muscle twitching, cramps, nausea, numbness, swelling in the hands, feet, skin changes and vomiting.	Hunger	Skunks
Cluster Headaches: that can awaken you in the middle of the night causing penetrating pain around one eye on one side of your head.	Agonizing pain generally located in or around the eye but may radiate to other areas of your face, head, neck and shoulders, a one-sided pain.	Serenity	skunks
Cocaine Dependence: also called coke or blow that is a dangerous stimulant that is in both powdered and crack rock (hard) appearance. Powdered cocaine can be snorted by melting the power and injecting it. Crack cocaine is consumed by heating the stone in a pipe and inhaling the smoke. The high resulting from cocaine varies depending on the method used.	Anxiety, irritability, paranoia, restlessness, loss of the sense of smell, nosebleeds, difficulty swallowing, hoarseness and chronically runny nose.	Happiness	Fruity
Colitis Inflammation: that affects the large intestine. After a period of remission of months or even years. You could experience what's commonly known as a flare.	Constant urge to have a bowel movement. Tenesmus may exist with abdominal pain may come in waves building diarrhea and continuous pain.	Upliftedness	Woody

Conjunctivitis also called (Pinkeyes): redness and infection of the thin tissues layer of the whites of the eyes. The membranes on the inner part of the eyelids. Pinkeye is most often caused by a virus or by a bacterial infection.	Pink Eye is commonly caused by a bacterial or viral infection. An allergic in one or both eyes, also redness, itchiness and discharge.	Focus	Hash
Constipation: is when stools are hard and hard to pass.	Hard Stool to pass	Happiness	Minty
Cohn Disease an inflammatory bowel disease (IBD): Inflammation of the digestive tract that often spreads deep into layers of affected bowel tissue. That leads to abdominal pain, diarrhea, fatigue, malnutrition and weight loss.	Abdominal pain or cramping, blood in stool, diarrhea, fatigue, fever. Inflammation of the bile ducts, eyes, joints, liver and skin. Mouth sores, weight loss and pain around the anus due to swelling from a tunnel into the skin (fistula).	Hunger	Pink
Cystic Fibrosis (CF): is a disorder that mainly genetic that affects the lungs, pancreas, liver, kidneys and intestine.	Breathlessness coug that produces thick mucus (sputum). Exercise intolerance, stuffy nose, lung infections and wheezing.	Serenity	Skunks
Damage to Spinal Cord: is a collection of nerves that travels from the bottom of the brain down your back. Injuries can cause weakness or complete loss of muscle function.	Damage to spinal cord, bladder or bowels control. Problem moving arms or legs, headache, numbness, tingling in extremities. Pain, pressure or stiffing in the back and neck area.	Sleepiness	Spicy
Darier Disease: is a genetic disorder characterized by skin changes.	Darier's disease has bleeding under the skin, wart like blemishes on the arms, back, chest, elbows and behind the ears and scalp.	Focus	Hash
Degenerative Arthritis: is often called (Osteoarthritis or degenerative changes) joint disease. Narrow the space between vertebrae and bone spurs can develop.	Degenerative arthritis is with age, inflammation, joints and increases swelling.	Hunger	Pink

Delirium Tremens: is also known as alcohol withdrawal delirium (AWD) is the most severe form of alcohol withdrawal. It causes sudden and severe problems in your brain and nervous system.	Anxiety, chest pain, delusion, fatigue, increased breathing or heart rate. Sweating, restlessness and mood swings.	Sleepiness	Spicy
Dermatomyositis: an uncommon incendiary disease. Condition that occurs when muscles become inflamed (inflammatory myopathy). It is one of only three known inflammatories.	Weakness in the muscles, tenderness, problems in swallowing, lung problems and hard calcium deposits underneath the skin	Happiness	Minty
Diabetes Adult Onset: is a metabolic disorder that can be characterized by hyperglycemia (high blood sugar). The lack of insulin resistance and relative lack of insulin. Diabetes is in contrast to diabetes mellitus type 1.	Excess thirst and frequent urination. Type 2 diabetes makes up about 90 percent of cases.	Hunger	Pink
Diabetes Insulin-Dependent diabetes mellitus (IDDM): also known as type 1 diabetes. Usually starts before fifteen years of age but can occur in adults also. Diabetes involves the pancreas gland which is located behind the stomach.	Weight loss poor weight gain even if eating large amounts of food. More thirst than usual. Enuresis (bedwetting), frequent urination, feeling tired all the time. Later signs of diabetes are dry skin, urine sugar and acetone will be active.	Happiness	Minty
Diabetes Peripheral Arterial Disease also called (PAD): occurs when blood vessels in the legs are narrowed or blocked by fatty deposits and blood flow to your feet and legs decreases.	Leg pain can occur especially when walking or exercising, numbness, tingling or coldness in the lower legs.	Sleepiness	Spicy
Diarrhea: is caused by an increased flow of water into the intestine. Reduced absorption of fluid from the organ or rapid passage of stool through the body.	Bowel movements are frequent and watery.	Upliftedness	Woody

Diverticulitis: is a bulging pouch or sac that can form on internal organs. Diverticula can occur anywhere in the colon but most commonly develop near the end of the colon on the left side (sigmoid colon).	Diverticulitis can go unnoticeable for quite a while before complications start to occur. Most people live their whole lives without the knowledge that they have diverticulitis until a doctor orders tests for an unrelated condition.	Happiness	Minty
Dysthymic Disorder: materializes as depression, can last at least two years or longer.	Loss of interest in activities, sadness or feeling down, hopelessness, tiredness, lack of energy, low self-esteem, self-criticism. Feeling incapable, trouble concentrating and making decisions, irritability or excessive anger	Hunger	Pink
Eczema (Atopic Dermatitis): is a condition that can make your skin red and itchy. Can flare up periodically and then subside. Most common in children but can occur at any age with symptoms of hay fever and asthma.	Severe itching red to brownish-gray patches on ankles, eyelids, feet, hands, wrists, neck, upper chest, inside the bend of the elbows and knees.	Serenity	Skunks
Emphysema: can gradually damage the air sacs (alveoli) in your lungs, making you progressively more short of breath. Emphysema is one of the several diseases known collectively as the chronic obstructive pulmonary disease (COPD).	Some people have emphysema for many years without symptoms. The primary symptom of emphysema is shortness of breath which begins gradually.	Sleepiness	Spicy
Endometrial Cancer: a form of cancer that began in the uterus (a hollow pear-shaped pelvic organ) where fetal development occurs. Endometrial cancer is sometimes called uterine sarcoma.	An abnormal watery or blood-tinged discharge from your vagina, pelvic pain, pain during intercourse and painful periods (dysmenorrhea). Pelvic pain and cramping may begin several days before and into your period with lower back and abdominal pain.	Focus	Hash

Endometriosis: is the materialization of uterine-lining tissue outside the uterus.	Painful periods (dysmenorrhea), pelvic, abdominal pain, heavy periods, infertility. Cramping may begin until several days into your period. Lower back and abdominal pain with intercourse.	Happiness	Minty
Epidermolysis Bullosa: is confirmed by the appearance of thin white bumps appearing on the skin.	Blisters inside the mouth (dental) and throat, difficulty swallowing (dysphasia), blisters on skin, feet, and hands. Thin white bumps or pimples (milia), Thin-appearing skin (atrophic scarring) and thin-appearing skin (atrophic scarring).	Hunger	Pink
Epididymitis: is red swollen or warm scrotum with testicle pain or tenderness usually on one side. Painful urination and frequent urinate discharge from the penis. Painful intercourse or ejaculation. A lump on the penis also discomfort in the lower abdomen also pelvic area blood in the semen.	Warmth in the scrotum area with low-grade fever, chills, pain, pressure, enlarged lymph nodes, urination, bowel movements, pain in the pelvic area during intercourse and ejaculation.	Serenity	Skunks
Epilepsy: is a neurological disease in which the brain seem clusters and abnormal signals causing seizures.	Abnormal body posturing a repetitive movement like rocking, bicycle pedaling, pelvic thrusting, eye and head movement.	Sleepiness	Spicy
Felty Syndrome: is of long standing rheumatoid arthritis. Felty syndrome is defined by three conditions rheumatoid arthritis, an enlarged spleen (splenomegaly), and an abnormally low white blood cell count. Felty syndrome is uncommon. It affects less than 1 percent of patients with rheumatoid arthritis.	Sleep difficulties, pain all over, eye discharge, burning in eye, morning stiffness, digestive disorders, muscle knots and cramping.	Focus	Hash

Fibromyalgia: is enormous pain in the muscles. But this syndrome causes many other symptoms.	pain in abdomen, back, neck, circumstance pain, gastrointestinal, mood swings, difficulty sleeping, depression and headache.	Happiness	Fruity
Friedreich Ataxia (FRDA): is a genetic, progressive, neurodegenerative movement disorder, with a mean age of onset between ten and fifteen years.	The initial symptom of FRDA is progressive ataxia of the limbs during walking. Ataxia involves poor muscle coordination that results in an unsteady gait and poor control of subtle movements.	Hunger	Hash
Gastritis: is inflammation of the lining of the stomach. The swelling of gastritis is most often the result of infection with the same bacterium that causes most stomach ulcers. Injury and drinking too much alcohol also can contribute to gastritis.	Nausea or recurrent upset stomach, abdominal bloating, abdominal pain, vomiting, indigestion. Burning or gnawing feeling in the stomach between meals or at night, hiccups and loss of appetite	Serenity	Minty
Genital Herpes: there's no cure for genital herpes. Genital herpes is a sexually transmitted infection called herpes simplex virus (HSV).Genital herpes lies dormant in your body and can reactivate several times a year.	Pain and itching with no visible sores in your genital area. You may have no sign or symptoms.	Sleepiness	Spicy
Glaucoma: is an eye condition that damages the optic nerve that is often caused by an abnormally high pressure in the eye.	Acute angle-closure glaucoma, blurred vision, eye redness and pain. Halos around lights, nausea, tunnel vision and vomiting.	Focus	Earthy
Glioblastoma Multiforme (GBM): is classification name is glioblastoma also known as grade IV astrocytoma the most common and most aggressive.	Drowsiness, headaches, nausea and vomiting also difficulty with memory and speech. Weakness on one side of the body and changes in vision.	Happiness	Fruity
Graves' Disease: also known as toxic diffuse goiter and Flajani-Basedow-Graves disease. Autoimmune disease that affects the thyroid.	Increased appetite, diarrhea, excessive sweating, hair loss, hand tremor, heat intolerance, hyperactivity, itching, muscle weakness, moistness, muscle weakness, palpitations and skin warmth.	Hunger	Hash

Hemophilia A: is when you bleed your body typically pools blood cells together to form a clot to stop the bleeding. The clotting process is encouraged by certain blood particles (platelets and plasma proteins). Hemophilia occurs when you have a deficiency in one of these clotting factors. Hemophilia is inherited. However, about 30 percent of people with hemophilia have no family history of the disorder.	Bleeding in stool, urine, bruising, heavy periods, internal bleeding, nosebleed or swollen joints.	Happiness	Minty
Henoch-Schonlein Purpura: a disorder that causes inflammation and bleeding in the small blood vessels in your skin, joints, intestines and kidney.	Blood in stool, diarrhea, vomiting, rash or spots, blood in urine or fever.	Sleepiness	Spicy
Hepatitis C: is a liver disease. The virus causes acute and chronic hepatitis infection. Hepatitis C ranges from severe to a mild illness from a few weeks to a lifelong disease. Hepatitis C transfusion of unscreened blood and blood products.	Acute liver failure, decreased appetite, fatigue, joint pain, muscle pain, nausea and weight loss	Focus	Earthy
Hereditary Spinal Ataxia: also known as spinocerebellar atrophy (SCA) or spinocerebellar degeneration. Progressive genetic disease with multiple types. Each of which could be considered a disease in its own right.	The symptoms of an ataxia vary with the specific type and with the individual patient. In general a person with ataxia retains full mental capacity but progressively loses physical control.	Happiness	Fruity
HIV/AIDS (Human Immunodeficiency Virus): is a condition caused by infection. Stages of HIV are complicated by a disease of the lung known as pneumocystis pneumonia. Severe weight loss, a type of cancer known as Kaposi sarcoma or other AIDS-defining conditions.	Fever, headache, large tender lymph nodes, sores of the mouth and genitals and throat inflammation.	Woody	Earthy

Hospice: is patient care that focuses on the palliation of a chronically ill, terminally ill or seriously ill patient's pain and symptoms. Attending to their emotional and spiritual needs, for the sick, wounded or dying as well.	Hospice is for a terminally ill person who's expected to have six months or less to live.	Hunger	Happiness
Huntington Disease: an inherited disease that causes the progressive breakdown (degeneration) of nerve in the brain cells. Huntington disease has a substantial impact on a person's functional abilities and usually results in movement, thinking (cognitive) and psychiatric disorders.	Behavioral irritability, depression, mood swings, anxiety and hallucination.	Hunger	Hash
Hypertension: is a high blood pressure. A common condition in which there is long-term force of the blood against your artery walls such as heart disease.	Weakness, fainting, dizziness, confusion, agitation, a feeling of being outside yourself.	Sleepiness	Spicy
Hyperventilation Syndrome: is more accurate and relates to an overbreathing pattern that happens under certain conditions. This overbreathing results in a group of symptoms.	Bleeding, feeling anxious, pain, fever and yawning.	Upliftedness	Woody
Hypoglycemia: also known as low blood glucose or low blood sugar. Occurs when blood glucose drops below normal levels. Glucose is a vital source of energy for the body. Carbohydrates are the primary dietary source of glucose. Rice, potatoes, bread, tortillas, cereal, milk, fruit and sweets are all carbohydrate-rich foods.	Clamminess, drowsiness, dizziness, includes hunger, irritability, low blood sugar, paleness, rapid heartbeat, shakiness, sweating and weakness.	Woody	Earthy

Impotence: is a common problem among men and is characterized by the consistent inability to sustain an erection sufficient for sexual intercourse or the inability to achieve.	Anxiety, diabetes, alcoholism, impotence, medical conditions, (diabetes, alcoholism), medications, trauma, and outside influences can contribute to impotence.	Happiness	Fruity
Inflammatory Bowel Disease (IBD): is a combination of gut-brain axis problems, gut motility disorders, pain sensitivity, infections including small intestinal bacterial overgrowth.	Abdominal pain and cramping. Blood in your stool, diarrhea, fever, fatigue, reduced appetite and unintended weight loss.	Sleepiness	Spicy
Intermittent Explosive Disorder (IED): behavioral disorder. Repeated, sudden episodes of impulsive, aggressive, violent behavior or angry verbal outbursts. Overreacting grossly out of proportion to the situation, road rage, domestic abuse, throwing or breaking objects or other temper tantrums.	Energy changes, mood changes and tension.	Upliftedness	Woody
Lipomatosis: is believed to be an autosomal dominant condition in which multiple lipomas are present on the body (fatty tumors). Condition is benign. Many discrete encapsulated lipomas form on the trunk and extremities. This is one of the most commonly found mutations in solitary lipomatous tumors.	Abdominal pain containing the mass decreased function (range of motion), enlargement of varicose veins, fatigue, numbness, painful swelling and weight loss. Damaged to spinal cord and rare causes urinary bladder or bowel is affected.	Focus	Earthy
Lou Gehrig Disease: also known as amyotrophic lateral sclerosis (ALS); a rapidly progressive, uniformly fatal neurodegenerative disease. It is characterized by the loss of motor neurons in the spinal cord, brainstem and cerebral cortex, leading to a decline in muscular function.	Cramps, chewing, difficulty with writing or buttoning a shirt, leg or arm weakness. Causing an awkward gait or stumbling, twitching or stiff muscles, difficulty swallowing and slurred speech.	Happiness	Fruity

Lyme Disease:(Borrelia burgdorferi) is caused by the most common tick-borne illness (tick bite) in North America and Europe. Lyme disease is transmitted by the bite of an infected black-legged tick.	Lyme disease is often a bite mark that often becomes red, swollen and very tender. As the bacteria spread in the body severe headaches and neck stiffness and rash on other parts of the body. Particularly the knees and others large joints of the body with facial palsy.	Hunger	Hash
Lymphoma Hodgkin: is cancer that affects the immune system. It is a cancer of immune cells called lymphocytes.	Cancer that affects the immune system. It is a cancer of immune cells called lymphocytes.	Upliftedness	Woody
Malignant Melanoma: is a kind of cancer that can develop from the pigment-containing cells known as melanocytes. Melanomas usually occur in the skin but may rarely occur in the mouth, intestines or eye or sometimes develops from a mole.	Melanomas usually occur in the skin but may rarely occur in the mouth, intestines or eye. Sometimes develop from a mole.	Focus	Earthy
Mania: abnormally elevated mood arousal energy level. A state of heightened overall activation with enhanced practical expression together with a liability of effect.	Disconnected and speedy (racing) thoughts, grandiose beliefs, inappropriate happiness or euphoria. Inappropriate irritability, markedly increased energy, inappropriate social behavior, increased talking speed or volume and increased sexual desire	Happiness	Fruity
Melorheostosis: also known as Leri disease, unusual mesenchymal dysplasia manifesting as regions of sclerosing bone with the unique dripping wax appearance, or flowing candle appearance that began in childhood.	Absent or abnormal muscles, irregular bone growth, dripping candle wax appearance on x-ray. Imaging, cortical thickening unequal length of limbs, joint swelling, soft tissue abnormalities, subcutaneous calcification, tendon and ligament shortening	Hunger	Hash

Condition	Symptoms		
Meniere Disease: is a disarrange of the inner ear that causes spontaneous episodes of vertigo with a sensation of a spinning motion.	Feeling of fullness in the ear, hearing loss, ringing in the ear (tinnitus) and recurring episodes of vertigo	Serenity	Minty
Migraine Headaches: neurological disease characterized by recurrent moderate to severe headaches.	Constipation, food cravings, frequent yawning, increased thirst, mood changes from depression to euphoria, neck stiffness and urination	Minty	Spicy
Motion Sickness or Ketosis: also known as travel sickness. Condition in which a disagreement exists between visually perceived movement and the vestibule's sense of movement. Depending on the cause it can also be referred to as seasickness, car sickness, simulation sickness or airsickness.	Motion sickness can strike suddenly, feeling of uneasiness to cold sweat, dizziness and vomiting. Any form of transportation (car, ship, plane and train) can cause motion sickness.	Spicy	Woody
Mucopolysaccharidosis (MPS): is a collection of metabolic disorders caused by the absence or malfunctioning of lysosomal enzymes that needed to break down molecules. Glycosaminoglycans' long chains of sugar carbohydrates in each of our cells.	Enlarged cheeks, head, lips, tongue and nose. Deep voice, sleep apnea and carpal tunnel.	Focus	Earthy
Multiple sclerosis (MS): is a disease that attacks the protective sheath (myelin) that covers your nerves in your immune system. Myelin can disrupt communication between your brain and the rest of your body.	Constipation, depression, headache, whole body fatigue, muscular pain, tremor, mod swings, urinary leaking and blurred vision.	Happiness	Fruity
Muscle Esophageal Spasms: painful muscle contractions that affect your esophagus, the hollow tube between your throat and your stomach; sudden, severe chest pain that may last for few minutes to an hour.	Difficulty swallowing liquids such as red wine or extremely hot or cold liquids; the feeling that an object is stuck in your throat and the return of food and fluids back up your esophagus (regurgitation).	Hunger	Hash

Condition	Symptoms		
Muscular Dystrophy: collection of diseases that cause increasing weakness with loss of muscle mass. In irregular muscular dystrophy, progressive genes (mutations) interfere with the production of proteins needed to form healthy tissue.	Hard to get up from a lying or sitting position, frequent falls, large calf muscles, learning disabilities, muscle pain and stiffness, trouble running and jumping, waddling gait, and walking on the toes	Serenity	Minty
Myeloid Leukemia, Acute Myelogenous Leukemia (AML): cancer of the blood and bone marrow tissue inside bones where blood cells are made.	Early stages of acute leukemia may mimic the flu or other common diseases: fever, bone pain, lethargy, fatigue, shortness of breath, pale skin, frequent infection, easy bruising, and unusual bleeding.	Sleepiness	Spicy
Nail–Patella Syndrome: also known as HOOD syndrome; genetic disorder that results in small, poorly developed nails and kneecaps, elbows, chest, and hips. The name nail-patella can be misleading because the syndrome often affects other areas of the body, including a production of specific proteins.	Fingernail and toenail absence (aplasia), abnormally increased fluid pressure in eyes (glaucoma). The toenail is less often affected. Kneecap abnormalities are the second most common signs associated with this disorder.	Upliftedness	Woody
Nightmares: troubling dreams associated with negative feelings such as anxiety or fear.	The dream may seem vivid, real, and very upsetting, often becoming disturbing as the dream unfolds, leaving you feeling anxious, angry, scared, sad, or disgusted, with pounding heartbeats, and sweaty. Upon awakening, you can recall details of your dream.	Focus	Focus
Obesity: is a complicated disorder involving an excessive amount of body fat. Obesity isn't just a cosmetic concern. BMI is calculated by dividing your weight in kilograms (kg) by your height in meters squared (m²).	Obesity can be a concern with overweight-related health problem.	Happiness	Fruity

Obsessive-Compulsive Disorder (OCD): is irrational thought and anxieties (compulsions) that will lead you to do repetitive compulsions or behaviors. A person can have just one obsession or compulsions and still have OCD.	Fear of uncleanness or dirt. Needing things methodical and symmetrical, aggressive or horrific thoughts about harming yourself or others. Useless reflections including aggression or sexual or religious subjects.	Serenity	Minty
Opiate Dependence: is morphine injection is used to relieve direct to severe pain. It may also be used before or during surgery with an anesthetic (medicine that puts you to sleep).	Opiates development of tolerance (meaning the need to use more significant amounts). Withdrawal symptoms after reducing or stopping use can cause depression, upset stomach, insomnia, muscle aches and difficulty meeting social or work obligations.	Sleepiness	Spicy
Osteoarthritis: is the most common form of arthritis affecting millions of people worldwide. It occurs when the protective cartilage on the ends of your bones wears down over time.	Joint pain and stiffness. Treatment of affected joint, including the hand, wrist, neck, back, knee and hip involves medication and exercise.	Upliftedness	Woody
Panic Disorder: is a sudden episode of intense fear that triggers severe physical reactions when there is no real danger or apparent cause. Panic attacks can be very frightening. When panic attacks occur, you might think you're losing control or having a heart attack or even dying.	Palpitations, pounding heart or accelerated heart rate, sweating, trembling, shaking, sensations, shortness of breath, smothering, or feeling of choking.	Focus	Hash
Parkinson Disease: is progressive disorder of the nervous system that affects movement. It develops gradually. Sometimes starting with a barely noticeable tremor in just one hand. But while a tremor may be the most well-known sign of Parkinson disease, the disorder also commonly causes stiffness or slowing of movement.	Resting tremors, slow movement (bradykinesia), stiff muscles, lack of balance or falling, being stuck in place while walking, reduced arm swings on one side of your body, dragging foot, small voice, loss of automatic movements. Like blinking, swallowing, speech, writing, smell and taste.	Happiness	Fruity

Peripheral Neuropathy: is the result of damage to your peripheral nerves. Often causes weakness, numbness and pain usually in your hands and feet. It can also affect other areas of your body.	Gradual feeling of numbness, prickling or tingling in your feet or hands that spreads upward into your legs and arms. Sharp, jabbing, throbbing, freezing or burning pain, sensitivity to touch, lack of coordination, falling, muscle weakness or paralysis.	Hunger	Hash
Peritoneal Pain: is associated with peritoneal dialysis. Caused by germs around the catheter if you're receiving peritoneal dialysis.	Results in damage to your peripheral nerves. Often causes weakness, numbness and pain usually in your feet, hands and other areas of your body.	Serenity	Minty
Persistent Insomnia: is a persistent disorder that can make it hard to fall asleep, hard to stay asleep or both despite the opportunity for adequate sleep. With insomnia, you usually awaken feeling unrefreshed.	Anxiety, depression and stress are some of the most common causes of chronic insomnia.	Sleepiness	Spicy
Post-Polio Syndrome (PPS): polio or poliomyelitis is an infectious viral disease that can strike at any age and affects a person's nervous system.	Muscle weakness, extreme fatigue, joint pain, skeletal deformities, such as scoliosis. PPS symptoms copy those of the disorder known as Lou Gehrig disease.	Arousal	Dank
Post-Traumatic Arthritis: is a common form of osteoarthritis. Osteoarthritis is the wearing away of cartilage in the joint. This condition can occur in any joint, including the shoulder, elbow, wrist, hip, knee and ankle.	Joint pain; fluid accumulation in the joint, swelling, decreased tolerance for walking, sports, stairs and other activities that stress the joint.	Creativity	Earthy
Post-Traumatic Stress Disorder (PTSD): is a anxiety disorder that can develop after a person is exposed to one or more traumatic events such as major stress, sexual assault, warfare or other threats on the person's life.	Emotional numbness, difficulty concentrating and sleeping, feeling jumpy, flashbacks, nightmares, avoidance activities, people, places easily being irritated and angered.	Energy	Fruity

Premenstrual Syndrome (PMS): refers to physical and emotional symptoms that occur in the one to two weeks before a woman's period.	Common symptoms include acne, tender breasts, bloating, feeling tired, irritability and mood changes. Often symptoms are present for around six days.	Happiness	Minty
Prostate Cancer: also known as carcinoma of the prostate. The development of cancer in the prostate that's a gland in the male reproductive system. Prostate cancers are slow growing. Some grow relatively quickly. The cancer cells may spread from the prostate to other parts of the body.	Blood in semen, trouble urinating, decreased force in the stream of urine, discomfort in the pelvic area, bone pain erectile dysfunction	Hunger	Pink
Prostatitis Glands: all men have it is the size of a walnut that is found below the bladder and in front of your rectum. The prostatitis is to protect the sperm when traveling toward a female's egg.	Blood in the urine, or cloudy urine, flu-like symptoms, pain in abdomen, groin, genitals, lower back pelvic and painful or difficult urination(dysuria).	Serenity	Skunks
Psoriasis: is a long-lasting disease characterized by patches of abnormal skin. These skin patches are typically red, itchy and scaly. They may vary in severity from small and localized to complete body coverage. Injury to the skin can trigger psoriatic skin changes at that spot, which is known as Koebner phenomenon.	Inflammation and exfoliation of the skin over most of the body surface. It may be accompanied by severe itching, swelling and pain.	Sleepiness	Spicy
Pulmonary Fibrosis: a respiratory disease in which scars are formed in the lung tissues, leading to serious breathing problems.The accumulation of excess fibrous connective tissue (the process called fibrosis), leads to thickening of the walls. Causes reduced oxygen supply in the blood. As a consequence patients suffer from perpetual shortness of breath.	Shortness of breath, particularly with exertion, chronic dry, hacking coughing, fatigue and weakness, chest discomfort, including chest pain, loss of appetite and rapid weight loss.	Upliftedness	Woody

Quadriplegia: also known as tetraplegia paralysis caused by illness or injury that results in the partial or total loss of use of all their limbs and torso. Paraplegia is similar but does not affect the arms. The loss is usually sensory and motor which means that both sensation and control are lost.	Symptom is impairment to the limbs functioning is also impaired in the torso. This can mean a loss or impairment in controlling bowel, bladder, sexual function, digestion, breathing and other autonomic functions. Furthermore sensation is usually impaired in affected areas. This can manifest as numbness, reduced sensation or burning.	Arousal	Dank
Radiation Therapy: is a type of cancer treatment that uses beams of intense energy to kill cancer cells. Radiation therapy most often gets its power from x-rays but the power can also come from protons or other types of energy.	Late side effects such as lung or heart problems, may take years to develop and are often permanent when they do. The most common early side effects from radiation therapy are fatigue and skin problems. Other early side effects such as hair loss and nausea are typically specific to the site being treated.	Energy	Fruity
Raynaud Disease (ray-NOHZ): causes some areas of your body such as your fingers and toes to feel numb and cold in response to cold temperatures or stress. In Raynaud disease smaller arteries that supply blood to your skin narrow limiting blood circulation to affected areas (vasospasm).	Duration and severity of the blood vessel spasms underline the disorder. Raynaud disease signs and symptoms include cold fingers or toes. Color changes in your skin in response to cold or stress, numb, prickly feeling or stinging pain upon warming or stress relief.	Focus	Minty
Reiter Syndrome: inflammatory reaction to an infection somewhere in the body. It usually follows a urogenital or intestinal infection.	Symptoms of the disorder primarily involve three body systems: the joints, the eyes and the urinary or genital tract.	Happiness	Pink

Restless Legs Syndrome (RLS): not entirely known, can be related to genetic factors. Low iron levels in the brain or diseases such as chronic kidney or diabetes.	The condition causes an uncomfortable, itchy, pins and needles, or creepy crawly feeling in the legs. The sensations are usually worse at rest, especially when lying or sitting.	Focus	Hash
Rheumatoid Arthritis (RA): a form of arthritis that causes pain, swelling, stiffness and loss of function in your joints. It can affect any joint but is common in the wrist and fingers.	Joint inflammation sometimes affecting other joints, including the neck, shoulders, elbows, hips, knees, ankles, and feet; fatigue; occasional fevers; loss of energy.	Happiness	Minty
Rosacea: chronic (long-term) disease that affects the skin and sometimes the eyes. The disorder is characterized by redness, pimples and in advanced stages thickened skin. Rosacea usually affects the face.	Redness of the face, or blushing or flushing efficiently. Spiderlike blood vessels (telangiectasia) of the face, red nose, acne skin, sores, burning or stinging in the face, bloodshot and watery eyes.	Hunger	Pink
Schizoaffective Disorder: is a mental disorder that causes both a loss of contact with reality (psychosis) and mood problems (depression or mania). A person may experience psychosis and mood disturbances separately or simultaneously and will have periods of severe symptoms followed by improvement.	Changes in appetite and energy, disorganized speech, false beliefs (delusions), thinking someone is trying to harm (paranoia), changes in hygiene or grooming. Mood swing from too good to depressed or irritable, problems with concentration and sleeping, hopelessness, seeing things or hearing voices social isolation.	Serenity	Skunks
Schizophrenia: is a severe mental disorder in which people interpret reality abnormally. Schizophrenia may result in some combination of hallucinations, delusions and extremely disordered thinking and behavior that impairs daily functioning and can be disabling.	Symptoms of schizophrenia may vary but typically include delusions, hallucinations, disorganized thinking or speaking. Abnormal motor behavior or other negative cognitive behaviors. Having two or more of these symptoms for thirty days or more is typically indicative of schizophrenia.	Sleepiness	Spicy

Scoliosis: lateral (toward the side) curvature in the usually straight vertical line of the spine. When viewed from the front, the spine should show a mild roundness in the upper back and shows a degree of swayback.	A person's shoulder blade may stick out more than others and the hip may appear higher than the other. A child's head is not centered on its body. The child's rib may be higher on one side and waistline may be flat one side.	Upliftedness	Woody
Sedative-Dependent Seizures: Propofol with excitatory motor activity, such as myoclonic jerking and opisthotonus in humans and in animals. Suggests that it may aggravate clinical seizure activity in some circumstances.	Overstimulation of the central nervous system such as anxiety, agitation, grimacing, sleep disturbance, increased muscle tension and movement disorder. Reflecting gastrointestinal dysfunction diarrhea and gastric retention were most frequently seen.	Arousal	Dank
Seizures: based on the type of behavior and brain activity. Seizures are divided into two broad categories: generalized and partial (also called local or focal). Classifying the type of seizure helps doctors diagnose whether a patient has epilepsy.	Violent shaking and a loss of control. A sudden feeling of fear or anxiousness, feeling sick to your stomach. Dizziness and vision change. A jerking of the arms and legs that may cause you to drop things. An out of body sensation and headache.	Creativity	Earthy
Senile Dementia: a broad category of brain diseases that cause a long-term and often gradual decrease in the ability to think and remember such that a person's daily functioning is affected.	Other common symptoms include emotional problems, problems with language and a decrease in motivation. A person's consciousness is not affected. For the diagnosis to be present, it must be a change from a person's usual mental functioning and a greater decline than one would expect because of aging.	Euphoria	Hash

Severe Nausea: uneasiness of the stomach that often comes before vomiting. Vomiting is the forcible voluntary or involuntary emptying (throwing up) of stomach contents through the mouth.	Motion sickness or seasickness, early stages of pregnancy, medication induced vomiting, intense pain, emotional stress. Gallbladder disease, food poisoning, infections (such as the stomach flu).	Focus	Minty
Shingles (Herpes Zoster): common and highly contagious infection usually spread through sex. This infection is usually caused by the herpes simplex virus-2 (HSV-2) or the herpes simplex virus-1 (HSV-1). The virus usually responsible for cold sores.	When symptoms occur soon after a person is infected they tend to be severe. They may start as small blisters that eventually break open and produce raw painful sores that scab and heal over within a few weeks. The blisters and sores may be accompanied by flu-like symptoms with fever and swollen lymph nodes.	Happiness	Pink
Sinusitis: inflammation or swelling of the tissue lining the sinuses. Normally sinuses are filled with air. But when sinuses become blocked and filled with fluid, germs (bacteria, viruses and fungi) can grow and cause an infection.	Facial pain, pressure, nasal stuffiness, nasal discharge, loss of smell, cough and congestion. Additional symptoms may include fever, bad breath, fatigue and dental pain.	Happiness	Minty
Skeletal Muscular Somatic Nervous System (SoNS or voluntary nervous system): part of the peripheral nervous system.	Pain, fatigue, sleep disturbances.	Hunger	Pink
Sleep Apnea: your breathing often is blocked or partly blocked during sleep. The problem can be mild to severe based on how often your lungs don't get enough air. This may happen from five to more than fifty times an hour.	Excessive daytime sleepiness, waking with an unrepressed feeling after sleep, having problems with memory and concentration, feeling tired. Experiencing personality changes morning or night headaches. About half of all people with sleep apnea report headaches, heartburn or a sour taste in the mouth at night, sweating and chest pain while sleeping.	Serenity	Skunks

Spasticity: a form of muscle overactivity that occurs when communication between your brain and spinal cord is disrupted by a spinal cord injury other injury or illness.	Increased muscle tone, overactive reflexes, involuntary movements. Which may include spasms (brisk and or sustained involuntary muscle contraction). Clonus (series of fast involuntary contractions), pain, decreased functional abilities and delayed motor development. Difficulty with care and hygiene, abnormal posture.	Sleepiness	Spicy
Spinal Stenosis: narrowing of the open spaces within your spine that can put pressure on your spinal cord and the nerves. Pain that travel through the spine to your arms and legs. Spinal stenosis occurs most often in the lower back and the neck.	Numbness, weakness, cramping or pain in the legs, feet or buttocks. These symptoms get worse when you walk, stand straight or lean backward. The pain gets better when you sit down or lean forward. Stiffness in the legs and thighs, low back pain and in severe cases loss of bladder and bowel control.	Upliftedness	Woody
Surge-Weber Syndrome (SWS): sometimes referred to as encephalotrigeminal angiomatosis, rare congenital neurological and skin disorder. Associated with port-wine stains of the face, glaucoma, seizures, mental retardation and ipsilateral leptomeningeal angioma (cerebral malformations and tumors).	The birthmark can vary in color from light pink to deep purple and is caused by an overabundance of capillaries around the ophthalmic branch of the trigeminal nerve, just under the surface of the face.	Creativity	Earthy

Stuttering: speech disorder in which the flow of speech is disrupted by involuntary repetitions and prolongations of sounds, syllables, words or phrases as well as involuntary silent pauses or blocks in which the person who stutters is unable to produce sounds.	Difficulty starting a word, sentence, or phrase prolonging a word or sounds within a word. Repetition of a sound, syllable or word brief silence for certain syllables or pauses within a word (broken word). Addition of extra words such as "um" if difficulty moving to the next word is anticipated excess tension, tightness or movement of the face or upper body to produce a word. Anxiety about talking limited ability to effectively communicate.	Energy	Fruity
Tardive Dyskinesia (TD): is a neurological disorder characterized by involuntary uncontrollable movements especially of the mouth, tongue, trunk and limbs and occurring especially as a side effect of prolonged use of antipsychotic drugs (as phenothiazine).	Grimacing, tongue movements, lip smacking, lip puckering, pursing of the lips and excessive eye blinking	Euphoria	Hash
Temporomandibular Joint (TMJ) disorder: is your temporomandibular joint is a hinge that connects your jaw to the temporal bones of your skull. Which are in front of each ear. It lets you move your jaw up and down and side to side so you can talk, chew and yawn.	Aching, pain, and difficulty chewing pain around the ear, facial pain and jaw.	Focus	Minty
Tenosynovitis DeQuervain: painful condition affecting the tendons on the thumb side of your wrist. If you have deQuervain tenosynovitis it will probably hurt when you turn your wrist, grasp anything or make a fist.	Pain near the base of your thumb, swelling near the base of your thumb, difficulty moving your thumb and wrist. When you're doing something that involves grasping or pinching a "sticking" or "stop and go" sensation in your thumb when moving it.	Happiness	Minty

Tension Headache: generally a diffuse mild to moderate pain in your head that's often described as feeling like a tight band around your head. A tension headache (tension-type headache) is the most common type of headache and yet its causes aren't well understood.	Dull, aching head pain sensation of tightness or pressure across your forehead or on the sides and back of your head. Tenderness on your scalp, neck, and shoulder muscles.	Hunger	Pink
Terminal Illness Care: home based family-centered care for individuals facing a terminal illness. Hospice addresses these aspects of a terminal illness when appropriate.	A methodical process of denial, listen and accept. Ask person what they want.	Serenity	Skunks
Testicular Cancer: occurs in the testicles (testes), which are located inside the scrotum. A loose bag of skin underneath the penis. The testicles produce male sex hormones and sperm for reproduction.	A lump or enlargement in either testicles. Feeling of heaviness in the scrotum, a dull ache in the abdomen or groin. A sudden collection of fluid in the scrotum pain or discomfort in a testicle or the scrotum, enlargement or tenderness of the breasts and back pain.	Sleepiness	Spicy
Trigeminal Neuralgia: is a chronic pain disorder where blood vessels compress the nerves affecting the nerves that carry the sensation from your face to your brain. Brushing your teeth or putting on makeup can cause excruciating pain near the nose, lips, eyes or ears.	Pain in the area where that supplied by the trigeminal nerve causing spontaneous attacks of pain that is constant aching, burning, in cheek, jaw, teeth, gums, lips, eyes and forehead. Episodes of several attacks lasting days, weeks, months or longer.	Upliftedness	Woody
Tic Douloureux: also called trigeminal neuralgia the trigeminal nerve's function is disrupted. Usually the problem is the contact between a healthy blood vessel. One of the most painful illness to affect people.	Shooting or jabbing pain that can feel like an electric shock. Attacks of anxiety or attacks triggered by things such as touching the face, chewing, speaking and brushing teeth, constant aching, burning feeling in your jaw, teeth, gums, lips or less often the eye and forehead.	Arousal	Dank

Tietze Syndrome: rare musculoskeletal disease when the cartilage around the joints connecting the upper ribs to the breastbone swells up. Can be very painful but never severe. Sometimes it is the second or third bones that are most affected. No one knows what caused Tietze syndrome.	Can occur on the left side of your breastbone with aching, sharp or pressure-like effects on several ribs causing pain when you take a deep breath or a cough.	Creativity	Earthy
Tinnitus: cause of tinnitus is inner ear cell damage. Tiny delicate hairs in your hidden ear move about the tension of the sound waves in the ear. This can trigger the listener to release an electrical signal through a nerve from the ear to the brain. If the hair inside the ear is bent or broken. The ear can leak random electrical impulses to the mind causing tinnitus.	Ringing, buzzing, roaring, clicking and hissing	Energy	Fruity
Tobacco Dependence : also called nicotine dependence. An addiction to tobacco products and nicotine. Nicotine dependence means you can't stop using the substance even though it's causing you harm.	Can't stop smoking. You've made one or more dangerous but unsuccessful attempts to quit. With withdrawal symptoms with physical and mood-related cravings, anxiety, irritability, restlessness, difficulty concentrating, depressed mood, frustration, anger, increased hunger, insomnia, constipation or diarrhea	Euphoria	Happiness
Tourette Syndrome: is a nervous system (neurological) disorder that starts in childhood. It involves unusual repetitive movements or unwanted sounds that can't be controlled (tics).	Tics, brief and repetitive, involving a limited number of distinct muscle groups. Complex tics which are coordinated patterns of movements that require several muscle groups.	Focus	Minty

Trichotillomania: is also known as hair pulling disorder. Compulsive urge to pull out one's hair leading to hair loss and balding, distress and impairment.	Trichotillomania may be confined to one or two sites but can involve multiple locations. The scalp is the most common pulling site. Followed by the eyebrows, eyelashes, face, arms and legs. Some less-common areas can include the pubic area, underarms, beard and chest.	Happiness	Pink
Uterine Cancer: that begins in the uterus. The uterus is the hollow pear-shaped pelvic organ in women where fetal development occurs.	Vaginal bleeding after menopause, bleeding between periods an abnormal watery or blood-tinged discharge from your vagina and pelvic pain.	Focus	Hash
Viral Hepatitis: is an infection caused by a virus that attacks the liver and leads to inflammation. Most people are infected with the hepatitis C virus (HCV).	Some people have no symptoms. Others may have yellow discoloration of the skin and whites of the eyes. Abdominal diarrhea pain, reduced appetite, vomiting, or tiredness.	Happiness	Minty
Wasting Syndrome: AIDS patients are said to have it when they have lost at least 10 percent of their body weight. Because of diarrhea for at least a month and extreme weakness and fever that are not related to an infection especially muscle.	Depression, opportunistic infections, like a painful throat or feeling full, lack of energy. Medication side effects like nausea, changes in taste or mouth tingling.	Serenity	Skunks
Wittmaack-Ekbom Syndrome: also known as restless legs syndrome (RLS) or Willis-Ekbom disease (WED). Neurological disorder with irresistible urge to move one's body to stop uncomfortable or odd sensations. Commonly affects the legs but can affect the arms, torso and head.	An urge to move, leg twitching during sleep and motor restlessness.	Sleepiness	Spicy
Whiplash: neck injury because of forceful, rapid back-and-forth movement of the neck. Can occur during a rear-end auto accident, but the damage can also result from a sports accident or physical abuse.	Tendons and muscles in the neck to stretch and tear leaving you with a painful sore and stiff neck.	Upliftedness	Woody

The Bud Tender reference guide informs patients and the public of the psychoactive effects of different varieties of herbal alternatives and how each can affect you as well as the therapeutic benefits, conditions, symptoms and desired results though flavoring and scents.

GLOSSARY

Acquired Hypothyroidism sometimes called Hashimoto thyroiditis a disorder that does not allow the thyroid gland to make enough thyroid hormone.

Acute Gastritis (ACC) is a rare disease sudden inflammation or swelling of the lining of the stomach. It causes severe and irritating pain. Usually, the pain only lasts for a short time.

Adrenal Cortical Cancer (ACC) a rare disease. It is caused by a cancerous growth in the adrenal cortex.

Agoraphobia is a Phobia is defined as the severe, unrelenting fear of an activity or situation. Agoraphobia is fear of being outside or in a position from which one either cannot get away or from which escaping would be painful or humiliating.

AIDS-Related Illness people with AIDS have weakened immune systems, they're more prone to opportunistic infections. These organisms attack when there's an opportunity to infect.

Alcohol Abuse with previous psychiatric diagnosis where there is a recurring harmful use of ethanol despite its adverse consequences.

Alcoholism also is known as alcohol use disorder (AUD) alcohol dependence syndrome is a broad term for any drinking of alcohol that results in problems.

Alzheimer Disease is a progressive mental deterioration that may occur in middle or old age causing premature senility.

Amphetamine Dependency is a frequent long-term use of drugs. Some people become dependent faster than others.

Amyloidosis a rare disease that results from an accumulation of inappropriately folded proteins. These misfiled proteins are called amyloids.

Amyotrophic Lateral Sclerosis (ALS) also known as Lou Gehrig disease and Charcot disease. A particular disorder that involves the death of neurons.

Angina Pectoris was also known as stable angina. The medical term for chest pain or discomfort because of coronary heart disease.

Ankylosis Immobility can be caused by the destruction of the membranes that line the joint or weak bone structure. It is most often a result of lingering rheumatoid arthritis.

Anorexia an eating disorder characterized by low weight. Fear of gaining weight a strong desire to be thin and food restriction.

Anorexia Nervosa has physical and emotional components that require the attention of different healthcare providers. Primary care physicians, mental health counselors, psychologists, and psychiatrists.

Arteriosclerotic Health Disease is thickening and hardening of the walls of the coronary arteries is the results of infiltration and accumulation of white blood cells.

Arthritis Joints associates with bones that allow flexibility and movement. Joint pain will occur if there is damage because of disease or trauma. The illness or injury will interfere with the normal movement of the joint and produce pain.

Arthritis Rheumatoid is a chronic inflammatory disorder that typically affects the small joints in your hands and feet. Rheumatoid arthritis influences the lining of your joints causing a painful swelling that can eventually result in bone erosion and joint. Rheumatoid arthritis occurs when your immune system inadvertently attacks your own body's tissues. Rheumatoid arthritis sometimes can affect other organs of the body such as the skin, eyes, lungs and blood vessels.

Arthroplasty Gout Arthritis is a form of arthroplasty that involves inflammation of one or more joints. While the term "arthroplasty" may be used regardless of whether there is inflammation.

Asthma is the chronic inflammatory disease of the airways characterized by variable and recurring symptoms, such as reversible airflow obstruction and bronchospasm.

Attention-Deficit Hyperactivity Disorder (ADD/ADHD) similar to hyperkinetic disorder Neurodevelopmental. A Psychiatric disorder wherein there will be significant problems.

Autism/Asperger is a brain disorder that affects communication and interaction with others.

Autoimmune Disease can develop when your immune system infiltrates healthy cells. Depending on the type an autoimmune disease can affect one or many different types of body tissue. Also can also cause abnormal organ growth and changes in body function.

Back Pain felt in the back that usually originates from the bones, joints, muscles, nerves or other parts of the spine.

Back Strain is an injury to both a tendon or muscle. Cords are the hard fibrous bands of tissue that connect muscle to bone. With a back pressure spine is twisted, pulled or torn. A sprain is the stretching or tearing of a ligament. Bands of tissue that connect two or more bones at a joint and prevent excessive movement of the joint.

Bulimia: also known as (bulimia nervosa) is one of many eating disorders. This mental illness is characterized by episodes of bingeing and somehow purging the food and associated calories in the pursuit of weight loss.

Cachexia (cancer) marked weight loss, muscular loss, resistance to traditional therapies and difficulties in performing routine activities and fatigue.

Cancer common types of cancer include breast, colon, lung, skin, prostate and ovarian cancer.

Carpal Tunnel Syndrome (pinched nerves) is a hand and arm condition that causes numbness, tingling, and other symptoms.

Cerebral Palsy: is a disrupt of movement of the muscle toning or posture that is caused by an insult to the immature developing the brain. Muscle tone or posture that is produced by an insult to the immature developing brain.

Cervical Disc Disease where degeneration is a common cause of neck pain most frequently felt like a firm neck.

Cervicobrachial Syndrome common cause of neck pain most frequently felt like a stiff neck. Cervical degenerative disc disease is far less common than disc degeneration in the lumbar spine.

Bells' Palsy is a form of facial paralysis after a dysfunction of the cranial nerve VII (the facial nerve) responsible for an inability to regulate facial muscles on the affected side. Often the altered front of the eye cannot be closed. The eye must be protected from drying up, or the cornea may be permanently damaged resulting in impaired vision. This condition is a rapid onset of partial or complete paralysis that often occurs overnight.

Bipolar Disorder affective is a disorder and manic-depressive illness which is a mental disorders, of periods of elevated moods and periods of depression. During mania, an individual feels or acts unusually happy, energetic or irritable. They often make poorly decisions thought-out their lives, with little regards to the consequences. The need for sleep is usually reduced. During periods of depression, there may be crying, poor eye contact with others and a negative outlook on life. The risk of suicide other mental health issues such as anxiety disorder and substance use disorder are commonly associated.

Brain Tumor Malignant is a disease of the brain in which there are Cancer cells in the brain tissue (malignant cells). Cancer cells will grow to form a mass (tumor) of cancer tissue that interferes with the brain that causes such as sensation, memory, muscle control and other standard body dysfunction.

Bruxism grinding and gnashing of the teeth. Bruxism can injure teeth and cause local pain in the mouth or jaw that may contribute to a temporomandibular joint (TMJ) syndrome.

Chemotherapy (often abbreviated to chemo) a category of cancer treatment that uses chemical substances, especially one or more anticancer drugs.

Chronic Fatigue Syndrome is a complex disorder characterized by enormous fatigue that can't be explained by any underlying medical condition. Fatigue worsens with mental or physical activity.

Chronic Pain often defined as pain lasting more than twelve weeks whereas; acute pain is a normal feeling that alerts us to possible injury.

Chronic Renal Failure is the gradual loss of kidney function. Your kidneys filter wastes and excess fluids from your blood which is then excreted in your urine. When chronic kidney disease reaches an advanced stage dangerous levels of fluid, electrolytes and wastes can build up in your body.

Cluster Headache that commonly awakens you in the middle of the night with intense pain in or proximal of one eye on one side of your head.

Cocaine Dependence also called coke or blow is a dangerous substance that can be found in both powdered and crack rock form. Powdered cocaine is used by snorting it or melting the powder and injecting it. Crack cocaine is disbursed by heating the rock in a pipe and inhaling the smoke. The subsequent high from cocaine varies depending on the method in which it is consumed.

Colitis is an inflammation that affects the large intestine. After a period of remission of months or even years, you can experience what's commonly known as a flare.

Conjunctivitis also called (pinkeye) with redness and inflammation of the transparent membranes. Causing the whites of the eyes and the tissues on the central part of the eyelids to be inflamed. Pinkeye is most often caused by an illness, bacterial infection, allergies or chemicals.

Crohn Disease can influence any portion of the GI tract from the mouth to the anus. It most frequently affects the end of the small intestine (the ileum) where it links the beginning of the colon. Crohn disease may develop in "patches" affecting some areas of the GI tract while outgoing other sections are entirely unaffected. In Crohn disease, the inflammation can extend through the entire thickness of the bowel wall of the affected area.

Cystic Fibrosis (CF) also recognized as mucoviscidosis genetic disorder that influences not only the lungs but also the Kidneys, Liver, Pancreas and Intestines. Long-term issues include difficulty breathing and coughing up sputum as a result of frequent lung infections.

Damage to the Spinal Cord is a collection of nerves that start from the brain (bottom) down your back. There are thirty-one pairs of nerves that leave the spinal cord and go to your arms, chest, legs and, gut. These nerves allow your brain to give instructions to your muscles and cause activities of your arms and legs.

Darier Disease is a dark, brittle patch on the skin sometimes containing pus. The crusty patches are also known as keratotic papules, follicular keratosis or follicular dyskeratosis.

Degenerative Arthritis of the disc can cause local pain in the affected area. Any level of the spine can be painful by disc degeneration. When disc degeneration influences the spine of the neck, it is introduced as cervical disc disease. When the mid back is pretentious, the condition is referred to as thoracic disc disease.

Delirium Tremens Alcohol removal delirium (AWD) is a severe form of alcohol withdrawal. It causes sudden and severe problems in your brain and nervous system.

Dermatomyositis is an uncommon incendiary disease. That occurs when muscles become inflamed (inflammatory myopathy). It is one of only three known inflammatories.

Diabetes Adult Onset is a metabolic disorder that is characterized by hyperglycemia (high blood sugar) in the context of insulin resistance and relative lack of insulin. This is in contrast to diabetes mellitus type 1 in which there is an absolute requirement of insulin because of the disintegration of islet cells in the pancreas.

Diabetes Insulin Dependent (IDDM) also known as type 1 diabetes usually starts before fifteen years of age but can occur in adults too. Diabetes involves the pancreas gland which is located behind the stomach. The particular cells (beta cells) of the pancreas produce a hormone called insulin.

Diabetes Peripheral Vascular also called (PAD) occurs when blood vessels in the legs are restricted or blocked by fatty deposits and blood flow to your feet and legs decreases.

Diarrhea caused by elevated secretion of fluid into the intestine. Reduced absorption of fluid from the intestine or quick passage of stool within the gut.

Diverticulitis is a bulging pouch or sac that can develop on internal organs. Which are bulging sacs that push outward on the colon wall. Diverticulitis can occur anyplace in the colon but most commonly from near the end of the colon on the left side (sigmoid colon).

Dysthymic Disorder is a form of depression symptoms normally last for at least two years and often for much longer than that. Dysthymia interferes with your faculty to function and enjoy life.

Eczema Atopic Dermatitis (eczema) is an appearance that makes your skin red and itchy. It is well known in children but can occur at any age. Atopic dermatitis is long-lasting (chronic) and tends to flare up periodically and then subside.

Emphysema Progressively is damaging to the air sacs (alveoli) in your lungs that build up progressively causing shortness of breath. Emphysema is one of the several diseases known collectively as the chronic obstructive pulmonary disease (COPD). Smoking is the leading cause of emphysema.

Endometrial Cancer is a kind of cancer that starts in the uterus. The uterus is a hollow, pear-shaped pelvic organ in women where fetal development occurs. Endometrial cancer is a layer of cells that form the lining of the uterus (endometrium). Endometrial cancer is sometimes called (uterine cancer).

Endometriosis is the occurrence of uterine-lining tissue outside the uterus. Symptoms may include abdominal pain, infertility and heavy periods. Treatment options include pain relievers, hormones and surgery.

Epidermolysis Bullosa is a combination of rare illnesses that cause blisters on the skin. Blisters can appear in response to minor injury, heat, rubbing, adhesive tape, friction or scratching. The blisters can occur inside the body such as the lining of the mouth and intestines.

Epididymitis (Epididymis) is inflammation of the coiled tube at the back of the testicle that stores and carries sperm. Epididymitis is caused by a bacterial infection including sexually transmitted diseases. Males of any age can get epididymitis.

Epilepsy (Neurological Disorder) is a central nervous system illness in which nerve cells in the brain become disrupted causing seizures.

Also periods of weird behavior, sensations and sometimes loss of consciousness.

Felty Syndrome a complication of rheumatoid arthritis. Felty syndrome is the presence of three conditions, rheumatoid arthritis, an enlarged spleen (splenomegaly) and an abnormally low white blood cell count. Felty syndrome is uncommon.

Fibromyalgia means extensive pain in the muscles, but this syndrome can cause many other symptoms.

Friedreich Ataxia (FRDA) genetic is a progressive neurodegenerative movement disorder. Also with a mean age of onset between ten and fifteen years.

Gastritis is inflammation of the lining of the stomach. The swelling of gastritis is most often the result of infection with the same bacterium that causes most stomach ulcers. Injury and drinking too much alcohol also can contribute to gastritis.

Genital Herpes is a common sexually transmitted virus that affects men and women. Features of genital herpes include pain, itching, and sores in your genital area. Sometimes there are no signs or symptoms of genital herpes. If infected you can be contagious even if you have no visible signs.

Glaucoma is an illness that causes damage to your optic nerve and can worsen over time. Glaucoma is pressure inside the eye. Glaucoma tends to be inherited and may not show up until later in life.

Glioblastoma Multiform (GBM) who classification name is (glioblastoma) also known as grade IV astrocytoma the most common and most destructive malignant primary brain tumor in humans.

Graves Disease (Toxic Diffuse Goiter) and Flajani-Basedow-Graves' is an autoimmune disease that affects the thyroid system.

Hemophilia A when you bleed your body typically groups blood cells together to form a clot to stop the bleeding. The clotting process is determined by individual blood particles (platelets and plasma proteins). Hemophilia occurs when you have a deficiency and is inherited.

Henoch-Schonlein Purpura is a disorder that causes inflammation and bleeding in the small blood vessels in your skin, joints, intestines and kidney.

Hepatitis C Virus is a liver disease. The hepatitis C virus is a blood-borne virus the most modern models of infection are through unsafe injection practices, unscreened blood transfusion, blood products and inadequate sterilization of medical equipment.

Hereditary Spinal Ataxia is known as spinocerebellar atrophy (SCA) or spinocerebellar degeneration. A progressive degenerative genetic disease with multiple types each of which could be considered a disease in its right.

Human Immunodeficiency Virus (HIV/AIDS) is an infection and acquired as a spectrum of conditions. Infection of the lung known as pneumocystis pneumonia severe weight loss. A type of cancer known as (Kaposi sarcoma) or other AIDS-defining conditions.

Hospice Patient Care that focus on the palliation of a chronically terminally ill or seriously ill patient's. Pain and symptoms and attending to their emotional and spiritual needs.

Huntington Disease is an inherited and progressive disease that causes breakdown (degeneration) of nerve cells in the brain. Huntington disease has a significant impact on a person's functional abilities and usually results in movement, thinking (cognitive) and psychiatric disorders.

Hypertension is known as high blood pressure; it is a condition in which the long-term force of the blood forced into your artery walls causing heart disease. The more frequently your heart pumps, the narrower your arteries creating high blood pressure.

Hypertension Sleep is a disorder and low levels of sleep that has a significant risks of heart disease, obesity, and even reduced lifespan.

Hyperventilation Syndrome is more accurate and relates to a breathing pattern that happens under certain conditions with a group of another symptom.

Hypoglycemia is low blood sugar that occurs when blood glucose drops below normal levels. Glucose is a vital source of energy for the body that comes from food. Carbohydrates are the primary dietary source of glucose. Rice, potatoes, bread, tortillas, cereal, milk, fruit and sweets are all carbohydrate-rich foods.

Impotence is a common problem among men consistent inability to sustain an erection sufficient for sexual intercourse or the inability to achieve or both.

Inflammatory Bowel Disease involves chronic inflammation of all or portion of the digestive tract. Both usually include severe diarrhea, pain, fatigue, and weight loss. IBD can be debilitating and leads to life-threatening complications.

Intermittent Explosive Disorder (IED) is an explosive disorder involves repeated abrupt incidents of aggressive, impulsive, angry verbal outbursts, violent behavior or in which you react entirely out of proportion to the situation. Road rage, domestic abuse, throwing or breaking objects or other temper tantrums may be signs of an intermittent explosive disorder.

Intractable Vomiting is repeated vomiting that resists medical treatment.

Lipomatosis is believed to be an autosomal dominant condition in which multiple lipomas are present on the body (fatty tumors). The disease is benign. Many discrete encapsulated lipomas form on the trunk and extremities. This is most commonly found mutations in solitary lipomatous tumors, but lipomas often have multiple variations. Reciprocal translocations involved have been observed.

Lou Gehrig Disease is a lateral sclerosis or (ALS) is a nervous system (neurological) disease that causes muscle weakness and impacts physical function.

Lyme Disease because of the bacterium *(Borrelia burgdorferi)*. The most common tick-borne illness in North America and Europe. Lyme disease is transmitted by the bite of an infected black-legged tick.

Lymphoma Hodgkin was previously known as Hodgkin disease that is cancer of the lymphatic system. Which is part of the immune system. In Hodgkin lymphoma cells in the lymphatic organism grow irregularly and can spread beyond the lymphatic system.

Major Depression is also known as clinical depression, unipolar depression or unipolar disorder. Or as recurrent depression in the case of repeated episodes. Which is a disorder characterized by a pervasive and persistent low mood that is accompanied by low self-esteem also loss of interest or pleasure in normally enjoyable activities. The term "depression" is used in different ways.

Malignant Melanoma is a type of cancer that develops from the pigment-containing organism recognized as melanocytes. Melanomas typically happen in the skin but may rarely occur in the mouth or eye. In women most frequently occur on the legs while in men they are most generally on the back. Sometimes they develop from a mole with relating changes including a shift in the color, increase in size, irregular edges, itchiness and skin breakdown.

Mania is the mood of an abnormally visible energy level or a state of heightened overall activation with enhanced practical expression together with a liability of effect. Although it is a mirror image of depression, the heightened mood can be either irritable or euphoric. Indeed as the mania progresses irritability that becomes more prominent and can ensure violence. Even though bipolar disorder is by far the most common cause of desire it is an essential component of other psychiatric conditions (bipolar type schizoaffective disorder).

Melorheostosis is a rare and progressive disease caused by thickening (hyperostosis) of the outer layers of bone (cortical bone). Melorheostosis affects both soft tissue growth and bone and development. While the disorder is benign, it often results in severe functional limitation, significant pain, malformed or immobilized muscles, ligaments, tendons, limb, hand and foot deformity.

Meniere Disease is the inner ear causes spontaneous episodes of vertigo. A feeling of a spinning motion, fluctuating hearing loss, ringing in the ear (tinnitus) and occasionally a sense of fullness or pressure in your ear. In many cases, Meniere Disease affects only one ear.

Migraine Headaches is a neurological disorder characterized by recurrent moderate to severe headaches.

Motion Sickness (Ketosis) is also known as travel sickness is a condition in which a disagreement exists between visually perceived movement and the vestibule's sense of movement. Depending on the cause it can also be referred to as seasickness, car sickness, simulation illness or airsickness.

Mucopolysaccharidosis is a disorder that divided into three separate syndromes

1. Hurler syndrome (MPS I-H)
2. Hurler-Scheie syndrome (MPS I-H/S)
3. Scheie syndrome (MPS I-S)

These are metabolic disorders caused by the malfunctioning of the liposomal enzymes needed to break down molecules called Glycosaminoglycans.

Multiple Sclerosis (MS) Myelin is damage disrupts communication between your brain and the rest of your body. Ultimately the nerves themselves may deteriorate a process that's currently irreversible.

Muscle Spasm Esophageal are painful muscle contractions that affect your esophagus. The hollow tube between your throat and your stomach. Esophageal spasms can feel like sudden rigid chest pain that lasts for a few minutes to hours.

Muscular Dystrophy is a disease that offset progressive weakness and loss of muscle mass. In Muscular Dystrophy, abnormal genes (mutations) interfere with the construction of proteins needed to form healthy tissue.

Myeloid Leukemia Acute myelogenous leukemia (AML) is a cancer of the blood and bone marrow. The spongy tissue inside bones where blood cells are made.

Nail–Patella Syndrome is also recognized as hood syndrome a Genetic Disorder that results in small poorly developed kneecaps and fingernails. It can also affect many other local areas of the body such as the chest, elbows, and hips. The name nail-patella can be incredibly misleading because the syndrome often affects any other locals of the body including particular proteins production.

Nervous Tissue is the central primary of the two parts of the nervous system. The brain and spinal cord of the (CNS) central nervous system. The peripheral nervous system (PNS) regulates and controls bodily functions and activity. It is collected from neurons or nerve cells which receive and transmit impulses and neuralgias. Also known as glial cells.

Nightmare is a troubling dream associated with negative feelings such as anxiety or fear. Nightmares are common and random ideas usually are nothing to worry about. However, they may become a problem if you have them often and they disrupt your sleep or cause fear when going to sleep.

Obesity Complex Disorder connected to an excessive amount of body fat. Obesity isn't just an enhancing concern. It grows your risk of health problems and diseases such as heart disease, diabetes, and high blood pressure.

Obsessive-Compulsive Disorder is characterized pathologically thoughts and fears (obsessions) that lead you to do repetitive behaviors (compulsions).

Opiate Dependence morphine injection is used to relieve moderate to severe pain. It may also be used before or during surgery with an anesthetic (medicine that puts you to sleep). Morphine belongs to the group of medications called narcotic analgesics (pain medicines). It acts on the Central Nervous System (CNS) to relieve pain.

Osteoarthritis is a common form of arthritis. Osteoarthritis can occur when the protective cartilage on the ends of your bones wears down over time.

Panic Disorder or panic attack is an abrupt episode of intense fear that triggers severe physical reactions when there is no real apparent or danger cause. Panic attacks can be terrifying when panic attacks occur you might think you're losing control, having a heart attack or even dying.

Parkinson Disease progressive disorder is of the nervous system that changes movements. It develops gradually, sometimes starting with a hardly visible tremor in just one hand. Tremors may be the most familiar sign of Parkinson disease the disorder also usually causes stiffness or slowing of movement.

Peripheral Neuropathy is an effect of damage to your peripheral nerves frequently cause numbness, pain, and weakness usually in your feet and hands.

Peritoneal Pain is associated with peritoneal dialysis caused by germs around the catheter.

Persistent Insomnia is a persistent disorder that can make it hard to fall asleep or to stay asleep. With insomnia, you awaken feeling unrefreshed. Insomnia can zap your energy level, mood, work performance, health and quality of life.

Porphyria refers to a collection of disorders that result from an accumulation of common chemicals that produce porphyrin in your body. Porphyrins are fundamental for the function of hemoglobin. A protein in your red blood cells that links to porphyrin bind to iron and carries oxygen to your organs and tissue.

Post-Polio Syndrome (PPS) or poliomyelitis is an infectious viral disease that can strike at any age and affects a person's nervous system.

Post-Traumatic Arthritis is a mutual form of osteoarthritis (OA) that is caused by a previous injury or another type of trauma. Osteoarthritis is a long absence of cartilage in the joint. This condition can occur in any joint including the shoulder, elbow, wrist, hip, knee and ankle.

Post-Traumatic Stress Disorder (PTSD) is an anxiety disorder that can develop after a person is exposed to one or more traumatic events such as significant stress, sexual assault, warfare or threats on the person's life.

Premenstrual Syndrome (PMS) also known as physical and emotional symptoms that happen one to two weeks before a woman's menstrual.

Prostate Cancer is recognized as carcinoma of the prostate that develops in the prostate. A gland in the male reproductive system, most prostate cancers are slow-growing whereas some grow relatively quickly. The cancer cells may spread from the prostate to other parts of the body particularly the bones and lymph nodes.

Psoriasis is a long-lasting disease characterized by patches of abnormal skin. These skin patches are typically red, scaly and itchy. They may fluctuate in severity from small and localized to complete body coverage. Injury to the skin can activate psoriatic skin changes at that spot which is known as (Koebner Phenomenon). Psoriasis is linked to an increased risk of lymphomas, psoriatic, cardiovascular disease, Crohn Disease, and depression. Psoriatic arthritis influences up to 30 percent of individuals with psoriasis.

Pulmonary Fibrosis is a respiratory disease in which scars are formed in the lung tissues leading to severe scar formation and breathing problems. The addition of excess Fibrous Connective Tissue (called Fibrosis) results in reduced oxygen supply in the blood and thickening of the walls.

Quadriplegia is also known as tetraplegia paralysis originating from injury or illness that results in the partial or entire loss of use of torso and all limbs. Paraplegia is similar but does not affect the arms. The damage is typically sensory and motor which means that both sensation and control are lost. Quadriparesis or tetraparesis, on the other hand, implies muscle weakness affecting all four limbs. It may be flaccid or spastic.

Radiation Therapy is a type of cancer regimen that uses streams of penetrating energy to kill cancer cells. Radiation therapy most often gets its power from x-rays.

Raynaud Disease (Ray-NOHZ) is caused by some areas of your body such as your toes and fingers to feel cold and numb in response to stress and cold temperatures. In Raynaud disease smaller arteries that supply blood to your skin narrow limiting blood circulation to affected areas (vasospasm).

Reiter Syndrome is an inflammatory response to an infection someplace in the body. It usually follows a urogenital or intestinal disease.

Restless Legs Syndrome (RLS) is an unpleasant feeling or sensation when trying to fall asleep and a strong urge to move.

Rheumatoid Arthritis (RA) is a development of arthritis that causes swelling pain, stiffness, and loss of performance in your joints. It can affect any joint in the wrist and fingers.

Rosacea is a chronic (long-term) disease that sometimes changes the eyes. Pimples and redness characterize the disorder and in advanced stages thickened the skin. Rosacea usually affects the face.

Schizoaffective Disorder is a mental state that causes mood problems (depression or mania) and a loss of contact with reality (psychosis). A person may experience psychosis and mood disturbances separately or simultaneously and will have periods of harsh symptoms followed by improvement.

Scoliosis is where one hip may appear higher than the other. The child's head is not concentric over their body. Also, the shoulder may occur higher than the other. The ribs occur on one side when the child bends forward from the waist. The waistline may be flat on the one hand.

Scoliosis is when lateral (toward the side) curvature in the usually straight vertical line of the spine. If viewed from the side of the spine should show a mild roundness in the upper back and shows a degree of sway back (inward curvature) in the lower back. When a person with a healthy spine is viewed from the front or back the spine appears to be straight. When a person with scoliosis is examined from the back or front of the spine seems to be curved.

Sedative-Dependent Seizures is a propofol with excitatory motor activity. Such as myoclonic jerking and opisthotonus in humans and animals suggests it may aggravate clinical seizure activity.

Seizures are based on the input of behavior and brain activity. Seizures are divided into two broad categories widespread and partial (also called local or focal). Classifying the type of seizure helps doctors diagnose whether a patient has epilepsy.

Senile Dementia is also known as (Senility) broad category of brain diseases that cause a long-term and often gradual decrease in the capability to remember and think where daily functioning is affected.

Severe Nausea is an uneasiness of the stomach that often comes before vomiting. Vomiting is the forcible voluntary or involuntary emptying (throwing up) of stomach contents through the mouth.

Shingles (Herpes Zoster) is a common and highly contagious infection usually spread through sex. This disease is caused by the various herpesvirus-2 (HSV-2) or the herpes simplex virus-1 (HSV-1).

Sinusitis is swelling of the tissue liner of the sinuses. Typically filled with air but when sinuses becomes congested and filled with bacteria, viruses, fungi, fluid and germs can grow and cause an infection.

Skeletal Muscular Somatic Nervous System (SoNS or voluntary nervous system) is associated with skeletal muscular optional control of body movements.

Spasticity is a muscle regulator disorder that is characterized by tight or stiff muscles. Also, reflexes may persist for too long and maybe too strong (hyperactive reflexes). An infant with a hyperactive grasp response may keep his or her hand in a tight fist.

Sleep Apnea is breathing often is partly or blocked during sleep. The problem can be mild to severe. If your lungs don't get, enough air sleep apnea may happen from five to more than fifty times an hour.

Spasticity is a muscle control disorder when the muscles are tight or stiff inability to control those muscles. Also, reflexes may persist for long periods and may be too high (hyperactive reflexes).

Spinal Stenosis of the lower back and lumbar area. If you need information on spinal stenosis of the neck see the topic cervical spinal stenosis.

Surge-Weber Syndrome (SWS) is sometimes referred to as encephalotrigeminal angiomatosis a rare congenital neurological and skin disorder. It is one of the phakomatoses frequently associated with port-wine stains.

Stuttering is not uncommon for children between the ages of two and five. For a lot of children, it's purely part of learning a language of putting words together to develop sentences. It may come and go, or it can last for a few weeks or a couple of years. But for some stuttering can evolve into a lifelong condition that causes problems in school and in functioning as an adult.

Tardive Dyskinesia (TD) is difficult-to-treat and often deadly form of dyskinesia. Tardive Dyskinesia is a disorder resulting in involuntary, repetitive body movements. In this type of Dyskinesia, the involuntary movements are tardive meaning they have a slow or belated onset.

Temporomandibular Joint Disorder (TMJ) is a hinge that connects your jaw to the temporal bones of a person's skull which are in front of each ear so you can move your jaw up and down and side to side chew, talk and yawn.

Tenosynovitis DeQuervain is a condition distressing the tendons on the thumb side of your wrist. Having deQuervain tenosynovitis it will almost certainly hurt when you turn your wrist to grasp anything or make a fist.

Tension Headache is a diffuse mild to moderate pain in your head that's frequently described as feeling like having a tight band around your head. A Tension Headache is a common type of headache, and yet its causes aren't well understood.

Terminal Illness care is home-based family-centered care for individuals facing a terminal illness. Hospice addresses these aspects of a terminal illness when appropriate.

Testicular Cancer occurs in the (testes) testicles which are found inside the scrotum a moveable bag of skin beneath the penis.

Thyroiditis Neuralgia is a chronic pain condition that affects the trigeminal nerve.

TIC Douloureux also called (Trigeminal Neuralgia) when the trigeminal nerve's function is disrupted. Usually, the problem is the contact between a healthy blood vessel in this circumstance a vein or an artery and the trigeminal nerve at the base of your brain. This connection puts pressure on the nerve and causes it to malfunction.

Tietze Syndrome costochondritis is a swelling of the cartilage that connects a rib to the breastbone (sternum). Pain caused by costochondritis might mime that of a heart attack or other heart conditions.

Tinnitus is when the inner ear cell is damaged tiny, fragile hairs in your inner ear move about the pressure of sound waves. Tinnitus triggers ear cells to release an electrical signal through a nerve from your ear to your brain. Your brain interprets these indications as sound. When the hairs inside your inner ear are broken or bent they can "leak."

Tobacco Dependence also called (Nicotine Dependence) addiction to tobacco products and nicotine. Nicotine dependence means you can't quit using the substance even though it's causing you harm.

Tourette Syndrome is a nervous system (neurological) disorder that beginnings in childhood. It involves unusual repetitive movements or unnecessary sounds that can't be controlled (tics).

Trichotillomania is a comprehensive overview covers risk factors for hair-pulling disorder.

Uterine Cancer is the hollow, pear-shaped pelvic organ in women where fetal development occurs. Uterine cancer has been known to begin in the womb.

Viral Hepatitis is an infection caused by a virus that attacks the liver and gets inflamed.

Wasting Syndrome is the thoracic outlet syndrome is a collection of disorders that occur when the nerves or blood vessels in the space between your collarbone and your first rib (thoracic outlet) become compressed. Wasting syndrome can cause pain in your shoulders and neck and numbness in your fingers.

Whiplash is a neck injury that's caused by a dynamic rapid back-and-forth movement of the neck like the cracking of a whip. Whiplash injury can also result from a sports accident, auto accident, physical abuse or other trauma.

Wittmaack-Ekbom Syndrome also known as (Restless Legs Syndrome) (RLS) or (Willis-Ekbom Disease) (WED) is a neurological disorder represented by an overwhelming urge to change one's body to stop odd or uncomfortable sensations. It most generally affects the legs but can affect the head, arms, torso and even missing limbs moving the affected body part.

Writer's Cramp also called Mogigraphia and Scrivener's Palsy, is a disorder caused by cramps or spasms. Certain muscles of the hand and forearm and presents itself while performing fine motor tasks such as writing or playing an instrument. Writer's cramp is a task-specific focal dystonia of the hand.

APPENDIX

A

Acrotrophodynia - see Immersion
ACTH Ectopic Syndrome - E24.3 - Hybrid Cannabis
Actinic - see condition
Actinobacillosis, actinobacillus - A28.8 - Indica Cannabis
Actinomyces, infection - see actinomycosis
Actinomycetoma, foot - B47.1 - Salvia Cannabis
Actinomycosis, actinomycotic - A42.9 - Salvia Cannabis
Actinoneuritis - G62.82 - Indica Cannabis
Action, heart
Activated Protein C resistance - D68.51 - Salvia Cannabis
Active - see condition
Acute - see also condition
Acyanotic Heart Disease, congenital - Q24.9 - Salvia Cannabis
Acystia - Q64.5 - Salvia Cannabis
Adamantinoblastoma - see ameloblastoma
Adamantinoma - see also cyst, calcifying odontogenic
Adamantoblastoma - see ameloblastoma
Adams-Stokes, Morgagni - I45.9 - Salvia Cannabis
Addiction - see also dependence - F19.20 - Indica Cannabis
Addisonian Crisis - E27.2 - Indicia Cannabis
Addison's
Addison-Biermer Anemia, pernicious - D51.0 - Indica Cannabis
Addison-Schilder Complex - E71.528 - Hybrid Cannabis
Additional - see also accessory
Adenoacanthoma - see neoplasm, malignant, by site
Adenoameloblastoma - see cyst, calcifying odontogenic
Adenocarcinoma, tumor
Adenocarcinoma - see also malignant neoplasm, by site
Adenocarcinoma in Situ - also neoplasm in situ, by site
Adenofibroma
Adenofibrosis
Adenoiditis, chronic - J35.02 - Hybrid Cannabis

Adenoids - see condition
Adenolipoma - see also neoplasm, in situ, benign, by site
Adenolipomatosis - E88.89 - Salvia Cannabis
Adenolymphoma
Adenomatosis
Adenomatous
Adenomyoma - see also neoplasm, by site
Adenomyometritis - N80.0 - Hybrid Cannabis
Adenomyosis - N80.0 - Indica Cannabis
Adenopathy, lymph gland - R59.9 - Indicia Cannabis
Adenosalpingitis - see salpingitis
Adenosarcoma - see neoplasm, malignant by site
Adenosclerosis - I88.8 - Hybrid Cannabis
Adenosis, sclerosing - see fibroadenosis, breast
Adenovirus, as cause of disease classified
    elsewhere - B97.0 - Hybrid Cannabis
Adherent - see also adhesions
Adhesions, adhesive, Post-infective - K66.0 - Indica Cannabis
Adiaspiromycosis - B48.8 - Indicia Cannabis
Adie, Holmes - see anomaly, pupil, function, tonic pupil
Adiponecrosis Neonatorum - P83.8 - Indica Cannabis
Adiposis - see also obesity
Adiposity - see also obesity
Adiposogenital Dystrophy - E23.6 - Cannabidiol (CBD)
Adjustment
Administration of TPA, RTPA - Z92.82 - Indica Cannabis
Admission (for) - see also encounter
Adnexitis, suppurative - see salpingo-oophoritis
Adolescent X-linked adrenoleukodystrophy - E71.521 - Indica Cannabis
Adrenal, gland - see condition
Adrenalism, tuberculous - A18.7 - Hybrid Cannabis
Adrenalitis, adrenitis - E27.8 - Indicia Cannabis
Adrenarche, premature - E27.0 - Cannabidiol (CBD)
Adrenocortical Syndrome - see cushing's, syndrome
Adrenogenital Syndrome - E25.9 - Hybrid Cannabis
Adrenogenitalism, congenital - E25.0 - Indicia Cannabis
Adrenoleukodystrophy - E71.529 - Hybrid Cannabis
Adrenomyeloneuropathy - E71.522 - Hybrid Cannabis
Adventitious Bursa - also see bursopathy, specified type NEC

Adverse Effect - see table of drugs and chemicals, categories - T36-T50 - Hybrid Cannabis
Advice - see counseling
Adynamia, episodic, hereditary, periodic - G72.3 - Hybrid Cannabis
Aeration Lung Imperfect, newborn - see atelectasis
Aerobullosis - T70.3 - Hybrid Cannabis
Aerocele - see embolism, air
Aerodermectasia
Aerodontalgia - T70.29 - Indicia Cannabis
Aeroembolism - T70.3 - Cannabidiol (CBD)
Aerogenes Capsulatus Infection - A48.0 - Hybrid Cannabis
Aero-Otitis Media - T70.0 - Hybrid Cannabis
Aerophagy, aerophagia, psychogenic - F45.8 - Hybrid Cannabis
Aerophobia - F40.228 - Cannabidiol (CBD)
Aerosinusitis - T70.1 - Indicia Cannabis
Aerotitis - T70.0 - Hybrid Cannabis
Afibrinogenemia - defect, coagulation - D68.8 - Cannabidiol (CBD)
African
Aftercare - see also care - Z51.89 - Cannabidiol (CBD)
After-Cataract - see cataract, secondary
Agalactia, primary - O92.3 - Salvia Cannabis
Agammaglobulinemia, acquired, secondary, no familial - D80.1 - Hybrid Cannabis
Aganglionosis, bowel, colon - Q43.1 - Cannabidiol (CBD)
Age, old - see senility
Agenesis
Ageusia - R43.2 - Cannabidiol (CBD)
Agitated - see condition
Agitation - R45.1 - Cannabidiol (CBD)
Aglossia, congenital - Q38.3 - Hybrid Cannabis
Aglossia-Adactylia Syndrome - Q87.0 - Hybrid Cannabis
Aglycogenosis - E74.00 - Hybrid Cannabis
Amnesia, body image, other senses, tactile - R48.1 - Cannabidiol (CBD)
Agoraphobia - F40.00 - Cannabidiol (CBD)
Agrammatism - R48.8 - Indicia Cannabis
Agranulocytopenia - see agranulocytosis
Agranulocytosis: chronic, cyclical, genetic, infantile
Graphic, absolute - R48.8 - Cannabidiol (CBD)
Ague, dumb - see malaria

Agyria - Q04.3 - Indicia Cannabis
Ahumada-Del Castillo syndrome - E23.0 - Hybrid Cannabis
Aichmophobia - F40.298 - Cannabidiol (CBD)
AIDS, related complex - B20 - Hybrid Cannabis
Ailment Heart - see disease, heart
Ailurophobia - F40.218 - Cannabidiol (CBD)
Ainhum, disease - L94.6 - Hybrid Cannabis
AIPHI - Acute idiopathic pulmonary hemorrhage in infants over 28 days old - R04.81 - Cannabidiol (CBD)
Airplane Sickness - T75.3 - Cannabidiol (CBD)
Akathisia, drug-induced, treatment-induced - G25.71 - Cannabidiol (CBD)
Akinesia - R29.898 - Indica Cannabis
Akinetic Mutism - R41.89 - Saliva Cannabis
Akureyri's Disease - G93.3 - Hybrid Cannabis
Alactasia, congenital - E73.0 - Hybrid Cannabis
Alagille's Syndrome - Q44.7 - Indicia Cannabis
Alastrim - B03 - Saliva Cannabis
Albers-Schonberg Syndrome - Q78.2 - Hybrid Cannabis
Albert's Syndrome - see tendinitis
Albinism, albino - E70.30 - Saliva Cannabis
Albinismus - E70.30 - Hybrid Cannabis
Albright, McCune, Sternberg - Q78.1 - Hybrid Cannabis
Albuminous - see condition
Albuminuria, albuminuria, acute, chronic, subacute - see also proteinuria R80.9 - Indicia Cannabis
Albuminurophobia - F40.298 - Cannabidiol (CBD)
Alcaptonuria - E70.29 - Indica Cannabis
Alcohol, alcoholic, alcohol-induced
Alcoholism, chronic, without remission - F10.20 - Cannabidiol (CBD)
Alder, reilly, anomaly or syndrome, leukocyte granulation - D72.0 - Hybrid Cannabis
Aldosteronism - E26.9 - Indica Cannabis
Aldosteronoma - D44.10 - Indica Cannabis
Aldrich, Wiskott syndrome, eczema-thrombocytopenia - D82.0 - Hybrid Cannabis
Alektorophobia - F40.218 - Cannabidiol (CBD)
Aleppo Boils - B55.1 - Hybrid Cannabis
A leukemic - see condition
Aleukia

Alexia - R48.0 - Indicia Cannabis
Algoneurodystrophy - M89.00 - Hybrid Cannabis
Algophobia - F40.298 - Cannabidiol (CBD)
Alienation, mental - see psychosis
Alkalemia - E87.3 - Hybrid Cannabis
Alkalosis - E87.3 - Hybrid Cannabis
Alkaptonuria - E70.29 - Salvia Cannabis
Allen-Masters Syndrome - N83.8 - Hybrid Cannabis
Allergy, allergic, reaction - T78.40 - Cannabidiol (CBD)
Allescheriasis - B48.2 - Hybrid Cannabis
Alligator Skin Disease - Q80.9 - Cannabidiol (CBD)
Allochiria, allochiria - R20.8 - Hybrid Cannabis
Almeida's Disease - see paracoccidioidomycosis
Alopecia, hereditary, seborrheic - L65.9 - Cannabidiol (CBD)
Alpers' Disease - G31.81 - Hybrid Cannabis
Alpine Sickness - T70.29 - Indica Cannabis
Alport Syndrome - Q87.81 - Indicia Cannabis
Apparent Life-Threatening Event (ALTE) - R68.13 - Hybrid Cannabis
Altitude high, effects - see effect, adverse, high altitude
Aluminosis, of lung - J63.0 - Hybrid Cannabis
Alveoli are Alveolus, alveolar - see condition
Alymphocytosis - D72.810 - Hybrid Cannabis
Alymphoplasia, thymic - D82.1 - Hybrid Cannabis
Alzheimer's Disease - see disease
Alzheimer's - Q83.8 - Cannabidiol (CBD)
Amathophobia - F40.228 - Cannabidiol (CBD)
Amaurosis, acquired, congenital - see also blindness
Amaurotic idiocy, infantile, juvenile, late - E75.4 - Cannabidiol (CBD)
Amaxophobia - F40.248 - Indicia Cannabis
Ambiguous Genitalia - Q56.4 - Cannabidiol (CBD)
Amblyopia, congenital, ex anopsia, partial, suppression
Ameba, amebic, histolytic - see also amebiasis
Amebiasis - A06.9 - Indica Cannabis
Ameboma, of intestine - A06.3 - Saliva Cannabis
Amelia - Q73.0 - Indicia Cannabis
Ameloblastoma - see also cyst, calcifying odontogenic
Amelogenesis Imperfect - K00.5 - Indica Cannabis
Amenorrhea - N91.2 - Hybrid Cannabis
Amentia - see disability, intellectual

American
Ametropia - see disorder, refraction
Amianthosis - J61 - Hybrid Cannabis
Amimia - R48.8 - Cannabidiol (CBD)
Amino-Acid Disorder - E72.9 - Hybrid Cannabis
Aminoacidopathy - E72.9 - Hybrid Cannabis
Aminoaciduria - E72.9 - Hybrid Cannabis
Agnes (t)is Syndrome, post-traumatic - F04 Hybrid Cannabis
Amnesia - R41.3 - Cannabidiol (CBD)
Amnion, amniotic - see condition
Amnionitis - see pregnancy, complicated
Amok - F68.8 - Cannabidiol (CBD)
Amoral traits - F60.89 - Indicia Cannabis
Ampulla
Amputation - by site, acquired
Amputee, bilateral, old - Z89.9 - Hybrid Cannabis
Amsterdam Dwarfism - Q87.1 - Cannabidiol (CBD)
Amusia - R48.8 - Salvia Cannabis
Amyelencephalus, myelencephala - Q00.0 - Hybrid Cannabis
Amyelia - Q06.0 - Hybrid Cannabis
Amygdalitis - see tonsillitis
Amygdalolith - J35.8 - Salvia Cannabis
Amyloid Heart, disease - E85.4 - Cannabidiol (CBD)
Amyloidosis, generalized, primary - E85.9 - Salvia Cannabis
Amylopectinosis, brancher enzyme deficiency - E74.03 - Indica Cannabis
Amylophagia - see pica
Amyoplasia Congenital - Q79.8 - Indica Cannabis
Amyotonia - M62.89 - Indicia Cannabis
Amyotrophia, amyotrophy, amyotrophic - G71.8 - Hybrid Cannabis
Anacidity, gastric - K31.83 - Cannabidiol (CBD)
Anaerosis of Newborn - P28.89 - Indica Cannabis
Analbuminemia - E88.09 - Indica Cannabis
Analgesia - see anesthesia
Analphalipoproteinemia - E78.6 - Cannabidiol (CBD)
Anaphylactoid Syndrome of pregnancy - O88.01- Hybrid Cannabis
Anaphylaxis - see shock, anaphylactic
Anaplasia Cervix - see also dysplasia, cervix - N87.9 - Hybrid Cannabis
Anaplasmosis, human - A77.49 - Hybrid Cannabis
Anarthria - R47.1 - Cannabidiol (CBD)

Anasarca - R60.1 - Salvia Cannabis
Anastomosis
Anatomical Narrow Angle - H40.03- Salvia Cannabis
Ancylostoma, ancylostomiasis, brazilians', canine, duodenal - B76.0 - Cannabidiol (CBD)
Andersen's Disease, glycogen storage - E74.09 - Hybrid Cannabis
Anderson-Fabry Disease - E75.21 - Hybrid Cannabis
Andes Disease - T70.29 - Hybrid Cannabis
Andrews' Disease, bacteria - L08.89 - Cannabidiol (CBD)
Androblastoma Androgen - insensitivity syndrome - see also syndrome, androgen insensitivity - E34.50 - Indicia Cannabis
Androgen Resistance Syndrome - E34.50 - Hybrid Cannabis
Android Pelvis - Q74.2 - Cannabidiol (CBD)
Androphobia - F40.290 - Cannabidiol (CBD)
Anastasias, pulmonary, newborn - see atelectasis
Anemia, essential, general, hemoglobin deficiency, infantile, primary, profound - D64.9 - Cannabidiol (CBD)
Anemophobia - F40.228 - Cannabidiol (CBD)
Anencephalus, anencephaly - Q00.0 - Hybrid Cannabis
Anergasia - see psychosis, organic
Anesthesia, anesthetic - R20.0 - Hybrid Cannabis
Anetoderma, maculosum - L90.8 - Salvia Cannabis
Aneurin Deficiency - E51.9 - Cannabidiol (CBD)
Aneurysm, anastomotic, artery, cirsoid diffuse, false, fusiform - I72.9 - Hybrid Cannabis
Angelman Syndrome - Q93.5 - Hybrid Cannabis
Anger - R45.4 - Cannabidiol (CBD)
Angiectasis - I99.8 - Indicia Cannabis
Angiitis - I77.6 - Salvia Cannabis
Angina Attack - cardiac, chest, heart, pectoris, syndrome, vasomotor - pectoris,syndrome,vasomotor - I20.9 - Cannabidiol (CBD)
Angioblastoma - see neoplasm, connective tissue, uncertain behavior
Angiocholecystitis - see cholecystitis, acute
Angiocholitis - see also cholecystitis, acute - K83.0 - Hybrid Cannabis
Angiodysgenesis Spinalis - G95.19 - Cannabidiol (CBD)
Angiodysplasia, cecum, colon - K55.20 - Cannabidiol (CBD)
Angioedema, allergic, any site with urticaria - T78.3 - Cannabidiol (CBD)
Angioendothelioma - uncertain behavior
Angioendotheliomatosis - C85.8 - Cannabidiol (CBD)

Angiofibroma
Angiohemophilia (A) (B) - D68.0 - Cannabidiol (CBD)
Angioid Streaks, choroid, macula, retina - H35.33 - Hybrid Cannabis
Angiokeratoma - see neoplasm, skin, benign
Angioleiomyoma - see neoplasm, connective tissue, benign
Angiolipoma - see also lipoma
Angioma - see also hemangioma, by site
Angiomatosis - Q82.8 - Indicia Cannabis
Angiomyolipoma - see lipoma
Angiomyoliposarcoma - see neoplasm, connective tissue, malignant
Angiomyoma - see neoplasm, connective tissue, benign
Angioneurosis - F45.8 - Indicia Cannabis
Angioneurotic Edema - allergic any site with urticaria - T78.3 - Cannabidiol (CBD)
Angiopathia, angioplasty - I99.9 - Salvia Cannabis
Angiosarcoma - Connective tissue, malignant
Angiosclerosis - see arteriosclerosis
Angiosperm, peripheral, traumatic, vessel - I73.9 - Hybrid Cannabis
Angiospastic Disease or edema - I73.9 - Cannabidiol (CBD)
Angiostrongyliasis
Anguillulosis - see strongyloidiasis
Angulation
Angulus Infectious, lips - K13.0 - Cannabidiol (CBD)
Anhedonia - R45.84 - Salvia Cannabis
Anhidrosis - L74.4 - Indica Cannabis
An Hydration, anhydremia - E86.0 - Cannabidiol (CBD)
Anhydremia - E86.0 - Cannabidiol (CBD)
Anidrosis - L74.4 - Hybrid Cannabis
Anorexia, congenital - Q13.1 - Cannabidiol (CBD)
Anisakiasis, infection, infestation - B81.0 - Hybrid Cannabis
Anisakis Larvae Infestation - B81.0 - Hybrid Cannabis
Aniseikonia - H52.32 - Hybrid Cannabis
Anisocoria, pupil - H57.02 - Indicia Cannabis
Anisocytosis - R71.8 - Cannabidiol (CBD)
Anisometropia, congenital - H52.31 - Hybrid Cannabis
Ankle - see condition
Ankyloblepharon, eyelid, acquired - see also blepharophimosis
Ankyloglossia - Q38.1 - Hybrid Cannabis
Ankylosis, fibrous, osseous, joint - M24.60 - Cannabidiol (CBD)

Ankylostoma - see ancylostoma
Ankylostomiasis - see ancylostomiasis
Ankylurethria - see stricture, urethra
Annular - see also condition
Anodontia, complete, partial, vera - K00.0 - Hybrid Cannabis
Anomaly, anomalous, congenital, unspecified type - Q89.9 - Hybrid Cannabis
Anomia - R48.8 - Salvia Cannabis
Anonychia, congenital - Q84.3 - Cannabidiol (CBD)
Anophthalmos, anophthalmus, congenital, globe - Q11.1 - Cannabidiol (CBD)
Anopia, anopsia - H53.46- Hybrid Cannabis
Anorchia, anorchism, anorchidism - Q55.0 - Salvia Cannabis
Anorexia - R63.0 - Indicia Cannabis
Anorgasmy, psychogenic, female - F52.31 - Cannabidiol (CBD)
Anosmia - R43.0 - Indicia Cannabis
Anosognosia - R41.89 - Indicia Cannabis
Anosteoplasia - Q78.9 - Indicia Cannabis
Anovulatory Cycle - N97.0 - Hybrid Cannabis
Anoxemia - R09.02 - Cannabidiol (CBD)
Anoxia, pathological - R09.02 - Cannabidiol (CBD)
Anteflexion - see anteversion
Antenatal
Antepartum - see condition
Anterior - see condition
Antero-Occlusion - M26.220 - Hybrid Cannabis
Anteversion Circulating
Anthophobia - F40.228 - Indica Cannabis
Anthracosilicosis - J60 - Indica Cannabis
Anthracosis, lung, occupational - J60 - Cannabidiol (CBD)
Anthrax - A22.9 - Indicia Cannabis
Anthropoid Pelvis - Q74.2 - Cannabidiol (CBD)
Anthropophobia - F40.10 - Indicia Cannabis
Antibodies, maternal, blood group - see immunization, affecting
    management of pregnancy
Antibody
Anticardiolipin Syndrome - D68.61 - Cannabidiol (CBD)
Anticoagulant, circulating, intrinsic, disorder, hemorrhagic -
    D68.318 - Indicia Cannabis
Ant Diuretic Hormone Syndrome - E22.2 - Cannabidiol (CBD)
Antimonial Cholera - see poisoning, antimony

Antiphospholipid
Antisocial Personality - F60.2 - Cannabidiol (CBD)
Antithrombinemia - see circulating anticoagulants
Antithromboplastinemia - D68.318 - Hybrid Cannabis
Antithromboplastinogenemia - D68.318 - Hybrid Cannabis
Antitoxin complication or reaction - complications, vaccination
Antlophobia - F40.228 - Cannabidiol (CBD)
Antritis - J32.0 - Hybrid Cannabis
Antrum, antral - see condition
Anuria - R34 - Hybrid Cannabis
Anus, anal - see condition
Anusitis - K62.89 - Indicia Cannabis
Anxiety - F41.9 - Cannabidiol (CBD)
Aorta, aortic - see condition
Aortectasia - see ectasia, aorta
Aortitis, nonsyphilitic, calcific - I77.6 - Salvia Cannabis
Apathetic thyroid storm - see thyrotoxicosis
Apathy - R45.3 - Hybrid Cannabis
Aerophobia - F40.228 - Hybrid Cannabis
Apepsia - K30 - Salvia Cannabis
Aperistalsis, esophagus - K22.0 - Salvia Cannabis
Apertognathia - M26.29 - Salvia Cannabis
Apert's Syndrome - Q87.0 - Cannabidiol (CBD)
Aphasia - R13.0 - Indicia Cannabis
Aphasia, acquired, postoperative - H27.0- Indicia Cannabis
Aphasia, amnesic, global, nominal, semantic, syntactic - R47.01 - Indicia Cannabis
Aphonia, organic - R49.1 - Hybrid Cannabis
Apathies, pathos - see also condition
Apical - see condition
Apiphobia - F40.218 - Cannabidiol (CBD)
Aplasia - see also agenesis
Apnea, anemic (of), spells - R06.81- Cannabidiol (CBD)
Apneumatosis, newborn - P28.0 - Cannabidiol (CBD)
Apocrine Metaphase, breast - see dysplasia, mammary, specified type NEC
Apophysitis, bone - see also osteochondropathy
Apoplectiform Convulsions, cerebral ischemia - I67.82 - Cannabidiol (CBD)
Apoplexies, apoplexy, apoplectic
Appearance
Appendage

Appendicitis, pneumococcal, retrocecal - K37 - Indicia Cannabis
Appendicopathia Oxyurica - B80 - Indicia Cannabis
Appendix, appendicle - see also condition
Appetite
Apple Peel Syndrome - Q41.1 - Salvia Cannabis
Apprehension State - F41.1 - Indicia Cannabis
Apprehensiveness, abnormal - F41.9 - Cannabidiol (CBD)
Approximal Wear - K03.0 - Cannabidiol (CBD)
Apraxia - classic - ideational, ideomotor, motor, verbal - R48.2 - Salvia Cannabis
Aptyalism - K11.7 - Indicia Cannabis
Apudoma - see neoplasm, uncertain behavior - H40.83 - Cannabidiol (CBD)
Arabism Elephantiasis - see Infestation, filarial
Arachnids' - meningitis
Arachnodactyly - marfan's
Arachnoiditis - acute, adhesive, basal, brain, cerebrospinal - see meningitis
Arachnophobia - F40.210 - Hybrid Cannabis
Arboencephalitis, Australian - A83.4 - Cannabidiol (CBD)
Arborization Block, heart - I45.5 - Cannabidiol (CBD)
ARC, AIDS-Related Complex - B20 - Hybrid Cannabis
Arches - see condition
Arcuate Uterus - Q51.810 - Cannabidiol (CBD)
Arcuatus Uterus - Q51.810 - Cannabidiol (CBD)
Arcus, cornea - see degeneration, cornea, senile
Arc-welder's Lung - J63.4 - Cannabidiol (CBD)
Areflexia - R29.2 - Indicia Cannabis
Areola - see condition
Argentaffinoma - neoplasm, uncertain behavior, by site
Argininemia - E72.21 - Salvia Cannabis
Arginosuccinic Aciduria - E72.22 - Cannabidiol (CBD)
Argyll Robertson Phenomenon - pupil or syndrome, syphilitic - A52.19 - Cannabidiol (CBD)
Argyria, argyriasis
Argyrosis, conjunctiva - H11.13- - Indicia Cannabis
Arhinencephaly - Q04.1 - Hybrid Cannabis
Ariboflavinosis - E53.0 - Indicia Cannabis
Arm - see condition
Arnold-Chiari Disease - obstruction or syndrome, type II - Q07.00 - Cannabidiol (CBD)

Aromatic amino-acid metabolism disorder - E70.9 - Cannabidiol (CBD)
Arousals, confusional - G47.51 - Cannabidiol (CBD)
Arrest, arrested
Arrhenoblastoma
Arrhythmia - auricle,cardiac, juvenile, nodal, reflex, sinus, supraventricular, transitory, ventricle - I49.9 - Cannabidiol (CBD)
Arrillaga-Ayerza Syndrome, pulmonary sclerosis with pulmonary hypertension - I27.0 - Cannabidiol (CBD)
Arsenical Pigmentation - L81.8 - Indicia Cannabis
Arsenism - see poisoning, arsenic
Arterial - see condition
Arteriofibrosis - see arteriosclerosis
Arteriolar Sclerosis - see arteriosclerosis
Arteriolith - see arteriosclerosis
Arteriolitis - I77.6 - Indicia Cannabis
Arteriolosclerosis - see arteriosclerosis
Arterionephrosclerosis - see hypertension, kidney
Arteriopathy - I77.9 - Hybrid Cannabis
Arteriosclerosis, arteriosclerotic, diffuse, obliterans, senile with calcification - I70.90 - Cannabidiol (CBD)
Arteriospasm - I73.9 - Cannabidiol (CBD)
Arteriovenous - see condition
Arteritis - I77.6 - Indicia Cannabis
Artery, arterial - see also condition
Arthralgia, allergic - pain, joint
Arthritis, arthritic, acute, chronic, nonpyrogenic, subacute - M19.90 - Cannabidiol (CBD)
Arthrocele - see effusion, joint
Arthrodesis Status - Z98.1 - Indicia Cannabis
Arthrodynia - see also pain, joint
Arthrodysplasia - Q74.9 - Salvia Cannabis
Arthrofibrosis, joint - see ankylosis
Arthrogryposis, congenital - Q68.8 - Cannabidiol (CBD)
Arthrokatadysis - M24.7 - Indicia Cannabis
Arthropathy - see also arthritis - M12.9 - Indicia Cannabis
Arthropyosis - arthritis, pyogenic or pyemic
Arthrosis, degenerative, localized - osteoarthritis - M19.90 - Indicia Cannabis
Arthus' Phenomenon or reaction - T78.41 - Indicia Cannabis

Articular - see condition
Articulation, reverse, teeth - M26.24 - Cannabidiol (CBD)
Artificial
Arytenoid - see condition
Asbestosis, occupational - J61 - Indicia Cannabis
Ascariasis - B77.9 - Indicia Cannabis
Ascaridosis, ascaridiasis - see ascariasis
Ascaris, infection, infestation - see ascariasis
Ascending - see condition
Aschoff's Bodies - see myocarditis, rheumatic
Ascites, abdominal - R18.8 - Indicia Cannabis
Aseptic - see condition
Asherman's Syndrome - N85.6 - Cannabidiol (CBD)
Asialia - K11.7 - Salvia Cannabis
Asiatic Cholera - see cholera
Asimultagnosia, simultanagnosia - R48.3 - Hybrid Cannabis
Askin's Tumor -neoplasm, connective tissue, malignant
Asocial Personality - F60.2 - Indicia Cannabis
Asomatognosia - R41.4 - Indicia Cannabis
Aspartylglucosaminuria - E77.1 - Hybrid Cannabis
Asperger's Disease or syndrome - F84.5 - Cannabidiol (CBD)
Aspergilloma - see aspergillosis
Aspergillosis, with pneumonia - B44.9 - Cannabidiol (CBD)
Aspergillus, infection - aspergillosis
Aspermatogenesis - see azoospermia
Aspermia, testis - see azoospermia
Asphyxia, asphyxiation - R09.01 - Indicia Cannabis
Aspiration
Asplenia, congenital - Q89.01 - Cannabidiol (CBD)
Assam Fever - B55.0 - Cannabidiol (CBD)
Assault, sexual - see maltreatment
Assmann's Focus (NEC) - A15.0 - Hybrid Cannabis
Astasia, abasia, hysterical - F44.4 - Indicia Cannabis
Asteatosis Cutis - L85.3 - Hybrid Cannabis
Astereognosia, astereognosis - R48.1 - Indicia Cannabis
Asterixis - R27.8 - Cannabidiol (CBD)
Asteroid Hyalitis - see deposit, crystalline
Asthenia, asthenic - R53.1 - Indicia Cannabis
Asthenopia - see also discomfort, visual

Asthenospermia - abnormal, specimen, male genital organs
Asthma, asthmatic, bronchial, catarrh, spasmodic - J45.909 - Cannabidiol (CBD)
Astigmatism, compound, congenital - H52.20- Cannabidiol (CBD)
Astraphobia - F40.220 - Cannabidiol (CBD)
Astroblastoma
Astrocytoma, cystic
Astroglioma
Asymbolia - R48.8 Indicia Cannabis
Asymmetry - see also distortion
Asynergia, asynergy - R27.8 - Indicia Cannabis
Asystole, heart - see arrest, cardiac
At risk
Ataxia, ataxy, ataxic - R27.0 - Indicia Cannabis
Ataxia-telangiectasia, Louis-Bar - G11.3 - Hybrid Cannabis
Atelectasis, massive, partial, pressure, pulmonary - J98.11 - Cannabidiol (CBD)
Atelocardia - Q24.9 - Indicia Cannabis
Atelomyelia - Q06.1 - Cannabidiol (CBD)
Atheroembolism
Atheroma, atheromatous - I70.90 - Cannabidiol (CBD)
Atheromatosis - see arteriosclerosis
Atherosclerosis - see arteriosclerosis
Athetosis, acquired - R25.8 - Hybrid Cannabis
Athlete's
Athrepsia - E41 - Hybrid Cannabis
Athyrea, acquired - see hypothyroidism
Atonia, atony, atonic
Atopy - see history, allergy
Atransferrinemia, congenital - E88.09 - Salvia Cannabis
Atresia, atretic
Atrichia, atrichosis - see alopecia
Atrophia - see atrophy
Atrophie Blanche, en plaque, de milian - L95.0 - Hybrid Cannabis
Atrophoderma, atrophodermia - L90.9 - Salvia Cannabis
Atrophy, atrophic
Attack, attacks
Attention
Attrition

Atypical, atypism - see also condition
Auditory - see condition
Aujeszky's Disease - B33.8 - Indicia Cannabis
Aurantiasis, cutis - E67.1 - Cannabidiol (CBD)
Auricle, auricular - see condition
Auriculotemporal Syndrome - G50.8 - Cannabidiol (CBD)
Austin Flint Murmur, aortic insufficiency - I35.1 - Hybrid
Australian
Autism, autistic, childhood, infantile - F84.0 - Salvia Cannabis
Autodigestion - R68.89 - Hybrid
Autoerythrocyte Sensitization, syndrome - D69.2 - Hybrid Cannabis
Autographism - L50.3 - Indicia Cannabis
Autoimmune
Autointoxication - R68.89 - Hybrid Cannabis
Automatism - G93.89 - Hybrid Cannabis
Autonomic, autonomous
Autosensitivity, erythrocyte - D69.2 - Cannabidiol (CBD)
Autosensitization, cutaneous - L30.2 - Cannabidiol (CBD)
Autosome - see condition by chromosome involved
Autotopagnosia - R48.1 - Hybrid Cannabis
Autotoxemia - R68.89 - Indicia Cannabis
Autumn - see condition
Avellis' Syndrome
Aversion
Aviator's
Avitaminosis, multiple - deficiency, vitamin - E56.9 - Cannabidiol (CBD)
Avnrt, atrioventricular nodal re-entrant tachycardia - I47.1 - Hybrid Cannabis
Avrt, atrioventricular nodal re-entrant tachycardia - I47.1 - Hybrid Cannabis
Avulsion, traumatic
Awareness of Heart Beat - R00.2 - Indicia Cannabis
Axenfeld's
Axilla, axillary - see also condition
Axonotmesis - see Injury, nerve
Ayerza's Disease or syndrome, pulmonary artery sclerosis with pulmonary hypertension - I27.0 - Cannabidiol (CBD)
Azoospermia, organic - N46.01 - Indica Cannabis
Azotemia - R79.89 - Indicia Cannabis
Aztec Ear - Q17.3 - Hybrid Cannabis
Azygos

B

Baastrup's Disease - see kissing spine
Babesiosis - B60.0 - Cannabidiol (CBD)
Babington's Disease, familial hemorrhagic telangiectasia - I78.0 - Hybrid Cannabis
Babinski's Syndrome - A52.79 - Indicia Cannabis
Baby
Bacillary - see condition
Bacilluria - N39.0 - Hybrid Cannabis
Bacillus - see also Infection, bacillus
Back - see condition
Backache, postural - M54.9 - Indicia Cannabis
Backflow - see reflux
Backward Reading
Bacteria, bactericide, pustular - L40.3 - Indicia Cannabis
Bacterium, bacteria, bacterial
Bacteriuria, bacteriuria - N39.0 - Cannabidiol (CBD)
Bacteroides
Bad
Baez's Disease, cheilitis glandular is aposematism - K13.0 - Cannabidiol (CBD)
Baer a Sprung's Disease, eczema marginatum - B35.6 - Cannabidiol (CBD)
Bagasse Disease or pneumonitis - J67.1 - Salvia Cannabis
Bagassosis - J67.1 - Hybrid Cannabis
Baker's Cyst - see cyst, Baker's
Bakwin-Krida Syndrome, Cranial metaphyseal dysplasia - Q78.5 - Cannabidiol (CBD)
Balancing Side Interference - M26.56 - Indicia Cannabis
Balanitis, circinate, erosive, gangrenous, phagedenic, Vulgaris - N48.1 - Salvia Cannabis
Balanoposthitis - N47.6 - Indicia Cannabis
Blennorrhagia - see balanitis
Balantidiasis, Bal antibiosis - A07.0 - Cannabidiol (CBD)
Bald Tongue - K14.4 - Cannabidiol (CBD)
Baldness - see also alopecia
Balkan Grippe - A78 - Salvia Cannabis
Balloon Disease - adverse, high altitude
Balo's Disease, concentric sclerosis - G37.5 - Cannabidiol (CBD)
Bamberger-Marie Disease - see osteoarthropathy, hypertrophic, specified type NEC

Bancroft's filariasis - B74.0 - Indicia Cannabis
Band (s)
Bandemia - D72.825 - Cannabidiol (CBD)
Bandl's Ring, contraction - O62.4 - Hybrid Cannabis
Bangkok Hemorrhagic Fever - A91 - Salvia Cannabis
Bang's Disease, brucella abortus - A23.1 - Hybrid Cannabis
Bankruptcy, anxiety concerning - Z59.8 - Cannabidiol (CBD)
Bannister's Disease - T78.3 - Indicia Cannabis
Banti's Disease or Syndrome, with cirrhosis, with portal hypertension - K76.6 - Hybrid Cannabis
Bar, median, prostate - enlargement, enlarged, prostate
Barcoo Disease or rot - ulcer, skin
Barlow's Disease - E54 - Cannabidiol (CBD)
Barodontalgia - T70.29 - Hybrid Cannabis
Baron Münchausen syndrome - see disorder, fictitious
Barosinusitis - T70.1 - Indicia Cannabis
Barotitis - T70.0 - Indicia Cannabis
Barotrauma - T70.29 - Indicia Cannabis
Barraquer, Simons, disease, progressive lipodystrophy - E88.1 - Cannabidiol (CBD)
Barré-Guillain Disease or syndrome - G61.0 - Cannabidiol (CBD)
Barré-Liéou Syndrome - posterior cervical sympathetic - M53.0 - Indicia Cannabis
Barrel Chest - M95.4 - Indicia Cannabis
Barrett's
Bársony, Polgár, Tischendorf, syndrome, corkscrew esophagus - K22.4 - Indicia Cannabis
Bartholinitis, suppurating - N75.8 - Cannabidiol (CBD)
Barth Syndrome - E78.71 - Cannabidiol (CBD)
Bartonellosis - A44.9 - Hybrid Cannabis
Barton's Fracture - S52.56- Salvia Cannabis
Bartter's Syndrome - E26.81 - Indicia Cannabis
Basal - see condition
Basan's, hidrotic - Q82.4 - Indicia Cannabis
Baseball Finger - see dislocation, finger
Basedow's Disease, exophthalmic goiter - hyperthyroidism, goiter
Basic - see condition
Basilar - see condition
Bason's, hidrotic - Q82.4 - Hybrid Cannabis

Basopenia - see agranulocytosis
Basophilia - D72.824 - Cannabidiol (CBD)
Basophils, cortico-adrenal, cushing's, pituitary - E24.0 - Hybrid Cannabis
Bassen-Kornzweig Disease or Syndrome - E78.6 - Hybrid Cannabis
Bat ear - Q17.5 - Indicia Cannabis
Bateman's
Bathing Cramp - T75.1 - Cannabidiol (CBD)
Bathophobia - F40.248 Cannabidiol (CBD) -
Batten, Mayou - E75.4 - Salvia Cannabis
Batten-Steinert Syndrome - G71.11 - Indicia Cannabis
Battered - see maltreatment
Battey Mycobacterium Infection - A31.0 - Cannabidiol (CBD)
Battle Exhaustion - F43.0 - Indicia Cannabis
Battledore Placenta - O43.19- Salvia Cannabis
Baumgarten-Cruveilhier Cirrhosis, disease or syndrome - K74.69 - Hybrid Cannabis
Bauxite Fibrosis, of lung - J63.1 - Cannabidiol (CBD)
Bayle's Disease, general paresis - A52.17 - Hybrid Cannabis
Bazin's Disease, primary, tuberculous - A18.4 - Cannabidiol (CBD)
Beach Ear - see swimmer's, ear
Beaded Hair, congenital - Q84.1 - Indicia Cannabis
Béal Conjunctivitis or syndrome - B30.2 - Cannabidiol (CBD)
Beard's Disease, neurasthenia - F48.8 - Cannabidiol (CBD)
Beat (s)
Beau's
Bechtel Rev's Syndrome - spondylitis, ankylosing
Beck's Syndrome - anterior spinal artery occlusion - I65.8 - Hybrid Cannabis
Becker's
Beckwith-Wiedemann Syndrome - Q87.3 - Salvia Cannabis
Bed Confinement Status - Z74.01 - Indicia Cannabis
Bedsore - see ulcer, pressure, by site
Bedbug Bite (s) - bite(s), by site, superficial, insect
Bedclothes, asphyxiation or suffocation by - see asphyxia, traumatic, due to, mechanical, trapped
Bednar's
Bedridden - Z74.01 - Hybrid Cannabis
Bedsore - Bite(s), pressure
Bedwetting - enuresis
Bee sting - with allergic or anaphylactic shock - see toxicity, venom, arthropod, bee

Beer Drinker's Heart, disease - I42.6 - Indicia Cannabis
Begbie's Disease, exophthalmic goiter - hyperthyroidism, goiter
Behavior
Behçet's Disease or syndrome - M35.2 - Salvia Cannabis
Behr's Disease - or degeneration or macula
Beigel's Disease or morbus, white piedra - B36.2 - Cannabidiol (CBD)
Bejel - A65 - Indicia Cannabis
Bekhterev's Syndrome - see spondylitis, ankylosing
Belching - see eructation
Bell's
Bence Jones Albuminuria or proteinuria NEC - R80.3 - Indicia Cannabis
Bends - T70.3 - Indicia Cannabis
Benedikt's Paralysis or syndrome - G46.3 - Cannabidiol (CBD)
Benign - see also condition
Bennett's Fracture, displaced - S62.21- Cannabidiol (CBD)
Benson's Disease - see deposit, crystalline
Bent
Bereavement, uncomplicated - Z63.4 - Salvia Cannabis
Bergeron's Disease, hysterical chorea - F44.4 - Hybrid Cannabis
Berger's Disease - see nephropathy, IgA
Beriberi, dry - E51.11 - Indicia Cannabis
Berlin's Disease or edema, traumatic - S05.8X - Cannabidiol (CBD)
Bullock, baroque - L56.2 - Hybrid Cannabis
Bernard-Horner Syndrome - G90.2 - Cannabidiol (CBD)
Bernard-Soulier Disease or thrombopenia - D69.1 - Cannabidiol (CBD)
Bernhardt, Roth - see mononeuropathy, lower limb, meralgia parenthetical
Bernheim's Syndrome - see failure, heart, congestive
Bertielliasis - B71.8 - Hybrid Cannabis
Berylliosis, lung - J63.2 - Indicia Cannabis
Besnier-Boeck, Schaumann - see sarcoidosis
Besnier's
Bestiality - F65.89 - Salvia Cannabis
Best's Disease - H35.50 - Cannabidiol (CBD)
Beta-Mercapto Lactate-cysteine disulfuric - E72.09 - Cannabidiol (CBD)
Betting and Gambling - Z72.6 - Cannabidiol (CBD)
Bezoar - T18.9 - Cannabidiol (CBD)
Bezold's Abscess - see mastoiditis, acute
Bianchi's Syndrome - R48.8 - Indicia Cannabis
Bicornate or bicorn is uterus - Q51.3 - Salvia Cannabis

Bicuspid Aortic Valve - Q23.1 - Cannabidiol (CBD)
Biedl-Bardet Syndrome - Q87.89 - Hybrid Cannabis
Bielschowsky, jansky - E75.4 - Cannabidiol (CBD)
Biemer's, Pernicious - D51.0 - Indicia Cannabis
Brett's Disease - L93.0 - Cannabidiol (CBD)
Bifid, congenital
Bifurcation, congenital
Big Spleen Syndrome - D73.1 - Cannabidiol (CBD)
Bigeminal Pulse - R00.8 - Salvia Cannabis
Bilateral - see condition
Bile
Bilharziasis - see also schistosomiasis
Biliary - see condition
Bilirubin Metabolism Disorder - E80.7 - Cannabidiol (CBD)
Bilirubinemia, familial nonhemolytic - E80.4 - Indicia Cannabis
Bilirubinuria - R82.2 - Cannabidiol (CBD)
Biliuria - R82.2 - Salvia Cannabis
Bilocular Stomach - K31.2 - Indicia Cannabis
Binswanger's Disease - I67.3 - Indicia Cannabis
Bipartite, bipartite
Bird
Birt-Hogg-Dube Syndrome - Q87.89 - Hybrid Cannabis
Birth
Birthmark - Q82.5 - Hybrid Cannabis
Bisalbuminemia - E88.09 - Indicia Cannabis
Biskra's Button - B55.1 - Salvia Cannabis
Bite(s), animal, human
Biting, cheek or lip - K13.1 - Cannabidiol (CBD)
Biventricular Failure, heart - I50.9 - Cannabidiol (CBD)
Björck, Thorson, syndrome, malignant carcinoid - E34.0 - Cannabidiol (CBD)
Black
Blackfan-Diamond Anemia or syndrome congenital hypoplastic anemia, - D61.01 - Indicia Cannabis
Blackhead - L70.0 - Cannabidiol (CBD)
Blackout - R55 - Cannabidiol (CBD)
Bladder - see condition
Blast, air, hydraulic, immersion underwater
Blastoma - see neoplasm, malignant by site
Blastomycosis, blastomycotic - B40.9 - Hybrid Cannabis

Bleb (s) - R23.8 - Indicia Cannabis
Blebitis, post-procedural - H59.40 - Salvia Cannabis
Bleeder, familial, hereditary - see neoplasm,
Bleeding - see also hemorrhage
Blennorrhagia, blennorrhagic - see gonorrhea
Blennorrhea, acute, chronic - see also gonorrhea
Blepharoptosis - see entropion
Blepharitis, angular, ciliates, eyelid, marginal, nonulcerative - H01.009 - Salvia Cannabis
Blepharochalasis - H02.30 - Indicia Cannabis
Blepharoclonus - H02.59 - Cannabidiol (CBD)
Blepharoconjunctivitis - H10.50 - Cannabidiol (CBD)
Blepharophimosis, eyelid - H02.529 - Cannabidiol (CBD)
Blepharoptosis - H02.40 - Indicia Cannabis
Blepharopyorrhea, gonococcal - A54.39 - Hybrid Cannabis
Blepharospasm - G24.5 - Cannabidiol (CBD)
Blighted Ovum - O02.0 - Hybrid Cannabis
Blind - see also blindness
Blindness, acquired, congenital, both eyes - H54.0 - Hybrid Cannabis
Blister, nonthermal
Bloating - R14.0 - Indicia Cannabis
Bloch-Sulzberger Disease or syndrome - Q82.3 - Cannabidiol (CBD)
Block, blocked
Blockage - see obstruction
Blocq's Disease - F44.4 - Hybrid Cannabis
Blood
Blood-Forming Organs, disease - D75.9 - Cannabidiol (CBD)
Bloodgood's Disease - see mastopathy, cystic
Bloom, Machacek, Torre - Q82.8 - Salvia Cannabis
Blount's Disease - or osteochondrosis - see osteochondrosis, juvenile, tibia
Blue
Blueness - see cyanosis
Blues, postpartum - O90.6 - Indicia Cannabis
Blurring, visual - H53.8 - Cannabidiol (CBD)
Blushing, abnormal, excessive - R23.2 - Cannabidiol (CBD)
BMI - see body, mass index
Boarder, hospital NEC - Z76.4 - Hybrid Cannabis
B Lockhart's impetigo - L01.02 - Salvia Cannabis

Bodechtel-Guttman Disease, subacute sclerosing panencephalitis -
    A81.1 - Cannabidiol (CBD)
Border-Sedgwick Syndrome, ataxia-telangiectasia - G11.3 - Hybrid Cannabis
Body, bodies
Boeck's
Boerhaave's Syndrome, spontaneous esophageal rupture - K22.3 -
    Salvia Cannabis
Boggy
Boil - see also furuncle, by site
Bold hives - see urticaria
Bombé, iris - see membrane, pupillary
Bone - see condition
Bonnevie-Ullrich Syndrome - Q87.1 - Indicia Cannabis
Bonnier's Syndrome - H81.8 - Hybrid Cannabis
Bonvale Dam Fever - T73.3 - Cannabidiol (CBD)
Bony Block of Joint - see ankylosis
Boop, bronchiolitis obliterans organized pneumonia - J84.89 - Indicia Cannabis
Borderline
Borna Disease - A83.9 - Hybrid Cannabis
Bornholm Disease - B33.0 - Hybrid Cannabis
Boston Exanthem - A88.0 - Cannabidiol (CBD)
Bocelli, ductus, patent, persistent - Q25.0 - Cannabidiol (CBD)
Bothriocephalus Latus Infestation - B70.0 - Cannabidiol (CBD)
Botulism, foodborne intoxication - A05.1 - Indicia Cannabis
Bouba - see yaws
Bouchard's Nodes, with arthropathy - M15.2 - Cannabidiol (CBD)
Bouffée Délirante - F23 - Salvia Cannabis
Bouillaud's Disease or syndrome, rheumatic heart disease - I01.9 -
    Cannabidiol (CBD)
Bourneville's Disease - Q85.1 - Cannabidiol (CBD)
Boutonniere Deformity, finger - deformity, finger, boutonniere
Bouveret, Syndrome, Paroxysmal Tachycardia - I47.9 - Hybrid
    Cannabis
Bovine Heart - see hypertrophy, cardiac
Bowel - see condition
Bowen's
Bowing
Bowleg (s), acquired - M21.16- Indicia Cannabis
Boyd's Dysentery - A03.2 - Hybrid Cannabis

Brachial - see condition
Brachycardia - R00.1 - Indicia Cannabis
Brachycephaly - Q75.0 - Indicia Cannabis
Bradley's Disease - A08.19 - Hybrid Cannabis
Bradyarrhythmia, cardiac - I49.8 - Indicia Cannabis
Bradycardia, sinoatrial, sinus, vagal - R00.1 - Indicia Cannabis
Bradykinesia - R25.8 - Salvia Cannabis
Bradypnea - R06.89 - Indicia Cannabis
Bradytachycardia - I49.5 - Indicia Cannabis
Brailsford's Disease or osteochondrosis - osteochondrosis, juvenile, radius
Brain - see also condition
Branched-Chain Amino-Acid Disorder - E71.2 - Cannabidiol (CBD)
Branchial - see condition
Branchiogenic Remnant, in Neck - Q18.0 - Salvia Cannabis
Brandt's Syndrome, acrodermatitis enteropathica - E83.2 -
    Cannabidiol (CBD)
Brash, water - R12 - Hybrid Cannabis
Braves-Jacksonian Epilepsy - epilepsy, localization-related, symptomatic,
    with simple partial seizures
Braxton Hicks Contractions - see false, labor
Brazilian Leishmaniasis - B55.2 - Indicia Cannabis
BRBPR - K62.5 - Hybrid Cannabis
Break, retina, without detachment - H33.30- Hybrid Cannabis
Breakdown
Breast - see also condition
Breath
Breathing
Breathlessness - R06.81 - Cannabidiol (CBD)
Breda's Disease - see yaws
Breech Presentation, mother - O32.1 - Cannabidiol (CBD)
Brisky's Disease - N90.4 - Indicia Cannabis
Brennemann's Syndrome - I88.0 - Hybrid Cannabis
Brenner
Bretonneau's Disease or angina - A36.0 - Cannabidiol (CBD)
Breus' Mole - O02.0 - Salvia Cannabis
Brevicollis - Q76.49 - Cannabidiol (CBD)
Brickmakers' Anemia - B76.9 - Indicia Cannabis
Bridge, myocardial - Q24.5 - Salvia Cannabis
Bright Red Blood per rectum - BRBPK62.5

Bright's Disease - see also nephritis
Brill, Zinsser, Disease, recrudescent typhus - A75.1 Cannabidiol (CBD)
Brill-Symmes' Disease - C82.90 - Salvia Cannabis
Brion-Kayser Disease - see fever, parathyroid
Briquet's Disorder or syndrome - F45.0 - Hybrid Cannabis
Brissaud's
Brittle
Broad - see also condition
Broad - or floating-abetalipoproteinemia - E78.2 - Indicia Cannabis
Brock's Syndrome, atelectasis enlarged lymph nodes - J98.19 - Cannabidiol (CBD)
Brock-Duhring Disease, dermatitis herpetiformis - L13.0 - Cannabidiol (CBD)
Brodie's Abscess or disease - M86.8X - Hybrid Cannabis
Broken
Bromhidrosis, bromidrosis - L75.0 - Hybrid Cannabis
Bromidism, bromism - G92 - Hybrid Cannabis
Bromidrosiphobia - F40.298 - Cannabidiol (CBD)
Bronchi, bronchial - see condition
Bronchiectasis, cylindrical, diffuse, fusiform, localized, saccular - J47.9 - Cannabidiol (CBD)
Bronchiectasis - see bronchiectasis
Bronchiolitis, acute, infective, subacute - J21.9 - Cannabidiol (CBD)
Bronchitis, diffuse, fibrinous, hypostatic, infective, membranous - J40 - Cannabidiol (CBD)
Bronchoalveolitis - J18.0 - Indicia Cannabis
Bronchoaspergillosis - B44.1 - Cannabidiol (CBD)
Bronchocele meaning goiter - E04.0 - Indicia Cannabis
Broncholithiasis - J98.09 - Hybrid Cannabis
Bronchomalacia - J98.09 - Hybrid Cannabis
Bronchomycosis NOS - B49 - Indicia Cannabis
Bronchopleuropneumonia - see pneumonia, broncho
Bronchopneumonia - see pneumonia, broncho
Bronchopneumonia - see pneumonia, broncho
Bronchopulmonary - see condition
Bronchopulmonitis - see pneumonia, broncho
Bronchorrhea, see hemoptysis
Bronchorrhea - J98.09 - Cannabidiol (CBD)
Bronchospasm, acute - J98.01 - Hybrid Cannabis
Bronchospirochetosis - A69.8 - Hybrid Cannabis
Bronchostenosis - J98.09 - Indicia Cannabis

Bronchus - see condition
Brontophobia - F40.220 - Cannabidiol (CBD)
Bronze Baby Syndrome - P83.8 - Cannabidiol (CBD)
Brooke's Tumor - see neoplasm, skin, benign
Brown Enamel of teeth, hereditary - K00.5 - Cannabidiol (CBD)
Brown's Sheath Syndrome - H50.61- Salvia Cannabis
Brown-Séquard Disease, syndrome or paralysis - G83.81 Hybrid Cannabis
Bruce Sepsis - A23.0 - Indicia Cannabis
Brucellosis, infection - A23.9 - Cannabidiol (CBD)
Bruck-de Lange Disease - Q87.1 - Hybrid Cannabis
Bruck's Disease - see deformity, limb
Brugsch's Syndrome - Q82.8 - Indicia Cannabis
Bruise, skin surface intact - contusion
Bruit, arterial - R09.89 - Hybrid Cannabis
Brush Burn - see abrasion, by site
Bruton's X-linked agammaglobulinemia - D80.0 - Hybrid Cannabis
Bruxism
Bubbly Lung Syndrome - P27.0 - Cannabidiol (CBD)
Bubo - I88.8 - Salvia Cannabis
Bubonic Plague - A20.0 - Indicia Cannabis
Bubonocele - see hernia, inguinal
Buccal - see condition
Buchanan's Disease or osteochondrosis - M91.0 - Cannabidiol (CBD)
Buchem's Syndrome, hyperostosis cortical - M85.2 - Hybrid Cannabis
Bucket-Handle Fracture or tear - semilunar cartilage - see tear, meniscus
Budd-Chiari Syndrome - hepatic vein thrombosis - I82.0 - Cannabidiol (CBD)
Budgerigar Fancier's Disease or lung - J67.2 - Indicia Cannabis
Buds
Buerger's Disease, thrombi angiitis obliterans - I73.1 - Cannabidiol (CBD)
Bulbar - see condition
Bulbus Cordis, left ventricle, persistent - Q21.8 - Cannabidiol (CBD)
Bulimia - F50.2 - Cannabidiol (CBD)
Bulky
Bulla (e) - R23.8 - Salvia Cannabis
Bullet Wound - see also wound, open
Bundle
Bunion - see deformity, toe, hallux valgus
Buphthalmia, buphthalmos, congenital - Q15.0 - Cannabidiol (CBD)
Burdwan Fever - B55.0 - Indicia Cannabis

Bürger-Grütz Disease or syndrome - E78.3 - Hybrid Cannabis
Buried
Burke's Syndrome - K86.8 - Hybrid Cannabis
Burkitt
Burn - electricity, flame, hot gas, liquid or hot object, radiation, steam, thermal - T30.0 - Hybrid Cannabis
Burnett's Syndrome - E83.52 - Indicia Cannabis
Burning
Burn-out, state - Z73.0 - Salvia Cannabis
Burns' Disease or osteochondrosis
Bursa - see condition
Bursitis - M71.9 - Hybrid Cannabis
Bursopathy - M71.9 - Indicia Cannabis
Burst Stitches or sutures - T81.31 - Cannabidiol (CBD)
Buruli Ulcer - A31.1 - Cannabidiol (CBD)
Bury's Disease - L95.1 - Hybrid Cannabis
Buschke's
Busse-Buschke Disease - B45.3 - Indicia Cannabis
Bwamba Fever - A92.8 - Cannabidiol (CBD)
Byssinosis - J66.0 - Indicia Cannabis
Bywaters' Syndrome - T79.5 - Hybrid Cannabis

C

Cachexia - R64 - Cannabidiol (CBD)
Café, Lait Spots - L81.3 - Indicia Cannabis
Caffey's Syndrome - Q78.8 - Salvia Cannabis
Caisson Disease - T70.3 - Cannabidiol (CBD)
Cake Kidney - Q63.1 - Cannabidiol (CBD)
Caked Breast, puerperal, postpartum - O92.79 - Hybrid Cannabis
Calabar Swelling - B74.3 - Cannabidiol (CBD)
Calcaneal Spur - see spur, bone, calcaneal
Calcaneal-Apophysitis - M92.8 - Indicia Cannabis
Calcareous - see condition
Calcinosis - J62.8 - Salvia Cannabis
Calciferol, vitamin D - E55.9 - Indicia Cannabis
Calcification
Calcified - see calcification
Calcinosis, interstitial, tumoral, universal - E83.59 - Cannabidiol (CBD)
Calciphylaxis - calcification, - E83.59 - Indicia Cannabis

Calcium
Calciuria - R82.99 - Hybrid Cannabis
Calculi - see calculus
Calculosis, intrahepatic - see calculus, bile duct
Calculus, calculi, calculus
Calicectasis - N28.89 - Salvia Cannabis
Caliectasis - N28.89 - Indicia Cannabis
California
Caligo Cornea - see opacity, cornea, central
Callositas, callosity, infected - L84 - Hybrid Cannabis
Callus, infected - L84 - Cannabidiol (CBD)
Calorie Deficiency or malnutrition - see also malnutrition - E46 - Salvia Cannabis
Calvé-Perthes Disease - see Legg-Calvé-Perthes disease
Calvé's Disease - see osteochondrosis, juvenile, spine
Calvities - see alopecia, androgenic
Cameroon Fever - see malaria
Camptocormia, hysterical - F44.4 - Indicia Cannabis
Camurati-Engelmann Syndrome - Q78.3 - Salvia Cannabis
Canal - see also condition
Canaliculitis, lacrimal, acute, subacute - H04.33- Hybrid Cannabis
Canavan's Disease - E75.29 - Cannabidiol (CBD)
Canceled Procedure, surgical - Z53.9 - Indicia Cannabis
Cancer - Neoplasm, by site, malignant
Cancer (o) - F45.29 - Salvia Cannabis
Cancerous - see neoplasm, malignant, by site
Cancrum Oris - A69.0 - Salvia Cannabis
Candidiasis, candidal - B37.9 - Indicia Cannabis
Candidid - L30.2 - Hybrid Cannabis
Candidosis - see candidiasis
Candiru Infection or infestation - B88.8 - Cannabidiol (CBD)
Canities, premature - L67.1 - Cannabidiol (CBD)
Canker, mouth, sore - K12.0 - Cannabidiol (CBD)
Cannabinosis - J66.2 - Hybrid Cannabis
Canton Fever - A75.9 - Cannabidiol (CBD)
Cantrell's Syndrome - Q87.89 - Indicia Cannabis
Capillariasis, intestinal - B81.1 - Hybrid Cannabis
Capillary - see condition
Caplan's Syndrome - see rheumatoid, lung

Capsule - see condition
Capsulitis, joint - see also enthesopathy
Caput
Car Sickness - T75.3 - Indicia Cannabis
Carapata, disease - A68.0 - Hybrid Cannabis
Carate - see pinta
Carbon Lung - J60 - Cannabidiol (CBD)
Carbuncle - L02.93 - Indicia Cannabis
Carbunculus - see carbuncle
Carcinoid, tumor - see tumor, carcinoid
Carcinoidosis - E34.0 - Cannabidiol (CBD)
Carcinoma, malignant - see also neoplasm, malignant
Carcinoma-in-situ - neoplasm, in situ, by site
Carcinomaphobia - F45.29 - Indicia Cannabis
Carcinomatosis - C80.0 - Cannabidiol (CBD)
Carcinosarcoma - see neoplasm, malignant, by site
Cardia, cardial - see condition
Cardiac - see also condition
Cardialgia - see pain, precordial
Cardiectasis - see hypertrophy, cardiac
Cardiochalasia - K21.9 - Indicia Cannabis
Cardiomalacia - I51.5 - Hybrid Cannabis
Cardiomegalia Glycogenica Diffusa - E74.02 - Salvia Cannabis
Cardiomegaly - see also hypertrophy, cardiac
Cardiomyoliposis - I51.5 - Salvia Cannabis
Cardiomyopathy, familial, idiopathic - I42.9 - Hybrid Cannabis
Cardionephritis - see hypertension, cardiorenal
Cardionephropathy - see hypertension, cardiorenal
Cardionephrosis - see hypertension, cardiorenal
Cardiopathia Nigra - I27.0 - Indicia Cannabis
Cardiopathy - disease, heart - I51.9 - Cannabidiol (CBD)
Cardiopericarditis - see pericarditis
Cardiophobia - F45.29 - Hybrid Cannabis
Cardiorenal - see condition
Cardiorrhexis - see Infarct, myocardium
Cardiosclerosis - see disease, heart, ischemic, atherosclerotic
Cardiosis - see disease, heart
Cardiospasm, esophagus, reflex, stomach - K22.0 - Indicia Cannabis
Cardiostenosis - see disease, heart

Cardiosymphysis - I31.0 - Cannabidiol (CBD)
Cardiovascular - see condition
Carditis, acute, bacterial, chronic, subacute - I51.89 - Cannabidiol (CBD)
Care-of, for, following
Caries
Carious Teeth - see caries, dental
Carneous Mole - O02.0 - Cannabidiol (CBD)
Carnitine Insufficiency - E71.40 - Indicia Cannabis
Carotid Body or sinus syndrome - G90.01 - Indicia Cannabis
Carotidynia - G90.01 - Hybrid Cannabis
Carotinemia, dietary - E67.1 - Indicia Cannabis
Carotinosis, cutis, skin - E67.1 - Salvia Cannabis
Carpal Tunnel Syndrome - see syndrome, carpal tunnel
Carpenter's Syndrome - Q87.0 - Hybrid Cannabis
Carpopedal Spasm - see tetany
Carr-Barr-Plunkett Syndrome - Q97.1 - Cannabidiol (CBD)
Carrier, suspected
Carrion's Disease - A44.0 - Hybrid Cannabis
Carter's Relapsing Fever, asiatic - A68.1 - Indicia Cannabis
Cartilage - see condition
Caruncle, inflamed
Cascade Stomach - K31.2 - Cannabidiol (CBD)
Caseation Lymphatic Gland, tuberculous - A18.2 - Indicia Cannabis
Cassidy, Scholte, syndrome, malignant carcinoid - E34.0 - Cannabidiol (CBD)
Castellani's Disease - A69.8 - Hybrid Cannabis
Castration, traumatic, male - S38.231 - Salvia Cannabis
Casts in Urine - R82.99 - Cannabidiol (CBD)
Cat
Catabolism, senile - R54 - Cannabidiol (CBD)
Catalepsy, hysterical - F44.2 - Indicia Cannabis
Cataplexy, idiopathic - see narcolepsy
Cataract, cortical, immature, incipient - H26.9 - Indicia Cannabis
Cataracta - see also cataract
Catarrh, catarrhal, acute, febrile, infectious, inflammation - see also condition - J00 - Indicia Cannabis
Catatonia, schizophrenic - F20.2 - Hybrid Cannabis
Catatonic
Cat-scratch - see also abrasion
Cauda Equina - see condition

Cauliflower Ear - M95.1- Indicia Cannabis
Causalgia, upper limb - G56.4- Cannabidiol (CBD)
Cause
Caustic Burn - see corrosion, by site
Cavare's Disease, familial periodic paralysis - G72.3 - Cannabidiol (CBD)
Cave-in, injury
Cavernitis, penis - N48.29 - Indicia Cannabis
Cavernositis - N48.29 - Salvia Cannabis
Cavernous - see condition
Cavitation of Lung - tuberculosis, pulmonary
Cavities, dental - see caries, dental
Cavity
Cavovarus Foot, congenital - Q66.1 - Hybrid Cannabis
Cavus Foot, congenital - Q66.7 - Indicia Cannabis
Cazenave's Disease - L10.2 - Hybrid Cannabis
Cecitis - K52.9 - Hybrid Cannabis
Cecum - see condition
Celiac
Cell (s) - see also condition
Cellulitis, diffuse, phlegmonous, septic, suppurative - L03.90 - Salvia Cannabis
Cementoblastoma, benign - see cyst, calcifying odontogenic
Cementoma - see cyst, calcifying odontogenic
Cementoperiostitis - see periodontitis
Cementosis - K03.4 - Indicia Cannabis
Central Auditory Processing Disorder - H93.25 - Indicia Cannabis
Central Pain Syndrome - G89.0 - Cannabidiol (CBD)
Cephalematocele, cephal (o)
Cephalematoma, cephalhematoma, calcified
Cephalgia, cephalalgia - see also headache
Cephalic - see condition
Cephalitis - see encephalitis
Cephalocele - see encephalocele
Cephalomenia - N94.89 - Indicia Cannabis
Cephalopelvic - see condition
Cerclage, with cervical incompetence - see incompetence, cervix, in pregnancy
Cerebellitis - see encephalitis
Cerebellum, cerebellar - see condition
Cerebral - see condition
Cerebritis - see encephalitis

Cerebro-Hepato-Renal Syndrome - Q87.89 - Indicia Cannabis
Cerebromalacia - see softening, brain
Cerebroside Lipidosis - E75.22 - Cannabidiol (CBD)
Cerebrospasticity, congenital - G80.1 - Hybrid Cannabis
Cerebrospinal - see condition
Cerebrum - see condition
Ceroid-Lipofuscinosis, neuronal - E75.4 Indicia Cannabis
Cerumen, accumulation, impacted - H61.2- Salvia Cannabis
Cervical - see also condition
Cervicalgia - M54.2 - Salvia Cannabis
Cervicitis - acute, chronic, nonvenereal, senile, atrophic, subacute, with ulceration - N72 - Hybrid Cannabis
Cervicocolpitis, emphysematosa, see also cervicitis - N72 - Salvia Cannabis
Cervix - see condition
Cesarean Delivery, previous, affecting management of pregnancy - O34.21 - Cannabidiol (CBD)
Céstan, Chenais - G46.3 - Indicia Cannabis
Céstan-Raymond Syndrome - I65.8 - Cannabidiol (CBD)
Cestode Infestation - B71.9 - Cannabidiol (CBD)
Cestodiasis - B71.9 - Hybrid Cannabis
Chabert's Disease - A22.9 - Cannabidiol (CBD)
Chacaleh - E53.8 - Salvia Cannabis
Chafing - L30.4 - Indicia Cannabis
Chagas', Mazza, Disease, chronic - B57.2 Cannabidiol (CBD)-
Chagres Fever - B50.9 - Cannabidiol (CBD)
Chairridden - Z74.09 - Hybrid Cannabis
Chalasia, cardiac sphincter - K21.9 - Indicia Cannabis
Chalazion - H00.19 - Cannabidiol (CBD)
Chalcosis - see also disorder, globe, degenerative, chalcosis
Chalicosis, pulmonum - J62.8 - Hybrid Cannabis
Chancre - any genital site, hard, hunterian, mixed, primary - A51.0 - Cannabidiol (CBD)
Chancroid, anus, genital, penis, perineum, rectum, urethra, vulva - A57 - Hybrid Cannabis
Chandler's Disease, osteochondritis dissecans, hip - see osteochondritis, dissecans, hip
Change (s) (in) (of) - removal
Changing Sleep, work schedule, affecting sleep - G47.26 - Indicia Cannabis
Changuinola Fever - A93.1 - Indicia Cannabis

Chapping Skin - T69.8 - Cannabidiol (CBD)
Charcot-Marie-Tooth Disease, paralysis or syndrome - G60.0 - Cannabidiol (CBD)
Charcot's
Charge Association - Q89.8 - Salvia Cannabis
Charley-Horse, quadriceps - M62.831 - Indicia Cannabis
Charlouis' Disease - see yaws
Cheadle's Disease - E54 - Salvia Cannabis
Checking (of)
Check-up - examination
Chédiak-Higashi, Steinbrinck, syndrome, congenital - E70.330 - Indicia Cannabis
Cheek - see condition
Cheese Itch - B88.0 - Cannabidiol (CBD)
Cheese-Washer's Lung - J67.8 - Cannabidiol (CBD)
Cheese-Worker's Lung - J67.8 - Indicia Cannabis
Cheilitis, acute, angular, catarrhal, chronic, exfoliative - K13.0 - Cannabidiol (CBD)
Cheilodynia - K13.0 - Salvia Cannabis
Cheiloschisis - see cleft, lip
Cheilosis, angular - K13.0 - Indicia Cannabis
Cheiromegaly - M79.89 - Hybrid Cannabis
Cheiropompholyx - L30.1 - Hybrid Cannabis
Cheloid - see keloid
Chemical Burn - see corrosion, by site
Chemodectoma - see paraganglioma, nonchromaffin
Chemosis, conjunctiva - see edema, conjunctiva
Chemotherapy, session
Cherubism - M27.8 - Indicia Cannabis
Chest - see condition
Cheyne-Stokes breathing, respiration - R06.3 - Cannabidiol (CBD)
Chiari's
Chicago Disease - B40.9 - Cannabidiol (CBD)
Chickenpox - see varicella
Chiclero Ulcer or sore - B55.1 - Cannabidiol (CBD)
Chigger, infestation - B88.0 - Cannabidiol (CBD)
Chignon Disease - B36.8 - Hybrid Cannabis
Chilaiditi's Syndrome, subphrenic displacement, colon - Q43.3 - Hybrid Cannabis
Chilblain (s), lupus - T69.1 - Indicia Cannabis

Child
Childbirth - see delivery
Childhood
Chill (s) - R68.83 - Cannabidiol (CBD)
Chilomastigiasis - A07.8 - Hybrid Cannabis
Chimera 46,XX/46,XY - Q99.0 - Hybrid Cannabis
Chin - see condition
Chinese Dysentery - A03.9 - Indicia Cannabis
Chionophobia - F40.228 - Cannabidiol (CBD)
Chitral Fever - A93.1 - Cannabidiol (CBD)
Chlamydia, chlamydial - A74.9 - Cannabidiol (CBD)
Chlamydiosis - see chlamydia
Chloasma, skin, idiopathic, symptomatic - L81.1 - Indicia Cannabis
Chloroma - C92.3 - Salvia Cannabis
Chlorosis - D50.9 - Hybrid Cannabis
Chlorotic Anemia - D50.8 - Cannabidiol (CBD)
Chocolate Cyst, ovary - N80.1 - Cannabidiol (CBD)
Choked
Chokes, resulting from bends - T70.3 - Hybrid Cannabis
Choking Sensation - R09.89 - Indicia Cannabis
Cholangiectasis - K83.8 - Hybrid Cannabis
Cholangiocarcinoma
Cholangiohepatitis - K83.8 - Salvia Cannabis
Cholangiohepatoma - C22.0 - Indicia Cannabis
Cholangiolitis, acute, chronic, extrahepatic, gangrenous - K83.0 - Cannabidiol (CBD)
Cholangioma - D13.4 - Cannabidiol (CBD)
Cholangitis, ascending, primary, recurrent, sclerosing, secondary - K83.0 Cannabidiol (CBD)
Cholecystectasia - K82.8 - Salvia Cannabis
Cholecystitis - K81.9 - Cannabidiol (CBD)
Cholecystolithiasis - see calculus, gallbladder
Choledochitis, suppurative - K83.0 - Indicia Cannabis
Choledocholith - see calculus, bile duct
Choledocholithiasis, common duct, hepatic duct - calculus, bile duct
Cholelithiasis, cystic duct, gallbladder, impacted, multiple
Cholemia - see also jaundice
Choleperitoneum, choleperitonitis - K65.3 - Cannabidiol (CBD)
Cholera, asiatic, epidemic, malignant - A00.9 - Cannabidiol (CBD)

Cholerine - see cholera
Cholestasis NEC - K83.1 - Indicia Cannabis
Cholesteatoma, ear, middle, with reaction - H71.9- Indicia Cannabis
Cholesteatosis, diffuse - H71.3- Hybrid Cannabis
Cholesteremia - E78.0 Cannabidiol (CBD)
Cholesterin in vitreous - see deposit, crystalline
Cholesterol
Cholesterolemia, essential, familial, hereditary, pure - E78.0 - Cannabidiol (CBD)
Cholesterolosis, cholesterosis, gallbladder - K82.4 - Indicia Cannabis
Cholocolic Fistula - K82.3 - Indicia Cannabis
Choluria - R82.2 - Hybrid Cannabis
Chondritis - M94.8X9 - Salvia Cannabis
Chondroblastoma - see also neoplasm, bone, benign
Chondrocalcinosis - M11.20 - Hybrid Cannabis
Chondrodermatitis Nodularis Helicis or anthelicis
Chondrodysplasia - Q78.9 - Indicia Cannabis
Chondrodystrophy, chondrodystrophia, familial, fetalis - Q78.9 - Indicia Cannabis
Chondroectodermal Dysplasia - Q77.6 - Hybrid Cannabis
Chondrogenesis Imperfecta - Q77.4 - Indicia Cannabis
Chondrolysis - M94.35- Cannabidiol (CBD)
Chondroma - see also neoplasm, cartilage, benign
Chondromalacia, systemic - M94.20 - Indicia Cannabis
Chondromatosis - Neoplasm, cartilage, uncertain behavior
Chondro Myxosarcoma - see neoplasm, cartilage, malignant
Chondro-osteodysplasia, Morquio-Brailsford type - E76.219 - Cannabidiol (CBD)
Chondro-osteodystrophy - E76.29 - Salvia Cannabis
Chondro-osteoma - see neoplasm, bone, benign
Chondropathia tuberosa - M94.0 - Hybrid Cannabis
Chondrosarcoma - see neoplasm, cartilage, malignant
Chordee, nonvenereal - N48.89 - Indicia Cannabis
Chorditis, fibrinous, nodosa, tuberosa - J38.2 - Hybrid Cannabis
Chordoma - neoplasm, vertebral, column, malignant
Chorea, chronic, gravis, posthemiplegic, senile, spasmodic - G25.5 - Indicia Cannabis
Choreoathetosis, paroxysmal - G25.5 - Cannabidiol (CBD)
Chorioadenoma, destruens - D39.2 - Indicia Cannabis
Chorioamnionitis - O41.12- Salvia Cannabis

Chorioangioma - D26.7 - Hybrid Cannabis
Choriocarcinoma - see neoplasm, malignant, by site
Chorioencephalitis, acute, lymphocytic, serous - A87.2 - Cannabidiol (CBD)
Chorioepithelioma - see choriocarcinoma
Choriomeningitis, acute, lymphocytic, serous - A87.2 - Cannabidiol (CBD)
Chorionepithelioma - see choriocarcinoma
Chorioretinitis - see also Inflammation, chorioretinal
Chorioretinopathy, central serous - H35.71- Indicia Cannabis
Choroid - see condition
Choroideremia - H31.21 - Indicia Cannabis
Choroiditis - chorioretinitis
Choroidopathy - disorder, choroid
Choroidoretinitis - chorioretinitis
Choroidoretinopathy, central serous
Christian-Weber Disease - M35.6 - Indicia Cannabis
Christmas Disease - D67 - Cannabidiol (CBD)
Chromaffinoma - neoplasm, benign, by site
Chromatopsia - deficiency, color vision
Chromhidrosis, chromidrosis - L75.1 - Cannabidiol (CBD)
Chromoblastomycosis - chromomycosis
Chromoconversion - R82.91 - Cannabidiol (CBD)
Chromomycosis - B43.9 - Indicia Cannabis
Chromophytosis - B36.0 - Indicia Cannabis
Chromosome - see condition by chromosome involved
Chromotrichomycosis - B36.8 - Salvia Cannabis
Chronic - see condition
Churg-Strauss Syndrome - M30.1 - Cannabidiol (CBD)
Chyle Cyst, mesentery - I89.8 - Cannabidiol (CBD)
Chylocele, nonfilarial - I89.8 - Indicia Cannabis
Chylomicronemia, fasting, with hyperprebetalipoproteinemia - E78.3 - Cannabidiol (CBD)
Chylopericardium - I31.3 - Salvia Cannabis
Chylothorax, nonfilarial - I89.8 - Hybrid Cannabis
Chylous - see condition
Chyluria, nonfilarial - R82.0 - Hybrid Cannabis
Cicatricial, deformity - see cicatrix
Cicatrix, adherent, contracted, painful, vicious, scar - L90.5 - Hybrid Cannabis

Cidp, chronic inflammatory demyelinating polyneuropathy - G61.81 - Indicia Cannabis
Cin - see neoplasia, intraepithelial, cervix
Cinchonism - see deafness, ototoxic
Circle of Willis - see condition
Circular - see condition
Circulating Anticoagulants - see also, disorder, hemorrhagic - D68.318 - Indicia Cannabis
Circulation
Circulatory System - condition
Circulus Senilis, cornea - degeneration, cornea, senile
Circumcision - in absence of medical indication, ritual, routine - Z41.2 - Cannabidiol (CBD)
Circumscribed - see condition
Circumvallate Placenta - O43.11- Indicia Cannabis
Cirrhosis, cirrhotic, hepatic, liver - K74.60 - Cannabidiol (CBD)
Cistern, subarachnoid - R93.0 - Hybrid Cannabis
Citrullinemia - E72.23 - Cannabidiol (CBD)
Citrullinuria - E72.23 - Cannabidiol (CBD)
Civatte's Disease or poikiloderma - L57.3 - Indicia Cannabis
Clam Digger's Itch - B65.3 - Hybrid Cannabis
Clammy skin - R23.1 - Indicia Cannabis
Clap - see gonorrhea
Clarke-Hadfield Syndrome, pancreatic infantilism - K86.8 - Hybrid Cannabis
Clark's Paralysis - G80.9 - Salvia Cannabis
Clastothrix - L67.8 - Indicia Cannabis
Claude Bernard-Horner Syndrome - G90.2 - Salvia Cannabis
Claude's Disease or syndrome - G46.3 - Hybrid Cannabis
Claudication, intermittent - I73.9 - Indicia Cannabis
Claudicatio Venosa Intermittens - I87.8 - Hybrid Cannabis
Claustrophobia - F40.240 - Cannabidiol (CBD)
Clavus, infected - L84 - Cannabidiol (CBD)
Clawfoot, congenital - Q66.89 - Cannabidiol (CBD)
Clawhand, acquired - deformity, limb, clawhand
Clawtoe, congenital - Q66.89 - Cannabidiol (CBD)
Clay Eating - see pica
Cleansing of artificial opening - attention to, artificial, opening
Cleft, congenital - imperfect, closure
Cleidocranial Dysostosis - Q74.0 - Salvia Cannabis

Cleptomania - F63.2 - Cannabidiol (CBD)
Clicking Hip, newborn - R29.4 - Cannabidiol (CBD)
Climacteric, female - see also menopause
Clinical Research investigation, clinical trial, control subject, normal comparison, participant - Z00.6 - Indicia Cannabis
Clitoris - see condition
Cloaca, persistent - Q43.7 - Cannabidiol (CBD)
Clonorchiasis, clonorchis infection, liver - B66.1 - Hybrid Cannabis
Clonus - R25.8 - Hybrid Cannabis
Closed Bite - M26.29 - Indicia Cannabis
Clostridium (C.) - B96.7 - Indicia Cannabis
Closure
Clot, blood - see also embolism
Clouded State - R40.1 - Salvia Cannabis
Cloudy Antrum, antra - J32.0 - Cannabidiol (CBD)
Clouston's, hidrotic - Q82.4 - Cannabidiol (CBD)
Clubbed Nail Pachydermoperiostosis - M89.40 - Cannabidiol (CBD)
Clubbing of Finger (s), nails - R68.3 - Indicia Cannabis
Clubfinger - R68.3 - Cannabidiol (CBD)
Clubfoot, congenital - Q66.89 - Cannabidiol (CBD)
Clubhand, congenital, radial - Q71.4- Salvia Cannabis
Clubnail - R68.3 - Cannabidiol (CBD)
Clump, kidney - Q63.1 - Hybrid Cannabis
Clumsiness, clumsy child syndrome - F82 - Cannabidiol (CBD)
Cluttering - F80.81 - Indicia Cannabis
Clutton's Joints - A50.51 - Indicia Cannabis
Coagulation, intravascular, diffuse, disseminated - defibrination syndrome
Coagulopathy - see also defect, coagulation
Coalition
Coalminer's
Coalworker's Lung or pneumoconiosis - J60 - Cannabidiol (CBD)
Coarctation
Coated Tongue - K14.3 - Indicia Cannabis
Coats' Disease, exudative retinopathy - retinopathy, exudative
Cocainism - see dependence, drug, cocaine
Coccidioidomycosis - B38.9 - Cannabidiol (CBD)
Coccidioidosis - see coccidioidomycosis
Coccidiosis, intestinal - A07.3 - Cannabidiol (CBD)
Coccydynia, coccygodynia - M53.3 - Indicia Cannabis

Coccyx - see condition
Cochin-China diarrhea - K90.1 - Indicia Cannabis
Cockayne's Syndrome - Q87.1 - Hybrid Cannabis
Cocked up Toe - deformity, toe, specified NEC
Cock's Peculiar Tumor - L72.3 - Hybrid Cannabis
Codman's Tumor - see Neoplasm, bone, benign
Coenurosis - B71.8 - Cannabidiol (CBD)
Coffee-Worker's Lung - J67.8 - Indicia Cannabis
Cogan's Syndrome - H16.32- Hybrid Cannabis
Coitus, painful, female - N94.1 - Indicia Cannabis
Cold - J00 - Indicia Cannabis
Coldsore - B00.1 - Indicia Cannabis
Colibacillosis - A49.8 - Indicia Cannabis
Colic, bilious, infantile, intestinal, recurrent, spasmodic - R10.83 - Hybrid Cannabis
Colicystitis - Cystitis
Colitis, acute, catarrhal, chronic, noninfective, hemorrhagic - K52.9 - Indicia Cannabis
Collagenosis, collagen disease, nonvascular, vascular - M35.9 - Hybrid Cannabis
Collapse - R55 - Indicia Cannabis
Collateral - see also condition
Colles' fracture - S52.53- Indicia Cannabis
Collet, Sicard - G52.7 - Cannabidiol (CBD)
Collier's Asthma or lung - J60 - Cannabidiol (CBD)
Collodion Baby - Q80.2 - Cannabidiol (CBD)
Colloid Nodule, of thyroid, cystic - E04.1 - Salvia Cannabis
Coloboma, iris - Q13.0 - Indicia Cannabis
Coloenteritis - see enteritis
Colon - see condition
Colonization
Coloptosis - K63.4 - Salvia Cannabis
Color Blindness - see deficiency, color vision
Colostomy
Colpitis, acute - see vaginitis
Colpocele - N81.5 - Salvia Cannabis
Colpocystitis - see vaginitis
Colpospasm - N94.2 - Indicia Cannabis
Column, spinal, vertebral - see condition
Coma - R40.20 - Cannabidiol (CBD)

Comatose - see coma
Combat Fatigue - F43.0 - Salvia Cannabis
Combined - see condition
Comedo, comedones, giant - L70.0 - Indicia Cannabis
Comedocarcinoma - see also neoplasm, breast, malignant
Comedomastitis - see ectasia, mammary duct
Comminuted Fracture - code as fracture, closed
Common
Commotio, commotion, current
Communication
Compartment Syndrome, deep, posterior, traumatic - T79.A0 - Hybrid Cannabis
Compensation
Complaint - see also disease
Complete - see condition
Complex
Complication (s), from
Compressed Air Disease - T70.3 - Indicia Cannabis
Compression
Compulsion, compulsive
Concato's Disease, pericardial polyserositis - A19.9 - Cannabidiol (CBD)
Concavity Chest Wall - M95.4 - Hybrid Cannabis
Concealed Penis - Q55.69 - Cannabidiol (CBD)
Concern, normal - Z63.6 - Cannabidiol (CBD)
Concrescence, teeth - K00.2 - Indicia Cannabis
Concretio Cordis - I31.1 - Hybrid Cannabis
Concretion - see also calculus
Concussion, brain, cerebral, current - S06.0X - Cannabidiol (CBD)
Condition - see disease
Conditions Arising in the perinatal period - see newborn, affected by
Conduct Disorder - see disorder, conduct
Condyloma - A63.0 - Indicia Cannabis
Conflagration - see also burn
Conflict, with - see also discord
Confluent - see condition
Confusion, confused - R41.0 - Indicia Cannabis
Confusional Arousals - G47.51 - Salvia Cannabis
Congelation - T69.9 - Hybrid Cannabis
Congenital - see also condition
Congestion, congestive

Congestive - see congestion
Conical
Conjoined Twins - Q89.4 - Cannabidiol (CBD)
Conjugal Maladjustment - Z63.0 - Indicia Cannabis
Conjunctiva - see condition
Conjunctivitis, staphylococcal, streptococcal - H10.9 - Cannabidiol (CBD)
Conjunctivochalasis - H11.82- Cannabidiol (CBD)
Connective Tissue - see condition
Conn's Syndrome - E26.01 - Cannabidiol (CBD)
Conradi, Hunermann - Q77.3 - Indicia Cannabis
Consanguinity - Z84.3 - Indicia Cannabis
Conscious Simulation, of illness - Z76.5 - Cannabidiol (CBD)
Consecutive - see condition
Consolidation Lung, base - see pneumonia, lobar
Constipation, atonic, neurogenic, simple, spastic - K59.00 - Cannabidiol (CBD)
Constitutional - see also condition
Constitutionally Substandard - F60.7 - Indicia Cannabis
Constriction - see also stricture
Constrictive - see condition
Consultation
Consumption - see tuberculosis
Contact with - see also exposure, to
Contamination, food - see intoxication, foodborne
Contraception, contraceptive
Contraction (s)
Contusion, skin surface intact - T14.8 - Indicia Cannabis
Conus, congenital, any type - Q14.8 - Salvia Cannabis
Conversion Hysteria, neurosis or reaction - F44.9 - Hybrid Cannabis
Converter, tuberculosis, test reaction - R76.11 - Salvia Cannabis
Conviction, legal - Z65.0 - Hybrid Cannabis
Convulsions, idiopathic, seizure(s) - R56.9 - Hybrid Cannabis
Convulsive - see also convulsions
Cooley's Anemia - D56.1 - Indicia Cannabis
Coolie Itch - B76.9 - Cannabidiol (CBD)
Cooper's
Copra Itch - B88.0 - Cannabidiol (CBD)
Coprophagy - F50.8 - Indicia Cannabis
Coprophobia - F40.298 - Hybrid Cannabis
Coproporphyria, hereditary - E80.29 - Cannabidiol (CBD)

Cor
Corbus' Disease, gangrenous balanitis - N48.1 - Cannabidiol (CBD)
Cord - see also condition
Cordis Ectopia - Q24.8 - Hybrid Cannabis
Corditis, spermatic - N49.1 - Indicia Cannabis
Corectopia - Q13.2 - Hybrid Cannabis
Cori's Disease, glycogen storage - E74.03 - Cannabidiol (CBD)
Corkhandler's Disease or lung - J67.3 - Hybrid Cannabis
Corkscrew Esophagus - K22.4 - Cannabidiol (CBD)
Corkworker's Disease or lung - J67.3 - Cannabidiol (CBD)
Corn, Infected - L84 - Indicia Cannabis
Cornea - see also condition
Cornelia De Lange Syndrome - Q87.1 - Indicia Cannabis
Cornu Cutaneum - L85.8 - Salvia Cannabis
Cornual Gestation or pregnancy - O00.8 - Cannabidiol (CBD)
Coronary, artery - see condition
Coronavirus, as cause of disease classified elsewhere - B97.29 - Cannabidiol (CBD)
Corpora - see also condition
Corpulence - see obesity
Corpus - see condition
Corrected Transposition - Q20.5 - Indicia Cannabis
Corrosion, injury, acid, caustic, chemical, lime, external - T30.4 - Indicia Cannabis
Corrosive Burn - see corrosion
Corsican Fever - see malaria
Cortical - see condition
Cortico-Adrenal - see condition
Coryza, acute - J00 - Indicia Cannabis
Costen's Syndrome or complex - M26.69 - Indicia Cannabis
Costiveness - see constipation
Costochondritis - M94.0 - Hybrid Cannabis
Cotard's Syndrome - F22 - Hybrid Cannabis
Cot Death - R99 - Cannabidiol (CBD)
Cotia Virus - B08.8 - Cannabidiol (CBD)
Cotton Wool Spots, retinal - H35.81 - Indicia Cannabis
Cotugno's Disease - see sciatica
Cough, affected, chronic, epidemic, nervous - R05 - Indicia Cannabis
Counseling (for) - Z71.9 - Indicia Cannabis

Coupled Rhythm - R00.8 - Cannabidiol (CBD)
Couvelaire Syndrome or uterus - O45.8X - Hybrid Cannabis
Cowperitis - see Urethritis
Cowper's Gland - see condition
Cowpox - B08.010 - Indicia Cannabis
Coxa
Coxalgia, coxalgic, nontuberculous - Pain, joint, hip
Coxitis - see monoarthritis, hip
Coxsackie, virus, infection - B34.1 - Cannabidiol (CBD)
Crabs, meaning pubic lice - B85.3 - Indicia Cannabis
Crack Baby - P04.41 - Cannabidiol (CBD)
Cracked Nipple - N64.0 - Cannabidiol (CBD)
Cracked Tooth - K03.81 - Cannabidiol (CBD)
Cradle Cap - L21.0 - Cannabidiol (CBD)
Craft Neurosis - F48.8 - Hybrid Cannabis
Cramp (s) - R25.2 - Indicia Cannabis
Cranial - see condition
Craniofenestria, skull - Q75.8 - Cannabidiol (CBD)
Craniolacunia, skull - Q75.8 - Cannabidiol (CBD)
Craniopagus - Q89.4 - Hybrid Cannabis
Craniopathy, metabolic - M85.2 - Salvia Cannabis
Craniopharyngeal - see condition
Craniopharyngioma - D44.4 - Hybrid Cannabis
Craniorachischisis, totalis - Q00.1 - Hybrid Cannabis
Cranioschisis - Q75.8 - Indicia Cannabis
Craniostenosis - Q75.0 - Hybrid Cannabis
Craniosynostosis - Q75.0 - Hybrid Cannabis
Craniotabes, cause unknown - M83.8 - Indicia Cannabis
Cranium - condition
Craw-Craw - see Onchocerciasis
Creaking Joint - derangement, joint, specified type NEC
Creeping
Crenated Tongue - K14.8 - Cannabidiol (CBD)
Creotoxism - A05.9 - Hybrid Cannabis
Crepitus
Crescent or conus choroid, congenital - Q14.3 - Indicia Cannabis
Crest syndrome - M34.1 - Hybrid Cannabis
Cretin, cretinism, congenital, endemic, nongoitrous sporadic - E00.9 - Cannabidiol (CBD)

Creutzfeldt-Jakob Disease or syndrome, with dementia - A81.00 - Hybrid Cannabis
Crib Death - R99 - Cannabidiol (CBD)
Cribriform Hymen - Q52.3 - Cannabidiol (CBD)
Cri-du-Chat Syndrome - Q93.4 - Cannabidiol (CBD)
Crigler-Najjar Disease or syndrome - E80.5 - Hybrid Cannabis
Crime, victim of - Z65.4 - Cannabidiol (CBD)
Crimean Hemorrhagic Fever - A98.0 - Indicia Cannabis
Criminalism - F60.2 - Hybrid Cannabis
Crisis
Crocq's Disease, acrocyanosis - I73.89 - Hybrid Cannabis
Crohn's Disease - see enteritis, regional
Crooked Septum, nasal - J34.2 - Cannabidiol (CBD)
Cross Syndrome - E70.328 - Indicia Cannabis
Crossbite, anterior, posterior - M26.24 - Cannabidiol (CBD)
Cross-Eye - strabismus, convergent concomitant
Croup, croupous, catarrhal, infectious, inflammatory, non-diphtheritic - J05.0 - Hybrid Cannabis
Crouzon's Disease - Q75.1 - Hybrid Cannabis
Crowding, tooth, teeth, fully erupted - M26.31 - Cannabidiol (CBD)
Crest (CRST) Syndrome - M34.1 - Cannabidiol (CBD)
Cruchet's Disease - A85.8 - Indicia Cannabis
Cruelty in children - disorder, conduct
Crural Ulcer - see ulcer, lower limb
Crush, crushed, crushing - T14.8 - Indicia Cannabis
Crusta Lactea - L21.0 - Hybrid Cannabis
Crusts - R23.4 - Cannabidiol (CBD)
Crutch Paralysis - see injury, brachial plexus
Cruveilhier-Baumgarten Cirrhosis, disease or syndrome - K74.69 - Cannabidiol (CBD)
Cruveilhier's Atrophy or Disease - G12.8 - Cannabidiol (CBD)
Crying, constant, continuous, excessive
Cryofibrinogenemia - D89.2 - Cannabidiol (CBD)
Cryoglobulinemia - essential, idiopathic, mixed, primar, purpura, secondary,
 vasculitis - D89.1 - Indicia Cannabis
Cryptitis, anal, rectal - K62.89 - Cannabidiol (CBD)
Cryptococcus, cryptococcus, infection, neoformans - B45.9 - Cannabidiol (CBD)

Cryptopapillitis, anus - K62.89 - Indicia Cannabis
Cryptophthalmos - Q11.2 - Hybrid Cannabis
Cryptorchid, cryptorchism, cryptorchidism - Q53.9 - Cannabidiol (CBD)
Cryptosporidiosis - A07.2 - Hybrid Cannabis
Cryptostromosis - J67.6 - Cannabidiol (CBD)
Crystalluria - R82.99 - Cannabidiol (CBD)
Cubitus
Cultural Deprivation or shock - Z60.3 - Indicia Cannabis
Curling Esophagus - K22.4 - Hybrid Cannabis
Curling's Ulcer - see ulcer, peptic, acute
Curschmann, Batten, Steinert - G71.11 - Hybrid Cannabis
Curse, ondine's - see apnea, sleep
Curvature
Cushingoid due to Steroid Therapy - E24.2 - Indicia Cannabis
Cushing's
Cusp, Carabelli - omit code
Cut, external - see also laceration
Cutaneous - see also condition
Cutis - see also condition
Cyanosis - R23.0 - Hybrid Cannabis
Cyanotic Heart Disease - I24.9 - Indicia Cannabis
Cycle
Cyclical Vomiting - see also vomiting, cyclical - G43.A0 - Cannabidiol (CBD)
Cyclitis - see also iridocyclitis - H20.9 - Salvia Cannabis
Cyclencephaly - Q04.9 - Hybrid Cannabis
Cycloid Personality - F34.0 - Salvia Cannabis
Cyclophoria - H50.54 - Cannabidiol (CBD)
Cyclopia, cyclops - Q87.0 - Cannabidiol (CBD)
Cyclopism - Q87.0 - Hybrid Cannabis
Cyclosporiasis - A07.4 - Indicia Cannabis
Cyclothymia - F34.0 - Cannabidiol (CBD)
Cyclothymic Personality - F34.0 - Cannabidiol (CBD)
Cyclotropia - H50.41- Hybrid Cannabis
Cylindroma - neoplasm, malignant, by site
Cylindruria - R82.99 - Indicia Cannabis
Cynanche
Cynophobia - F40.218 - Hybrid Cannabis
Cynorexia - R63.2 - Hybrid Cannabis
Cyphosis - Kyphosis

Cyprus Fever - see brucellosis
Cyst, colloid, mucous, simple, retention
Cystadenocarcinoma - neoplasm, malignant,
Cystadenofibroma
Cystadenoma - see also neoplasm, benign
Cystathionine Synthase Deficiency - E72.11 - Indicia Cannabis
Cystathioninemia - E72.19 - Cannabidiol (CBD)
Cystathioninuria - E72.19 - Hybrid Cannabis
Cystic - see also condition
Cysticercosis, cysticerciasis - B69.9 - Cannabidiol (CBD)
Cysticercus Cellulose Infestation - see cysticercosis
Cystinosis (malignant) - E72.04 - Indicia Cannabis
Cystinuria - E72.01 - Indicia Cannabis
Cystitis, exudative, hemorrhagic, septic, suppurative - N30.90 - Indicia Cannabis
Cystocele, urethrocele
Cystolithiasis - N21.0 - Indicia Cannabis
Cystoma - neoplasm, benign, by site
Cystoplegia - N31.2 - Cannabidiol (CBD)
Cystoptosis - N32.89 - Hybrid Cannabis
Cystopyelitis - see pyelonephritis
Cystorrhagia - N32.89 - Indicia Cannabis
Cystosarcoma Phyllodes - D48.6 - Hybrid Cannabis
Cystostomy
Cystourethritis - see urethritis
Cystourethrocele - see also cystocele
Cytomegalic Inclusion Disease
Cytomegalovirus Infection - B25.9 - Cannabidiol (CBD)
Cytomycosis, reticuloendothelial - B39.4 - Indicia Cannabis
Cytopenia - D75.9 - Hybrid Cannabis
Czerny's Disease - periodic hydrarthrosis of the knee - effusion, joint, knee

D

Date, Finsen, disease, epidemic pleurodynia - B33.0 - Indicia Cannabis
Da Costa's Syndrome - F45.8 - Hybrid Cannabis
Dabney's Grip - B33.0 - Cannabidiol (CBD)
Dacryoadenitis, decry adenitis - H04.00 - Cannabidiol (CBD)
Dacryocystitis - H04.30 - Cannabidiol (CBD)
Dacryocystoblenorrhea - see inflammation, lacrimal, passages, chronic
Dacryocystocele - see disorder, lacrimal system, changes

Dacryolith, da cryo lithiasis - H04.51- Indicia Cannabis
Dacryoma - see disorder, lacrimal system, changes
Dacryopericystitis - see dacryocystitis
Dacryops - H04.11 - Sativa Cannabis
Dacryostenosis - see also stenosis, lacrimal
Dactylitis
Dactylolysis Spontaneous, ainhum - L94.6 - Indicia Cannabis
Dactylosymphysis - Q70.9 - Cannabidiol (CBD)
Damage
Dana-Putnam Syndrome, subacute combined sclerosis with pernicious anemia - see degeneration, combined
Danbolt, Cross, Syndrome, acrodermatitis, enteropathica - E83.2 - Hybrid Cannabis
Dandruff - L21.0 - Sativa Cannabis
Dandy-Walker Syndrome - Q03.1 - Hybrid Cannabis
Danlos' Syndrome - Q79.6 - Hybrid Cannabis
Darier, White, disease, congenital - Q82.8 - Indicia Cannabis
Darier-Roussy Sarcoid - D86.3 - Cannabidiol (CBD)
Darling's Disease or histoplasmosis - B39.4 - Cannabidiol (CBD)
Darwin's Tubercle - Q17.8 - Cannabidiol (CBD)
Dawson's, inclusion body - A81.1 - Cannabidiol (CBD)
De Beurmann, Gougerot - B42.1 - Hybrid Cannabis
De la Tourette's Syndrome - F95.2 - Indicia Cannabis
De Lange's Syndrome - Q87.1 - Cannabidiol (CBD)
De Morgan's Spots, senile angiomas - I78.1 - Cannabidiol (CBD)
De Quervain's
De Toni-Fanconi, Debré - E72.09 - Sativa Cannabis
Dead
Deaf Nonspeaking NEC - H91.3 - Indicia Cannabis
Deafmutism, acquired, congenital - H91.3 - Indicia Cannabis
Deafness, acquired, complete, hereditary, partial - H91.9- Indicia Cannabis
Death, cause unknown (of), unexplained, unspecified cause - R99 - Cannabidiol (CBD)
Debility, chronic, general, nervous - R53.81 - Caryophyllene (CB2) Cannabis
Débove's Disease, splenomegaly - R16.1 - Hybrid Cannabis
Decalcification
Decapsulation, kidney - N28.89 - Indicia Cannabis
Decay
Deciduous, acute

Decline, general - see debility - R41, 81 - Indicia Cannabis
Decompensation
Decompression Sickness - T70.3 - Indicia Cannabis
Decrease
Decubitus, ulcer, pressure, at site
Deepening Acetabulum - derangement, joint, specified type NEC, hip
Defect, defective - Q89.9 - Hybrid Cannabis
Deferentitis - N49.1 - Cannabidiol (CBD)
Defibrination Syndrome - D65 - Indicia Cannabis
Deficiency, deficient
Deficit - see also deficiency
Deflection
Defluvium
Deformity - Q89.9 - Cannabidiol (CBD)
Degeneration, degenerative
Deglutition
Degos' Disease - I77.89 - Hybrid Cannabis
Dehiscence (of)
Dehydration - E86.0 - Indicia Cannabis
Déjérine-Roussy Syndrome - G89.0 - Indicia Cannabis
Déjérine-Sottas Disease or neuropathy, hypertrophic - G60.0 - Sativa Cannabis
Déjérine-Thomas Atrophy - G23.8 - Hybrid Cannabis
Delay, delayed
Deletion (s)
Delhi Boil or button - B55.1 - Hybrid Cannabis
Delinquency, juvenile, neurotic - F91.8 - Cannabidiol (CBD)
Delinquent Immunization Status - Z28.3 - Cannabidiol (CBD)
Delirium, delirious ,acute or subacute, not alcohol or drug-induced, with dementia - R41.0 - Indicia Cannabis
Delivery, childbirth, labor
Delusions, paranoid - see disorder, delusional
Dementia, old age, degenerative, primary, persisting - F03.90 - Cannabidiol (CBD)
Demineralization, bone - see osteoporosis
Demodex Folliculorum, infestation - B88.0 - Hybrid Cannabis
Demophobia - F40.248 - Indicia Cannabis
Demoralization - R45.3 - Indicia Cannabis
Demyelination, demyelinization

Dengue, classical, fever - A90 - Indicia Cannabis
Dennie-Marfan Syphilitic Syndrome - A50.45 - Cannabidiol (CBD)
Dens Evaginatus, in dente or invaginatus - K00.2 - Cannabidiol (CBD)
Dense Breasts - R92.2 - Indicia Cannabis
Density
Dental - see also condition
Dementia Praecox - K00.6 - Cannabidiol (CBD)
Denticles, pulp - K04.2 - Hybrid Cannabis
Dentigerous Cyst - K09.0 - Cannabidiol (CBD)
Dentin
Dentinogenesis Imperfect - K00.5 - Cannabidiol (CBD)
Dentinoma - see cyst, calcifying odontogenic
Dentition, syndrome - K00.7 - Cannabidiol (CBD)
Dependence (on), syndrome - F19.20 - Indicia Cannabis
Dependency
Depersonalization, in neurotic state, neurotic, syndrome - F48.1 - Cannabidiol (CBD)
Depletion
Deployment, current, military - Z56.82 - Cannabidiol (CBD)
Depolarization, premature - I49.40 - Cannabidiol (CBD)
Deposit
Depraved Appetite - see pica
Depressed
Depression, acute, mental - F32.9 - Indicia Cannabis
Deprivation
Derangement
Dercum's Disease - E88.2 - Indicia Cannabis
Derealization, neurotic - F48.1 - Hybrid Cannabis
Dermal - see condition
Dermaphytid - see dermatophytosis
Dermatitis, eczematous - L30.9 - Indicia Cannabis
Dermatoarthritis, lipoid - E78.81 - Sativa Cannabis
Dermatochalasis, eyelid - H02.839 - Cannabidiol (CBD)
Dermatofibroma, lenticulare - neoplasm, skin, benign
Dermatofibrosarcoma, pigmented, protuberans) - neoplasm, skin, malignant
Dermatographia - L50.3 - Cannabidiol (CBD)
Dermatolysis, exfoliative, congenital - Q82.8 - Cannabidiol (CBD)
Dermatomegaly (NEC) - Q82.8 - Hybrid Cannabis
Dermatomucosomyositis - M33.10 - Indicia Cannabis

Dermatomycosis - B36.9 - Sativa Cannabis
Dermatomyositis, acute, chronic - see also dermatopolymyositis
Dermatoneuritis of Children - see poisoning, mercury
Dermatophilosis - A48.8 - Indicia Cannabis
Dermatophytid - L30.2 - Cannabidiol (CBD)
Dermatophytide - dermatophytosis
Dermatophytosis, epidermophyton, infection, microsporum, tinea, trichophyton - B35.9 - Cannabidiol (CBD)
Dermatopolymyositis - M33.90
Dermatopolyneuritis - see poisoning, mercury
Dermatorrhexis - Q79.6 - Hybrid Cannabis
Dermatosclerosis - see also scleroderma
Dermatosis - L98.9 - Hybrid Cannabis
Dermographia, dermographism - L50.3 - Indicia Cannabis
Dermoid, cyst - neoplasm, benign, by site
Dermopathy
Dermophytosis - see dermatophytosis
Descemetocele - H18.73 - Sativa Cannabis
Descemet's Membrane - see condition
Descending - see condition
Descensus Uteri - see prolapse, uterus
Desert
Desertion, newborn - see maltreatment
Desmoid, extra-abdominal, tumor - see neoplasm, connective tissue, uncertain behavior
Despondency - F32.9 - Indicia Cannabis
Desquamation, skin - R23.4 - Cannabidiol (CBD)
Destruction, destructive - see also damage
Destructiveness - see also disorder, conduct
Desultory Labor - O62.2 - Cannabidiol (CBD)
Detachment
Detergent Asthma - J69.8 - Cannabidiol (CBD)
Deterioration
Deuteranomaly, anomalous trichromat - H53.53 - Indicia Cannabis
Deuteranopia, complete, incomplete - H53.53 - Indicia Cannabis
Development
Developmental - see condition
Devergie's Disease, pityriasis rubra pilaris - L44.0 - Indicia Cannabis
Deviation (in)

Device
Devic's Disease - G36.0 - Sativa Cannabis
Devil's
Devitalized Tooth - K04.99 - Cannabidiol (CBD)
Devonshire Colic - see poisoning, lead
Dextraposition, aorta - Q20.3 - Cannabidiol (CBD)
Dextrinosis, limit, debrancher enzyme deficiency - E74.03 - Indicia Cannabis
Dextrocardia, true - Q24.0 - Hybrid Cannabis
Dextro Transposition, aorta - Q20.3 - Cannabidiol (CBD)
D-glycericacidemia - E72.59 - Indicia Cannabis
Dhat Syndrome - F48.8 - Hybrid Cannabis
Dhobi Itch - B35.6 - Cannabidiol (CBD)
Di George's Syndrome - D82.1 - Cannabidiol (CBD)
Di Guglielmo's Disease - C94.0- - Cannabidiol (CBD)
Diabetes, diabetic, mellitus, sugar - E11.9 - Sativa Cannabis
Diacyclothrombopathia - D69.1 - Indicia Cannabis
Diagnosis Deferred - R69 -- Hybrid Cannabis
Dialysis, intermittent, treatment
Diamond-Blackfan Anemia, congenital hypoplastic) - D61.01 - Sativa Cannabis
Diamond-Gardener Syndrome, autoerythrocyte sensitization - D69.2 - Sativa Cannabis
Diaper Rash - L22 - Cannabidiol (CBD)
Diaphoresis, excessive - R61 - Indicia Cannabis
Diaphragm - see condition
Diaphragmalgia - R07.1 - Indicia Cannabis
Diaphragmatitis, diaphragmitis - J98.6 - Hybrid Cannabis
Diaphysial Aclasis - Q78.6 - Hybrid Cannabis
Diaphysitis - see osteomyelitis, specified type NEC
Diarrhea, diarrheal, disease, infantile, inflammatory - R19.7 - Indicia Cannabis
Diastasis
Diastema, tooth, teeth, fully erupted - M26.32 - Cannabidiol (CBD)
Diastematomyelia - Q06.2 - Indicia Cannabis
Diataxia, cerebral - G80.4 - Cannabidiol (CBD)
Diathesis
Diaz's Disease or osteochondrosis, juvenile, talus, osteochondrosis, juvenile, tarsus
Dibothriocephalus, dibothriocephaliasis, latus, infection, infestation - B70.0 - Hybrid Cannabis
Dicephalus, dicephaly - Q89.4 - Indicia Cannabis

Dichotomy, teeth - K00.2 - Cannabidiol (CBD)
Dichromate, dichromatopsia, congenital - deficiency, color vision
Dichuchwa - A65 - Cannabidiol (CBD)
Dicroceliasis - B66.2 - Sativa Cannabis
Didelphia, didelphys - see double uterus
Didymytis - N45.1 - Sativa Cannabis
Dietary
Dietl's Crisis - N13.8 - Indicia Cannabis
Dieulafoy Lesion, hemorrhagic
Difficult, difficulty (in)
Diffuse - see condition
DiGeorge's Syndrome, thymic hypoplasia - D82.1 - Cannabidiol (CBD)
Digestive - see condition
Dihydropyrimidine Dehydrogenase Disease (DPD) - E88.89 - Hybrid Cannabis
Diktyoma - see neoplasm, malignant, by site
Dilaceration, tooth - K00.4 - Indicia Cannabis
Dilatation
Dilated, dilation - see dilatation
Diminished, diminution
Diminuta Taenia - B71.0 - Sativa Cannabis
Dimitri-Sturge-Weber Disease - Q85.8 - Hybrid Cannabis
Dimple
Dioctophyme Renalis, infection, infestation - B83.8 - Cannabidiol (CBD)
Dipetalonemiasis - B74.4 - Cannabidiol (CBD)
Diphallus - Q55.69 - Hybrid Cannabis
Diphtheria, diphtheritic, gangrenous, hemorrhagic - A36.9 - Cannabidiol (CBD)
Diphyllobothriasis, intestine - B70.0 - Indicia Cannabis
Diplacusis - H93.22- Hybrid Cannabis
Diplegia, upper limbs - G83.0 - Indicia Cannabis
Diplococcus, diplococcal - see condition
Diplopia - H53.2 - Hybrid Cannabis
Dipsomania - F10.20 - Cannabidiol (CBD)
Dipylidiasis - B71.1 - Cannabidiol (CBD)
Direction, teeth, abnormal, fully erupted - M26.30 - Cannabidiol (CBD)
Dirofilariasis - B74.8 - Hybrid Cannabis
Dirt-Eating Child - F98.3 - Indicia Cannabis
Disability, disabilities

Disappearance of Family Member - Z63.4 - Cannabidiol (CBD)
Disarticulation - see amputation
Discharge (from)
Discitis, diskitis - M46.40 - Indicia Cannabis
Discoid
Discoloration
Discomfort
Discontinuity, ossicles, ear - H74.2- Cannabidiol (CBD)
Discord (with)
Discordant connection
Discrepancy
Discrimination
Disease, diseased - see also syndrome
Disfigurement, due to scar - L90.5 - Indicia Cannabis
Disgerminoma - see dysgerminoma
Dish, diffuse idiopathic skeletal hyperostosis - see hyperostosis, ankylosing
Disinsertion, retina - see detachment, retina
Dislocatable Hip, congenital - Q65.6 - Cannabidiol (CBD)
Dislocation, articular
Disorder (of) - see also disease
Disorientation - R41.0 - Indicia Cannabis
Displacement, displaced
Disproportion
Disruptio uteri - see rupture, uterus
Disruption (of)
Dissatisfaction with
Dissecting - see condition
Dissection
Disseminated - see condition
Dissociation
Dissociative Reaction, state - F44.9 - Indicia Cannabis
Dissolution, vertebra - see osteoporosis
Distension, distention
Distoma Hepaticum Infestation - B66.3 - Hybrid Cannabis
Distomiasis - B66.9 - Hybrid Cannabis
Distomolar, fourth molar - K00.1 - Cannabidiol (CBD)
Disto-Occlusion, Division I, Division II - M26.212 - Sativa Cannabis
Distortion (s), congenital
Distress

Distribution Vessel, atypical - Q27.9 - Hybrid Cannabis
Districhiasis - L68.8 - Hybrid Cannabis
Disturbance (s) - see also disease
Diuresis - R35.8 - Indicia Cannabis
Diver's Palsy, paralysis or squeeze - T70.3 - Sativa Cannabis
Diverticulitis, acute - K57.92 - Cannabidiol (CBD)
Diverticulosis - K57.90 - Cannabidiol (CBD)
Diverticulum, diverticula, multiple - K57.90 - Indicia Cannabis
Division
Divorce, causing family disruption - Z63.5 - Cannabidiol (CBD)
Dix-Hallpike Neurolabyrinthitis - see neuronitis, vestibular
Dizziness - R42 - Indicia Cannabis
Dmac, also disseminated mycobacterium avium - intracellulare complex - A31.2 - Indicia Cannabis
DNR, do not resuscitate\ - Z66 - Hybrid Cannabis
Doan-Wiseman Syndrome, primary splenic neutropenia - agranulocytosis
Doehle-Heller Aortitis - A52.02 - Sativa Cannabis
Dog Bite - see bite
Dohle Body Panmyelopathic Syndrome - D72.0 - Indicia Cannabis
Dolichocephaly - Q67.2 - Indicia Cannabis
Dolichocolon - Q43.8 - Hybrid Cannabis
Dolichostenomelia - see syndrome, marfan's
Donohue's Syndrome - E34.8 - Hybrid Cannabis
Donor, organ or tissue - Z52.9 - Cannabidiol (CBD)
Donovanosis - A58 - Indicia Cannabis
Dorsalgia - M54.9 - Cannabidiol (CBD)
Dorsopathy - M53.9 - Cannabidiol (CBD)
Double
Douglas' Pouch, Cul-de-sac - see condition
Down Syndrome - Q90.9 - Indicia Cannabis
DPD, dihydropyrimidine dehydrogenase deficiency - E88.89 - Cannabidiol (CBD)
Dracontiasis - B72 - Sativa Cannabis
Dracunculiasis, dracunculosis - B72 - Sativa Cannabis
Dream State, hysterical - F44.89 - Cannabidiol (CBD)
Dreschlera, hawaiiensis, infection - B43.8 - Cannabidiol (CBD)
Drepanocytic Anemia - see disease, sickle-cell
Dresbach's Syndrome, elliptocytosis - D58.1 - Indicia Cannabis
Dressler's Syndrome - I24.1 - Hybrid Cannabis

Drift, ulnar - deformity, limb, specified type NEC, forearm
Drinking, alcohol
Drip, postnasal, chronic - R09.82 - Cannabidiol (CBD)
Droop
Drop (in)
Dropped Heart Beats - I45.9 - Indicia Cannabis
Dropsy, dropsical - see also hydrops
Drowned, drowning, near - T75.1 - Cannabidiol (CBD)
Drowsiness - R40.0 - Cannabidiol (CBD)
Drug
Drunkenness, without dependence - F10.129 - Indicia Cannabis
Drusen
Dry, dryness - see also condition
Disseminated Superficial Actinic Porokeratosis (DSAP) - L56.5 - Hybrid Cannabis
Duane's Syndrome - H50.81- Indicia Cannabis
Dubin-Johnson Disease or syndrome - E80.6 - Sativa Cannabis
Dubois' Disease, thymus gland - A50.59 - Indicia Cannabis
Dubowitz' Syndrome - Q87.1 - Cannabidiol (CBD)
Duchenne-Aran Muscular Atrophy - G12.21 - Cannabidiol (CBD)
Duchenne-Griesinger Disease - G71.0 - Indicia Cannabis
Duchenne's
Ducrey's Chancre - A57 - Indicia Cannabis
Duct, Ductus - see condition
Duhring's Disease, dermatitis herpetiformis - L13.0 - Hybrid Cannabis
Dullness, cardiac, decreased, increased - R01.2 - Indicia Cannabis
Dumb Ague - see malaria
Dumbness - see aphasia
Dumdum Fever - B55.0 - Indicia Cannabis
Dumping Syndrome, postgastrectomy - K91.1 - Hybrid Cannabis
Duodenitis, nonspecific, peptic - K29.80 - Hybrid Cannabis
Duodenocholangitis - cholangitis
Duodenum, duodenal
Duplay's Bursitis or periarthritis - tendinitis, calcific, shoulder
Duplication, duplex
Dupré's Disease, meningism - R29.1 - Indicia Cannabis
Dupuytren's Contraction or disease - M72.0 - Cannabidiol (CBD)
Durand-Nicolas-Favre Disease - A55 - Hybrid Cannabis
Durotomy, inadvertent, incidental - G97.41 - Sativa Cannabis
Duroziez's Disease, congenital mitral stenosis - Q23.2 - Hybrid Cannabis

Dutton's Relapsing Fever, West African - A68.1 - Hybrid Cannabis
Dwarfism - E34.3 - Indicia Cannabis
Dyke-Young Anemia, secondary, symptomatic - D59.1 - Cannabidiol (CBD)
Dysacusis - see abnormal, auditory perception
Dysadrenocortism - E27.9 - Cannabidiol (CBD)
Dysarthria - R47.1 - Cannabidiol (CBD)
Dysautonomia, familial - G90.1 - Cannabidiol (CBD)
Dysbarism - T70.3
Dysbasia - R26.2 - Indicia Cannabis
Dysbetalipoproteinemia, familial - E78.2 - Cannabidiol (CBD)
Dyscalculia - R48.8 - Hybrid Cannabis
Dyschezia - K59.00 - Hybrid Cannabis
Dyschondroplasia, with hemangiomata - Q78.4 - Cannabidiol (CBD)
Dyschromia, skin - L81.9 - Cannabidiol (CBD)
Dyscollagenosis - M35.9 - Cannabidiol (CBD)
Dyscranio-Pygo-Phalangy - Q87.0 - Indicia Cannabis
Dyscrasia
Dysendocrinism - E34.9 - Indicia Cannabis
Dysentery, catarrhal, diarrhea, epidemic, dysenteric, hemorrhagic, infectious, sporadic, tropical - A09 - Cannabidiol (CBD)
Dysequilibrium - R42 - Hybrid Cannabis
Dysesthesia - R20.8 - Hybrid Cannabis
Dysfibrinogenemia, congenital - D68.2 - Cannabidiol (CBD)
Dysfunction
Dysgenesis
Dysgerminoma
Dysgeusia - R43.2 - Indicia Cannabis
Dysgraphia - R27.8 - Hybrid Cannabis
Dyshidrosis, dysidrosis - L30.1 - Hybrid Cannabis
Dyskaryotic Cervical Smear - R87.619 - Cannabidiol (CBD)
Dyskeratosis - L85.8 - Hybrid Cannabis
Dyskinesia - G24.9 - Cannabidiol (CBD)
Dyslalia, developmental - F80.0 - Cannabidiol (CBD)
Dyslexia - R48.0 - Cannabidiol (CBD)
Dyslipidemia - E78.5 - Indicia Cannabis
Dysmaturity - see also light for dates
Dysmenorrhea, essential, exfoliative - N94.6 - Hybrid Cannabis
Dysmetabolic Syndrome X - E88.81 - Hybrid Cannabis
Dysmetria - R27.8 - Indicia Cannabis

Dysmorphism, due to
Dysmorphophobia, nondelusional - F45.22 - Cannabidiol (CBD)
Dysnomia - R47.01 - Cannabidiol (CBD)
Dysorexia - R63.0 - Cannabidiol (CBD)
Dysostosis
Dyspareunia, female - N94.1 - Cannabidiol (CBD)
Dyspepsia - R10.13 - Cannabidiol (CBD)
Dysphagia - R13.10 - Indicia Cannabis
Dysphagocytosis, congenital - D71 - Cannabidiol (CBD)
Dysphasia - R47.02 - Hybrid Cannabis
Dysphonia - R49.0 - Hybrid Cannabis
Dysphoria, postpartal - O90.6 - Indicia Cannabis
Dyspituitarism - E23.3 - Indicia Cannabis
Dysplasia - see also anomaly
Dyspnea, nocturnal, paroxysmal - R06.00 - Indicia Cannabis
Dyspraxia - R27.8 - Hybrid Cannabis
Dysproteinemia - E88.09 - Hybrid Cannabis
Dysreflexia, autonomic - G90.4 - Indicia Cannabis
Dysrhythmia
Dyssomnia - see disorder, sleep
Dyssynergia
Dysthymia - F34.1 - Indicia Cannabis
Dysthyroidism - E07.9 - Hybrid Cannabis
Dystocia - O66.9 - Cannabidiol (CBD)
Dystonia - G24.9 - Cannabidiol (CBD)
Dystonic Movements - R25.8 - Indicia Cannabis
Dystrophy, dystrophia
Dysuria - R30.0 - Hybrid Cannabis

E

Eales' Disease - H35.06 - Indicia Cannabis
Ear - see also condition
Earache - H92.0 - Hybrid Cannabis
Early Satiety - R68.81 - Cannabidiol (CBD)
Eaton-Lambert Syndrome (LEMS) - see syndrome, lambert-eaton
Eberth's Disease, typhoid fever - A01.00 - Cannabidiol (CBD)
Ebola Virus Disease - A98.4 - Cannabidiol (CBD)
Ebstein's Anomaly or syndrome, heart - Q22.5 - Indicia Cannabis
Eccentro-Osteochondrodysplasia - E76.29 - Indicia Cannabis

Ecchondroma - see neoplasm, bone, benign
Ecchondrosis - D48.0 - Cannabidiol (CBD)
Ecchymosis - R58 - Indicia Cannabis
Echinococcosis - see echinococcus
Echinococcosis - see echinococcus
Echinococcus, infection - B67.90 - Cannabidiol (CBD)
Echinorhynchiasis - B83.8 - Indicia Cannabis
Echinostomiasis - B66.8 - Cannabidiol (CBD)
Echolalia - R48.8 - Cannabidiol (CBD)
Echovirus, - cause of disease classified elsewhere - B97.12 - Hybrid Cannabis
Eclampsia, eclamptic, coma, convulsions, delirium, with hypertension - O15.9 -Indicia Cannabis
Economic Circumstances affecting care - Z59.9 - Sativa Strains
Economo's Disease - A85.8 - Indicia Cannabis
Ectasia, ectasis
Ecthyma - L08.0 - Cannabidiol (CBD)
Ectocardia - Q24.8 - Indicia Cannabis
Ectodermal Dysplasia, anhidrotic - Q82.4 - Hybrid Cannabis
Ectodermosis Erosive Periorificial's - L51.1 - Hybrid Cannabis
Ectopic, ectopia, congenital
Ectromelia - Q73.8 - Indicia Cannabis
Ectropion - H02.109 - Hybrid Cannabis
Eczema, acute, chronic, erythematous, issue, rub, squamous - L30.9 - Indicia Cannabis
Eczematoid - L30.2 - Indicia Cannabis
Eddowes Spurway - Q78.0 - Cannabidiol (CBD)
Edema, edematous, infectious, pitting, toxic - R60.9 - Cannabidiol (CBD)
Edentulism - see absence, teeth, acquired
Edsall's Disease - T67.2 - Hybrid Cannabis
Educational Handicap - Z55.9 - Indicia Cannabis
Edward's Syndrome - see trisomy - 758.2 - Hybrid Cannabis
Effect, adverse
Effect (s), of, from - see effect, adverse NEC
Effects, late - see sequelae
Effluvium
Effort Syndrome, psychogenic - F45.8 - Hybrid Cannabis
Effusion
Egg Shell Nails - L60.3 - Cannabidiol (CBD)
Egyptian Splenomegaly - B65.1 - Hybrid Cannabis

Ehrlichiosis - A77.40 - Tetrahydrocannabinol (THC)
Ehlers-Danlos Syndrome - Q79.6 - Indicia Cannabis
Eichstedt's Disease - B36.0 - Hybrid Cannabis
Eisenmenger's
Ejaculation
Ekbom's Syndrome, restless legs - G25.81 - Caryophyllene (CB2)
Ekman's Syndrome, brittle bones and blue sclera - Q78.0 - Cannabidiol (CBD)
Elastic Skin - Q82.8 - Caryophyllene (CB2)
Elastofibroma - see neoplasm, connective tissue, benign
Elastoma, juvenile - Q82.8 - Indicia Cannabis
Elastomyofibrosis - I42.4 - Cannabidiol (CBD)
Elastosis
Elbow - condition
Electric Current - electricity, effects, concussion, fatal, nonfatal, shock - T75.4 -Cannabidiol (CBD)
Electric Feet Syndrome - E53.8 - Cannabidiol (CBD)
Electrocution - T75.4 - Cannabidiol (CBD)
Electrolyte Imbalance - E87.8 - Tetrahydrocannabinol (THC)
Elephantiasis, nonfilarial - I89.0 - Indicia Cannabis
Elevated, elevation
Elliptocytosis, congenital, hereditary - D58.1 - Hybrid Cannabis
Ellison-Zollinger Syndrome - E16.4 - Hybrid Cannabis
Ellis-van Creveld Syndrome, chondroectodermal dysplasia - Q77.6 - Cannabidiol (CBD)
Elongated, elongation, congenital - see also distortion
Eltor Cholera - A00.1 - Hybrid Cannabis
Emaciation, due to malnutrition - E41 - Indicia Cannabis
Embadomoniasis - A07.8 - Hybrid Cannabis
Embedded Tooth, teeth - K01.0 - Indicia Cannabis
Embolic - see condition
Embolism, multiple, paradoxical - I74.9 - Indicia Cannabis
Embolus - see embolism
Embryoma - see also neoplasm, uncertain behavior, by site
Embryonic
Embryopathia (NOS) - Z599 - Hybrid Cannabis
Embryotoxon - Q13.4 - Indicia Cannabis
Emesis - see vomiting
Emotional Lability - R45.86 - Indicia Cannabis
Emotionality, pathological - F60.3 - Cannabidiol (CBD)

Emetogenic Disease - disorder, psychogenic
Emphysema - atrophic, bullous, chronic, interlobular, lung, obstructive, pulmonary, senile, vesicular - J43.9 - Salvia Cannabis
Empty Nest Syndrome - Z60.0 - Cannabidiol (CBD)
Empyema - acute, chest, double, pleura, supradiaphragmatic, thorax - J86.9 - Indicia Cannabis
En Coup De Saber Lesion - L94.1 - Indicia Cannabis
Enamel Pearls - K00.2 - Hybrid Cannabis
Enameloma - K00.2 - Hybrid Cannabis
Enanthema, viral - B09 - Cannabidiol (CBD)
Encephalitis - chronic, hemorrhagic, idiopathic, nonepidemic, spurious, subacute - G04.90 - Cannabidiol (CBD)
Encephalocele - Q01.9 - Indicia Cannabis
Encephalocystocele - see encephalocele
Encephalo Duro Arterio Synangiosis (EDAMS) - I67.5 - Cannabidiol (CBD)
Encephalomalacia, brain, cerebellar, cerebral - softening, brain
Encephalomeningitis - meningoencephalitis
Encephalomeningocele - encephalocele
Encephalo Meningomyelitis - meningoencephalitis
Encephalomyelitis - also encephalitis - G04.90 - Indicia Cannabis
Encephalo Myelo Cele - see encephalocele
Encephalo Myelo Meningitis - see meningoencephalitis
Encephalomyelopathy - G96.9 - Hybrid Cannabis
Encephalomyeloradiculitis, acute - G61.0 - Hybrid Cannabis
Encephalo Myelo Radiculoneuritis, acute, Guillain-Barré - G61.0 - Cannabidiol (CBD)
Encephalo Myeloradiculopathy - G96.9 - Indicia Cannabis
Encephalopathia hyperbilirubinemica, newborn - P57.9 - Caryophyllene (CB2)
Encephalopathy, acute - G93.40 - Hybrid Cannabis
Encephalorrhagia - see hemorrhage, intracranial, intracerebral
Encephalosis, posttraumatic - F07.81 - Hybrid Cannabis
Enchondroma - see also neoplasm, bone, benign
Enchondromatosis, cartilaginous, multiple - Q78.4 - Hybrid Cannabis
Encopresis - R15.9 - Hybrid Cannabis
Encounter, with health service, for - Z76.89 - Indicia Cannabis
Encystment - see cyst
Endarteritis, bacterial, subacute, infective - I77.6 - Cannabidiol (CBD)
Endemic - see condition

Endocarditis, chronic, marantic, nonbacterial, thrombotic, valvular - I38 - Salvia Cannabis
Endocardium, endocardial - see also condition
Endocervicitis - see also cervicitis
Endocrine - see condition
Endocrinopathy, pluriglandular - E31.9 - Indicia Cannabis
Endodontic
Endodontitis - K04.0 - Hybrid Cannabis
Endofibrosis - I42.3 - Cannabidiol (CBD)
Endomastoiditis - see mastoiditis
Endometrioma - N80.9 - Indicia Cannabis
Endometriosis - N80.9 - Indicia Cannabis
Endometritis - decidual, atrophic, non-specific, purulent, senile - N71.9 - Indicia Cannabis
Endometrium - condition
Endo Myocardiopathy, South African - I42.3 - Hybrid Cannabis
Endomyocarditis - endocarditis
Endomyometritis - also endometritis
Endopericarditis - also endocarditis
Endoperineuritis - disorder, nerve
Endophlebitis - also phlebitis
Endophthalmia - also endophthalmitis, purulent
Endophthalmitis, acute, infective, metastatic, subacute - H44.009 - Cannabidiol (CBD)
Endosalpingiosis - N94.89 - Indicia Cannabis
Endosteitis - also osteomyelitis
Endothelioma, bone - see neoplasm, bone, malignant
Endosalpingiosis, hemorrhagic infectional - D69.8 - Hybrid Cannabis
Endotoxemia - code to condition
Endotrachelitis - also cervicitis
Engelmann, camurati - Q78.3 - Indicia Cannabis
English Disease - see rickets
Engman's Disease - L30.3 - Hybrid Cannabis
Engorgement
Enlargement, enlarged - see also hypertrophy
Enophthalmos - H05.40- Cannabidiol (CBD)
Enostosis - M27.8 - Cannabidiol (CBD)
Entameba, entamebiasis - see amebiasis
Entanglement

Enteralgia - see pain, abdominal
Enteric - see condition
Enteritis, acute, diarrheal, hemorrhagic, noninfective, septic - K52.9 - Cannabidiol (CBD)
Enterobiasis - B80 - Cannabidiol (CBD)
Enterobius Vermicularis, infection, infestation - B80 - Indicia Cannabis
Enterocele - see also hernia, abdomen
Enterocolitis - see also enteritis - K52.9 - Cannabidiol (CBD)
Enterogastritis - see enteritis
Enteropathy - K63.9 - Indicia Cannabis
Enteric Peritonitis - see peritonitis
Enteroptosis - K63.4 - Hybrid Cannabis
Enterorrhagia - K92.2 - Hybrid Cannabis
Enterospasm - also syndrome, irritable, bowel
Enterostenosis - also obstruction, intestine - K56.69 - Hybrid Cannabis
Enterostomy
Enterovirus, as cause of disease classified elsewhere - B97.10 - Tetrahydrocannabinol (THC)
Enthesopathy, peripheral - M77.9 - Indicia Cannabis
Entomophobia - F40.218 - Cannabidiol (CBD)
Entomophthoromycosis - B46.8 - Hybrid Cannabis
Entrance, air into vein - also embolism, air
Entrapment, nerve - also neuropathy, entrapment
Entropion, eyelid, paralytic - H02.009 - Cannabidiol (CBD)
Enucleated Eye, traumatic, current - S05.7- Indicia Cannabis
Enuresis - R32 - Hybrid Cannabis
Eosinopenia - see agranulocytosis
Eosinophilia, allergic, hereditary, idiopathic, secondary - D72.1 - Cannabidiol (CBD)
Eosinophilia-Myalgia Syndrome - M35.8 - Hybrid Cannabis
Ependymitis, acute, cerebral, chronic, granular - also encephalomyelitis
Ependymoblastoma
Ependymoma, epithelial, malignant
Ependymopathy - G93.89 - Hybrid Cannabis
Ephelis, ephelides - L81.2 - Saliva cannabis
Epiblepharon, congenital - Q10.3 - Saliva cannabis
Epicanthus, epicanthic fold, eyelid, congenital - Q10.3 - Cannabidiol (CBD)
Epicondylitis, elbow
Epicystitis - see cystitis

Epidemic - see condition

Epidermidalization, cervix - see dysplasia, cervix

Epidermis, epidermal - see condition

Epidermodysplasia Verruciformis - B07.8 - Indicia Cannabis

Epidermolysis

Epidermophytid - see dermatophytosis

Epidermophytosis, infected - see dermatophytosis

Epididymis - see condition

Epididymitis, acute, nonvenereal, recurrent, residual - N45.1 - Tetrahydrocannabinol (THC)

Epididymo-orchitis - see also epididymitis - N45.3 - Cannabidiol (CBD)

Epidural - also condition

Epigastrium, epigastric - see condition

Epigastrocele - see hernia, ventral

Epiglottis - see condition

Epiglottitis, epiglottitis (acute) - J05.10 - Indicia Cannabis

Epignathus - Q89.4 - Cannabidiol (CBD)

Epilepsia Partial Continue - also kozhevnikof's epilepsy - G40.1 - Tetrahydrocannabinol (THC)

Epilepsy, epileptic attack, cerebral, convulsion, epilepsia - G40.909 - Indicia Cannabis

Epiloia - Q85.1 - Hybrid Cannabis

Epimenorrhea - N92.0 - Hybrid Cannabis

Epipharyngitis - also nasopharyngitis

Epiphora - H04.20 - Hybrid Cannabis

Epiphyseal Arrest - see arrest, epiphyseal

Epiphyseolysis, epiphysiolysis - see osteochondropathy

Epiphysitis - see also osteochondropathy

Epiplocele - see hernia, abdomen

Epiploitis - see peritonitis

Epiplosarcomphalocele - see hernia, umbilicus

Episcleritis, suppurative - H15.10 - Indicia Cannabis

Episode

Epispadias, female, male - Q64.0 - Cannabidiol (CBD)

Episplenitis - D73.89 - Cannabidiol (CBD)

Epistaxis, multiple - R04.0 - Cannabidiol (CBD)

Epithelioma, malignant - also neoplasm, malignant, by site

Epitheliomatous Pigmented - Q82.1 - Cannabidiol (CBD)

Epitheliopathy, multifocal placoid pigment - H30.14- Indicia Cannabis
Epithelium, epithelial - see condition
Epituberculosis, with atelectasis, allergic - A15.7 - Cannabidiol (CBD)
Eponychia - Q84.6 - Cannabidiol (CBD)
Epstein's
Epulis, gingiva, fibrous, giant cell - K06.8 - Sativa Strain
Equinia - A24.0 - Cannabidiol (CBD)
Equinovarus, congenital, talipes - Q66.0 - Indicia Cannabis
Equivalent
Erb, Duchenne, paralysis - newborn, birth injury - P14.0 - Cannabidiol (CBD)
Erb-Goldflam Disease or syndrome - G70.00 - Indicia Cannabis
Erb's
Erdheim's Syndrome, acromegalic macro spondylitis - E22.0 - Hybrid Cannabis
Erection, painful, persistent - see priapism
Ergosterol Deficiency, vitamin D - E55.9 - Indica Cannabis
Ergotism - see also poisoning, food, noxious, plant
Erosio interdigitalis blastomycetica - B37.2 - Indicia Cannabis
Erosion
Erotomania - F52.8 - Indicia Cannabis
Error
Eructation - R14.2 - Indicia Cannabis
Eruption
Erysipelas, gangrenous, infantile, newborn, phlegmonous, suppurative - A46 - Cannabidiol (CBD)
Erysipeloid - A26.9 - Indicia Cannabis
Erythema, erythematous, infection, inflammation - L53.9 - Hybrid Cannabis
Erythematous, erythematosus - see condition
Erythermalgia, primary - I73.81 - Indicia Cannabis
Erythralgia - I73.81 - Hybrid Cannabis
Erythrasma - L08.1 - Cannabidiol (CBD)
Erythredema, polyneuropathy - see poisoning, mercury
Erythremia, acute - C94.0- Cannabidiol (CBD)
Erythroblastopenia - also aplasia, red cell - D60.9 - Cannabidiol (CBD)
Erythroblastophthisis - D61.09 - Indicia Cannabis
Erythroblastosis, details, newborn - P55.9 - Cannabidiol (CBD)
Erythrocyanosis, curium - I73.89 - Cannabidiol (CBD)

Erythrocythemia - see erythremia
Erythrocytosis, megalosplenic, secondary - D75.1 - Indicia Cannabis
Erythroderma, secondary - see also erythema - L53.9 - Hybrid Cannabis
Erythrodysesthesia, palmar plantar (PPE) - L27.1 - Hybrid Cannabis
Erythrogenesis Imperfecta - D61.09 - Indicia Cannabis
Erythroleukemia - C94.0- Cannabidiol (CBD)
Erythromelalgia - I73.81 - Hybrid Cannabis
Erythrophagocytosis - D75.89 - Hybrid Cannabis
Erythrophobia - F40.298 - Indicia Cannabis
Erythroplakia, oral epithelium, and tongue - K13.29 - Cannabidiol (CBD)
Erythroplasia, Queyrat - D07.4 - Hybrid Cannabis
Escherichia Coli (E. coli) - B96.20 - Cannabidiol (CBD)
Esophagus - K22.4 - Cannabidiol (CBD)
Esophagitis, acute, alkaline, chemical, chronic, infection, necrotic, peptic, postoperative -K20.9 - Cannabidiol (CBD)
Esophagocele - K22.5 - Hybrid Cannabis
Esophagomalacia - K22.8 - Indicia Cannabis
Esophagospasm - K22.4 - Hybrid Cannabis
Esophagostenosis - K22.2 - Indicia Cannabis
Esophagostomiasis - B81.8 - Hybrid Cannabis
Esophagotracheal - see condition
Esophagus - see condition
Esophoria - H50.51 - Indicia Cannabis
Esotropia - see strabismus, convergent concomitant
Espundia - B55.2 - Hybrid Cannabis
Essential - see condition
Esthesioneuroblastoma - C30.0 - Cannabidiol (CBD)
Esthesioneurocytoma - C30.0 - Indicia Cannabis
Esthesioneuroepithelioma - C30.0 - Indicia Cannabis
Esthiomene - A55 - Indicia Cannabis
Estivoautumnal Malaria, fever - B50.9 - Cannabidiol (CBD)
Estrangement, marital - Z63.5 - Indicia Cannabis
Ethanol - alcoholism
Etherism - dependence, drug, inhalant
Ethmoid, ethmoidal - see condition
Ethmoiditis, chronic, nonpurulent, purulent - also sinusitis, ethmoidal
Ethyl - alcoholism
Eulenburg's Disease congenital paramyotonia - G71.19 - Cannabidiol (CBD)
Eumycetoma - B47.0 - Indicia Cannabis

Eunuchoidism - E29.1 - Cannabidiol (CBD)
European Blastomycosis - see cryptococcosis
Eustachian - see condition
Evaluation (for) (of)
Evans Syndrome - D69.41 - Indicia Cannabis
Event Apparent - life-threatening in newborn and infant (ALTE) - R68.13 - Cannabidiol (CBD)
Eventration - see also hernia, ventral
Eversion
Evidence
Evisceration
Evulsion - also avulsion
Ewing's Sarcoma or tumor - also neoplasm, bone, malignant
Examination (for), following, general, routine - Z00.00 - Hybrid Cannabis
Exanthem, exanthema - see also rash
Excess, excessive, excessively
Excitability, abnormal, under minor stress, personality disorder - F60.3 - Cannabidiol (CBD)
Excitation
Excitement
Excoriation, traumatic - see also abrasion
Exfoliation
Exfoliative - see condition
Exhaustion, exhaustive, physical (NEC) - R53.83 - Cannabidiol (CBD)
Exhibitionism - F65.2 - Indicia Cannabis
Exocervicitis - see cervicitis
Exomphalos - Q79.2 - Indicia Cannabis
Exophoria - H50.52 - Cannabidiol (CBD)
Exophthalmos - H05.2- Indicia Cannabis
Exostosis - see also disorder, bone
Exotropia - see strabismus, divergent concomitant
Explanation of
Exposure (to), also contact, with - T75.89 - Indicia Cannabis
Exsanguination - see hemorrhage
Exstrophy
Extensive - also condition
Extra - also accessory
Extrasystoles, supraventricular - I49.49 - Indicia Cannabis
Extrauterine Gestation or pregnancy - see pregnancy, by site

Extravasation
Extremity - see condition, limb
Extropy - also exstrophy
Extroversion
Extruded Tooth, teeth - M26.34 - Indicia Cannabis
Extrusion
Exudate
Exudative - also condition
Eye, eyeball, eyelid - see condition
Eyestrain - see disturbance, vision, subjective
Eyeworm Disease of Africa - B74.3 - Hybrid Cannabis

F

Faber's Syndrome, achlorhydric anemia - D50.9 - Salvia Cannabis
Fabry, Anderson - E75.21 - Indicia Cannabis
Faciocephalalgia, autonomic - also neuropathy, peripheral, autonomic - G90.09 - Hybrid Cannabis
Factor (s)
Fahr Disease, of brain - G23.8 - Hybrid Cannabis
Fahr Volhard Disease, of kidney - I12 - Hybrid Cannabis
Failure Failed
Fainting (fit) - R55 - Indicia Cannabis
Fallen Arches - also deformity, limb, flat foot
Falling Falls, repeated - R29.6 - Salvia Cannabis
Fallopian
Fallot's
False - see also condition
Family, familial - see also condition
Famine, effects of - T73.0 - Indicia Cannabis
Fanconi De Toni, Debré - E72.09 - Cannabidiol (CBD)
Fanconi's Anemia, congenital pancytopenia - D61.09 - Salvia Cannabis
Farber's Disease or syndrome - E75.29 - Cannabidiol (CBD)
Farcy - A24.0 - Indicia Cannabis
Farmer's
Farsightedness - see hypermetropia
Fascia - see condition
Fasciculation - R25.3 - Hybrid Cannabis
Fasciitis - M72.9 - Hybrid Cannabis

Fascioliasis - B66.3 - Indicia Cannabis
Fasciolopsis, fasciolopsiasis, intestinal - B66.5 - Hybrid Cannabis
Facioscapulohumeral Myopathy - G71.0 - Hybrid Cannabis
Fast pulse - R00.0 - Indicia Cannabis
Fat
Fatigue - R53.83 - Cannabidiol (CBD)
Fatness - see obesity
Fatty - see also condition
Fauces - see condition
Fauchard's Disease, periodontitis - see periodontitis
Faucitis - J02.9 - Hybrid Cannabis
Favism, anemia - D55.0 - Indicia Cannabis
Favus - see dermatophytosis
Fazio-Londe Disease or syndrome - G12.1 - Hybrid Cannabis
Fear Complex or reaction - F40.9 - Indicia Cannabis
Fear of - see phobia
Feared Complaint Unfounded - Z71.1 - Indicia Cannabis
Febris, febrile, see also fever
Fecal
Fecalith, impaction - K56.41 - Hybrid Cannabis
Fede's Disease - K14.0 - Hybrid Cannabis
Feeble Rapid Pulse - due to shock following injury - T79.4 - Hybrid Cannabis
Feeble-Minded - F70 - Indicia Cannabis
Feeding
Feeling (of)
Feer's Disease - see poisoning, mercury
Feet - see condition
Feigned Illness - Z76.5 - Salvia Cannabis
Feil-Klippel Syndrome, B Revi Collis - Q76.1 - Hybrid Cannabis
Feinmesser's, hidrotic - Q82.4 - Indicia Cannabis
Felinophobia - F40.218 - Cannabidiol (CBD)
Felon - see also cellulitis, digit
Felty's Syndrome - M05.00 - Indicia Cannabis
Female Genital cutting status - also female genital mutilation status (FGM)
Female Genital mutilation status (FGM) - N90.810 - Hybrid Cannabis
Femur, femoral - see condition
Fenestration, fenestrated - see also imperfect, closure
Ferrell's Disease, an aortic aneurysm - I71.9 - Hybrid Cannabis
Fertile Eunuch Syndrome - E23.0 - Salvia Cannabis

Fetid
Fetishism - F65.0 - Indicia Cannabis
Fetus, fetal - also condition
Fever, inanition, of unknown origin, persistent, with chill - R50.9 - Indicia Cannabis
Fibrillation
Fibrin
Fibrinogenolysis - see fibrinolysis
Fibrinogenopenia - D68.8 - Hybrid Cannabis
Fibrinolysis, hemorrhagic, acquired - D65 - Hybrid Cannabis
Fibrinogen, hereditary - D68.2 - Cannabidiol (CBD)
Fibrinopurulent - see condition
Fibrinous - see condition
Fibroadenoma
Fibroadenomas, breast, chronic, cystic, diffuse, periodic - N60.2 - Indicia Cannabis
Fibroangioma - see also neoplasm, benign, by site
Fibrochondrosarcoma - see neoplasm, cartilage, malignant
Fibrocystic
Fibrodysplasia Ossificans Progressiva - see myositis, ossifications, progressive
Fibroelastosis, Cordis, endocardial, endomyocardial - I42.4 - Cannabidiol (CBD)
Fibroid, tumor - also neoplasm connective tissue, benign
Fibrolipoma - also lipoma
Fibroliposarcoma - also neoplasm connective tissue, malignant
Fibroma - also neoplasm, connective tissue, benign
Fibromatosis - M72.9 - Indicia Cannabis
Fibromyalgia - M79.7 - Hybrid Cannabis
Fibromyoma - also neoplasm connective tissue, benign
Fibromyositis - M79.7 - Cannabidiol (CBD)
Fibro Myxo Lipoma - D17.9 - Indicia Cannabis
Fibromyxoma - see neoplasm connective tissue, benign
Fibromyxosarcoma - see neoplasm connective tissue, malignant
Fibro-Odontoma, ameloblastic - see cyst, calcifying odontogenic
Fibro-Osteoma - see neoplasm bone, benign
Fibroplasia, retrolental - H35.17- Indicia Cannabis
Fibrinopurulent - see condition
Fibrosarcoma - also neoplasm, connective tissue, malignant
Fibrosclerosis
Fibrosis, fibrotic
Fibrositis, periarticular - M79.7 - Indicia Cannabis

Fibrothorax - J94.1 - Hybrid Cannabis
Fibrotic - also fibrosis
Fibrous - also condition
Fibroxanthoma - also neoplasm, connective tissue, benign
Fibroxanthosarcoma - see neoplasm connective tissue, malignant
Fiedler's
Fifth Disease - B08.3 - Indicia Cannabis
Filaria, filarial, filariasis - see infestation, filarial
Filatov's Disease - see mononucleosis, infectious
File Cutter's Disease - see poisoning, lead
Filling Defect
Fimbrial Cyst - Q50.4 - Hybrid Cannabis
Financial Problem Affecting Care - (NOS) - Z59.9 - Indicia Cannabis
Findings, abnormal, inconclusive, without diagnosis - also abnormal
Finger - see condition
Fire, Saint Anthony's - see erysipelas
Fire-setting
Fish Hook Stomach - K31.89 - Cannabidiol (CBD)
Fishmeal-Workers Lung - J67.8 - Hybrid Cannabis
Fissure, fissured
Fistula, cutaneous - L98.8 - Salvia Cannabis
Fit - R56.9 - Tetrahydrocannabinol (THC)
Fitting, and adjustment (of)
Fitzhugh-Curtis Syndrome
Fitz's Syndrome, acute hemorrhagic pancreatitis - K85.8 - Salvia Cannabis
Fixation
Flabby Ridge - K06.8 - Indicia Cannabis
Flaccid - see also condition
Flail
Fla Jani's Disease - see hyperthyroidism, with, goiter, diffuse
Flap, Liver - K71.3 - Hybrid Cannabis
Flashbacks, residual to hallucinogen use - F16.283 - Cannabidiol (CBD)
Flat
Flatau-Schilder Disease 0 - G37.0 - Cannabidiol (CBD)
Flatback Syndrome - M40.30 - Hybrid Cannabis
Flattening
Flatulence - R14.3 - Indicia Cannabis
Flatus - R14.3 - Hybrid Cannabis
Flax-Dresser's Disease - J66.1 - Hybrid Cannabis

Flea Bite - also injury, bite, by site, superficial, insect
Flecks, glaucomatous, subcapsular - see cataract, complicated
Fleischer, Kayser ring, cornea - H18.04- Hybrid Cannabis
Fleshy Mole - O02.0 - Hybrid Cannabis
Flexibility Cereal - see catalepsy
Flexion
Flexner-Boyd Dysentery - A03.2 - Hybrid Cannabis
Flexner's Dysentery - A03.1 - Hybrid Cannabis
Flexure - see flexion
Flint Murmur, aortic insufficiency - I35.1 - Cannabidiol (CBD)
Floater, vitreous - see opacity, vitreous
Floating
Flooding - N92.0 - Indicia Cannabis
Floor - see condition
Floppy
Flu - see also Influenza
Fluctuating Blood Pressure - I99.8 - Cannabidiol (CBD)
Fluid
Flukes - see also infestation, fluke
Fluor, vaginitis - N89.8 - Indicia Cannabis
Fluorosis
Flush Syndrome - E34.0 - Cannabidiol (CBD)
Flushing - R23.2 - Cannabidiol (CBD)
Flutter
Febrile Nonhemolytic Transfusion Reaction (FNHTR) - R50.84 - Hybrid Cannabis
Fourier's Abscess - code by site under Abscess
Focus, Assmann's - see tuberculosis, pulmonary
Fogo Selvage - L10.3 - Indicia Cannabis
Foix-Alajouanine Syndrome - G95.19 - Hybrid Cannabis
Fold, folds, anomalous - also anomaly, by site
Folie a Deux - F24 - Hybrid Cannabis
Follicle
Follicular - see condition
Folliculitis, superficial - L73.9 - Cannabidiol (CBD)
Folliculome Lipidic
Følling's Disease - E70.0 - Indicia Cannabis
Follow-up - see examination, follow-up
Fong's Syndrome, hereditary poster-poncho - dysplasia - Q78.5 - Cannabidiol (CBD)

Food
Foot - see condition
Foramen Ovale, nonclosure, patent, persistent - Q21.1 - Cannabidiol (CBD)
Forbes' Glycogen Storage Disease - E74.03 - Indicia Cannabis
Fordyce-Fox Disease - L75.2 - Indicia Cannabis
Fordyce's Disease, mouth - Q38.6 - Salvia Cannabis
Forearm - see condition
Foreign Body
Forestier's Disease, rhizomelic pseudo polyarthritis - M35.3 - Indicia Cannabis
Formication - R20.2 - Cannabidiol (CBD)
Fort Bragg Fever - A27.89 - Indicia Cannabis
Fossa - see also condition
Foster-Kennedy Syndrome - H47.14- Indicia Cannabis
Fothergill's
Foul Breath - R19.6 - Cannabidiol (CBD)
Foundling - Z76.1 - Hybrid Cannabis
Fournier Disease or gangrene - N49.3 - Hybrid Cannabis
Fourth
Fonville's, peduncular - G46.3 - Salvia Cannabis
Fox-Fordyce Disease, apocrine miliaria - L75.2 - Cannabidiol (CBD)
Fracture, burst - also fracture, traumatic, by site
Breach, chronic - also fracture, pathological
Fracture, insufficiency - also fracture, pathologic by site
Fracture, pathological, pathologic - see also fracture - M84.40 - Indicia Cannabis
Fracture - abduction, traumatic, separation - see also fracture - T14.8 - Indicia Cannabis
Fragile, fragility
Fragility
Fragments, cataract, lens - H59.02 - Cannabidiol (CBD)
Frailty, frail - R54 - Salvia Cannabis
Frambesia, frambesia, tropical - see also yaws
From Beside
Frambesia - A66.1 - Hybrid Cannabis
Franceschetti-Klein, Wildervanck - Q75.4 - Cannabidiol (CBD)
Francis' Disease - see tularemia
Franklin Disease - C88.2 - Indicia Cannabis
Frank's Essential Thrombocytopenia - D69.3 - Cannabidiol (CBD)
Fraser's Syndrome - Q87.0 - Cannabidiol (CBD)
Freckle (s) - L81.2 - Salvia Cannabis

Frederickson's Hyperlipoproteinemia, type
Freeman Sheldon Syndrome - Q87.0 - Cannabidiol (CBD)
Freezing - see also effect, adverse, cold - T69.9 - Indicia Cannabis
Freiberg's Disease - infraction of metatarsal head or osteochondrosis
Frei's Disease - A55 - Cannabidiol (CBD)
Fremitus, friction, cardiac - R01.2 - Salvia Cannabis
Frenum, frenulum
Frequency Micturition, nocturnal - R35.0 - Hybrid Cannabis
Frey's Syndrome
Friction
Friderichsen-Waterhouse Syndrome or disease - A39.1 - Indicia Cannabis
Friedländer's B (Bacillus) - see also condition - A49.8 - Hybrid Cannabis
Friedreich's
Frigidity - F52.22 - Salvia Cannabis
Fröhlich's Syndrome - E23.6 - Cannabidiol (CBD)
Frontal - also condition
Frostbite, superficial - T33.90 - Cannabidiol (CBD)
Frotteurism - F65.81 - Salvia Cannabis
Frozen - also effect, adverse, cold - T69.9 - Indicia Cannabis
Fructokinase Deficiency - E74.11 - Cannabidiol (CBD)
Fructose, diphosphatase deficiency - E74.19 - Salvia Cannabis
Fructosemia, benign, essential - E74.12 - Hybrid Cannabis
Fructosuria, benign, essential - E74.11 - Hybrid Cannabis
Fuchs'
Fucosidosis - E77.1 - Hybrid Cannabis
Fugue - R68.89 - Indicia Cannabis
Fulminant, fulminating - see condition
Functional - see also condition
Functioning, intellectual, borderline - R41.83 - Cannabidiol (CBD)
Fundus - see condition
Fungemia - NOS - B49 - Indicia Cannabis
Fungus, fungus
Funiculitis, acute, chronic, endemic - N49.1 - Cannabidiol (CBD)
Funnel
Fever of unknown origin Fuo - R50.9 - Cannabidiol (CBD)
Furfur - L21.0 - Salvia Cannabis
Furrier's Lung - J67.8 - Cannabidiol (CBD)
Furrowed - K14.5 - Indicia Cannabis
Furuncle - L02.92 - Tetrahydrocannabinol (THC)

Furunculosis - see furuncle
Fused - see fusion, merged
Fusion, fused, congenital
Fusospirillosis, mouth, tongue, tonsil - A69.1 - Cannabidiol (CBD)
Fussy Baby - R68.12 - Cannabidiol (CBD)

G

Gain in Weight, abnormal, excessive - also weight, gain
Gaisböck's Disease, polycythemia hypertonic - D75.1 - Hybrid Cannabis
Gait Abnormality - R26.9 - Cannabidiol (CBD)
Galactocele, breast - N64.89 - Indica Cannabis
Galactokinase Deficiency - E74.29 - Cannabidiol (CBD)
Galactophorous - N61 - Salvia Cannabis
Galactorrhea - O92.6 - Salvia Cannabis
Galactosemia, classic, congenital - E74.21 - Hybrid Cannabis
Galactosemia - E74.29 - Cannabidiol (CBD)
Galacturia - R82.0 - Indica Cannabis
Galeazzi's Fracture - S52.37 - Hybrid Cannabis
Galen's Vein - see condition
Galeophobia - F40.218 - Hybrid Cannabis
Gall duct - see condition
Gallbladder - see also condition
Gallop Rhythm - R00.8 - Indica Cannabis
Gallstone - colic, cystic duct, gallbladder, impacted, multiple - see also calculus, gallbladder
Gambling - Z72.6 - Salvia Cannabis
Gammopathy, of undetermined significance (MGUS) - D47.2 - Cannabidiol (CBD)
Gamma's Disease, siderotic splenomegaly - D73.1 - Indica Cannabis
Gamophobia - F40.298 - Cannabidiol (CBD)
Gampsodactylia, congenital - Q66.7 - Salvia Cannabis
Gamestop's Disease, adynamia episodic hereditary - G72.3 - Hybrid Cannabis
Gandy-Nanta Disease, siderotic splenomegaly - D73.1 - Hybrid Cannabis
Gang
Gangliocytoma - D36.10 - Hybrid Cannabis
Ganglioglioma - also neoplasm, uncertain behavior, by site
Ganglion, compound, diffuse, joint, tendon, sheath - M67.40 - Cannabidiol (CBD)
Ganglioneuroblastoma - see neoplasm, nerve, malignant
Ganglioneuroma - D36.10 - Indica Cannabis

Ganglioneuromatosis - D36.10 - Cannabidiol (CBD)
Ganglionitis
Gangliosidosis - E75.10 - Hybrid Cannabis
Gangosa - A66.5 - Hybrid Cannabis
Gangrene - connective tissue, dropsical, dry, moist, skin, ulcer - also necrosis - I96 - Salvia Cannabis
Ganister Disease - J62.8 - Indicia Cannabis
Ganser's Syndrome, hysterical - F44.89 - Cannabidiol (CBD)
Gardner-Diamond Syndrome, auto, erythrocyte, sensitization - D69.2 - Cannabidiol (CBD)
Gargoylism - E76.01 - Salvia Cannabis
Garré's Disease - osteitis, sclerosing - also osteomyelitis, specified type NEC
Garrod's Pad, Knuckle - M72.1 - Indicia Cannabis
Gartner's Duct
Gas - R14.3 - Salvia Cannabis
Gastralgia - see also pain, abdominal
Gastrectasis - K31.0 - Salvia Cannabis
Gastric - see condition
Gastrinoma
Gastritis, simple - K29.70 - Indicia Cannabis
Gastrocarcinoma - see neoplasm, malignant, stomach
Gastrocolic - see condition
Gastrodisciasis, gastro discoid (ASIS) - B66.8 - Cannabidiol (CBD)
Gastroduodenitis - K29.90 - Indicia Cannabis
Gastrodynia - also, abdominal pain
Gastroenteritis, acute, chronic, noninfectious - also enteritis - K52.9 - Cannabidiol (CBD)
Gastroenteropathy - see also gastroenteritis - K52.9 - Hybrid Cannabis
Gastroenteroptosis - K63.4 - Hybrid Cannabis
Gastroesophageal Laceration - hemorrhage syndrome - K22.6 - Hybrid Cannabis
Gastrointestinal - see condition
Gastrojejunal - see condition
Gastrojejunitis - see also enteritis - K52.9 - Indicia Cannabis
Gastrojejunocolic - see condition
Gastroliths - K31.89 - Hybrid Cannabis
Gastromalacia - K31.89 - Cannabidiol (CBD)
Gastroparesis - K31.84 - Tetrahydrocannabinol (THC)
Gastroparesis - K31.84 - Cannabidiol (CBD)
Gastropathy - K31.9 - Cannabidiol (CBD)

Gastroptosis - K31.89 - Cannabidiol (CBD)
Gastrorrhagia - K92.2 - Indicia Cannabis
Gastroschisis, congenital - Q79.3 - Hybrid Cannabis
Gastrospasm, neurogenic, reflex - K31.89 - Hybrid Cannabis
Gastrostaxis - see gastritis, with bleeding
Gastrostenosis - K31.89 - Indicia Cannabis
Gastrostomy
Gastrosuccorrhea, continuous, intermittent - K31.89 - Hybrid Cannabis
Gatophobia - F40.218 - Indicia Cannabis
Gaucher's Disease or splenomegaly, adult, infantile - E75.22 - Cannabidiol (CBD)
Gee, Herter, Thaysen Disease - non-tropical sprue - K90.0 - Hybrid Cannabis
Gélineau's Syndrome - G47.419 - Indicia Cannabis
Gemination, tooth, teeth - K00.2 - Tetrahydrocannabinol (THC)
General, generalized - see condition
Genetic
Genital - see condition
Genito-Anorectal Syndrome - A55 - Cannabidiol (CBD)
Genitourinary System - see condition
Genu
Geographic Tongue - K14.1 - Indicia Cannabis
Geophagia - see pica
Geotrichosis - B48.3 - Hybrid Cannabis
Gephyrophobia - F40.242 - Cannabidiol (CBD)
Gerbode Defect - Q21.0 - Cannabidiol (CBD)
Gastroesophageal Reflux Disease Gerd - K21.9 - Indicia Cannabis
Gerhardt's
German Measles - see also rubella
Germinoma - see neoplasm, malignant by site
Gerontoxon - see degeneration, cornea, senile
Gerstmann-Sträussler-Scheinker Syndrome (GSS) - A81.82 - Hybrid Cannabis
Gerstmann's Syndrome - R48.8 - Hybrid Cannabis
Gestation, period - see also pregnancy
Gestational
Ghon Tubercle, primary infection - A15.7 - Cannabidiol (CBD)
Ghost
Ghoul Hand - A66.3 - Cannabidiol (CBD)
Gianotti-Crosti Disease - L44.4 - Indicia Cannabis
Giant

Giardiasis - A07.1 - Cannabidiol (CBD)
Gibert's Disease or Pityriasis - L42 - Hybrid Cannabis
Giddiness - R42 - Salvia Cannabis
Gierke's Disease, glycogenosis I - E74.01 - Hybrid Cannabis
Gigantism, cerebral, hypophyseal, pituitary - E22.0 - Cannabidiol (CBD)
Gilbert's Disease or syndrome - E80.4 - Indicia Cannabis
Gilchrist's Disease - B40.9 - Hybrid Cannabis
Gilford-Hutchinson Disease - E34.8 - Hybrid Cannabis
Gilles de la Tourette's Disease - or syndrome, motor-verbal tic - F95.2 - Hybrid Cannabis
Gingivitis - K05.10 - Cannabidiol (CBD)
Gingivoglossitis - K14.0 - Indicia Cannabis
Gingivopericementitis - see periodontitis
Gingivitis - see gingivitis, chronic
Gingivostomatitis - K05.10 - Cannabidiol (CBD)
Gland, glandular - see condition
Glanders - A24.0 - Cannabidiol (CBD)
Glanzmann, Naegeli - D69.1 - Salvia Cannabis
Glasgow Coma Scale
Glass-Blowers Disease, cataract - see cataract, specified NEC
Glaucoma - H40.9 - Indicia Cannabis
Glaucomatous Flecks, subcapsular - see cataract, complicated
Glazed Tongue - K14.4 - Salvia Cannabis
Gleet, Gonococcal - A54.01 - Indicia Cannabis
Glénard's Disease - K63.4 - Hybrid Cannabis
Glioblastoma, multiform
Glioma, malignant
Gliomatosis Cerebral - C71.0 - Cannabidiol (CBD)
Ganglioneuroma - neoplasm, uncertain behavior by site
Gliosarcoma
Gliosis, Cerebral - G93.89 - Salvia Cannabis
Glisson's Disease - see rickets
Globinuria - R82.3 - Hybrid Cannabis
Globus, hysterics - F45.8 - Hybrid Cannabis
Glomangioma - D18.00 - Salvia Cannabis
Glomangiomyoma - D18.00 - Indicia Cannabis
Glomangiosarcoma - see neoplasm connective tissue, malignant
Glomerular
Glomerulitis - see glomerulonephritis

Glomerulonephritis - see also nephritis - N05.9 - Tetrahydrocannabinol (THC)
Glomerulopathy - see glomerulonephritis
Glomerulosclerosis - see also sclerosis, renal
Glossagra - K14.6 - Indicia Cannabis
Glossalgia - K14.6 - Cannabidiol (CBD)
Glossitis - chronic superficial, gangrenous - K14.0 - Indicia Cannabis
Glossocele - K14.8 - Tetrahydrocannabinol (THC)
Glossodynia - K14.6 - Cannabidiol (CBD)
Glossoncus - K14.8 - Cannabidiol (CBD)
Glossopathy - K14.9 - Indicia Cannabis
Glossophobia - K14.3 - Tetrahydrocannabinol (THC)
Glossoplegia - K14.8 - Salvia Cannabis
Glossoptosis - K14.8 - Salvia Cannabis
Glossopyrosis - K14.6 - Tetrahydrocannabinol (THC)
Glossotrichia - PK14.3 - Salvia Cannabis
Glossy Skin - L90.8 - Indicia Cannabis
Glottis - see condition
Glottis - see also laryngitis - J04.0 - Cannabidiol (CBD)
Glucagonoma
Glucoglycinuria - E72.51 - Cannabidiol (CBD)
Glucose-Galactose Malabsorption - E74.39 - Cannabidiol (CBD)
Glue
Glutaric Aciduria - E72.3 - Indicia Cannabis
Glycinemia - E72.51 - Hybrid Cannabis
Glycinuria, renal, with ketosis - E72.09 - Salvia Cannabis
Glycogen
Glycogenosis, diffuse, generalized - also disease, glycogen storage
Glycopenia - E16.2 - Salvia Cannabis
Glycosuria - R81 - Salvia Cannabis
Gnathostoma Spinigerous, infection, infestation, gnathostomiasis - B83.1 - Indicia Cannabis
Goiter, plunging, substernal - E04.9 - Hybrid Cannabis
Goiter-Deafness Syndrome - E07.1 - Hybrid Cannabis
Goldberg Syndrome - Q89.8 - Hybrid Cannabis
Goldberg-Maxwell Syndrome - E34.51 - Hybrid Cannabis
Goldblatt's Hypertension or kidney - I70.1 - Indicia Cannabis
Goldenhar, Gorlin - Q87.0 - Indicia Cannabis

Goldflam-Erb Disease or syndrome - G70.00 - Cannabidiol (CBD)
Goldscheider's Disease - Q81.8 - Cannabidiol (CBD)
Goldstein's Disease, familial hemorrhagic telangiectasia - I78.0 - Hybrid Cannabis
Golfer's Elbow - see epicondylitis, media
Gonadoblastoma
Gonecystitis - see vesiculitis
Gongylonemiasis - B83.8 - Hybrid Cannabis
Goniosynechiae - see adhesions, iris, on to synechiae
Gonococcemia - A54.86 - Hybrid Cannabis
Gonococcus, gonococcal, disease, infection - A54.9 - Salvia Cannabis
Gonocytoma
Gonorrhea, acute, chronic - A54.9 - Indicia Cannabis
Goodall's Disease - A08.19 - Cannabidiol (CBD)
Goodpasture's Syndrome - M31.0 - Cannabidiol (CBD)
Gopalan's Syndrome, burning feet - E53.0 - Cannabidiol (CBD)
Gorlin-Chaudry-Moss Syndrome - Q87.0 - Indicia Cannabis
Gottron's Papules - L94.4 - Hybrid Cannabis
Gouge Rot's Syndrome, presymptomatic - L81.7 - Hybrid Cannabis
Gougerot-Blum Syndrome, pigmented, purpuric, lichenoid - L81.7 -Salvia Cannabis
Gougerot-Carteaud Disease - or syndrome, confluent reticulate papillomatosis - L83 - Cannabidiol (CBD)
Gouley's Syndrome, constrictive pericarditis - I31.1 - Indicia Cannabis
Goundou - A66.6 - Salvia Cannabis
Gout, gouty - acute, attack, flare - gout, chronic - M10.9 - Cannabidiol (CBD)
Gout, chronic - see also gout, gouty - M1A.9 - Cannabidiol (CBD)
Gower's
Gradenigo's Syndrome - also otitis, suppurative, acute
Graefe's Disease - strabismus, paralytic, ophthalmoplegia, progressive
Graft-Versus-Host Disease - D89.813 - Indicia Cannabis
Grain Handlers Disease or lung - J67.8 - Hybrid Cannabis
Grain Mite, Itch - B88.0 - Salvia Cannabis
Grand Mal - also epilepsy, generalized, specified NEC
Grand Multipara Status only, not pregnant - Z64.1 - Salvia Cannabis
Granite Worker's Lung - J62.8 - Indicia Cannabis
Granular - see also condition
Granulation Tissue Abnormal, excessive - L92.9 - Salvia Cannabis
Granulocytopenia Primary, malignant - see agranulocytosis
Granuloma - L92.9 - Cannabidiol (CBD)
Granulomatosis - L92.9 - Cannabidiol (CBD)

Granulomatous Tissue, abnormal, excessive - L92.9 - Salvia Cannabis
Granulosis - L74.8 - Salvia Cannabis
Graphite Fibrosis, of lung - J63.3 - Indicia Cannabis
Graphospasm - F48.8 - Cannabidiol (CBD)
Grating Scapula - M89.8X1 - Hybrid Cannabis
Gravel, Urinary - see calculus, urinary
Graves' Disease - see hyperthyroidism with, goiter
Gravis - see condition
Grawitz Tumor - C64 - Hybrid Cannabis
Gray Syndrome, newborn - P93.0 - Indicia Cannabis
Grayness, hair, premature - L67.1 - Salvia Cannabis
Green Sickness - D50.8 - Cannabidiol (CBD)
Greenfield's Disease
Greenstick Fracture - code also fracture, by site
Grey Syndrome, newborn - P93.0 - Cannabidiol (CBD)
Grief - F43.21 - Cannabidiol (CBD)
Griesinger's Disease - B76.9 - Hybrid Cannabis
Grinder's Lung or pneumoconiosis - J62.8 - Salvia Cannabis
Grinding, Teeth
Grip
Grippe Gripped - see also influenza
Grisel's Disease - M43.6 - Hybrid Cannabis
Groin - see condition
Grooved Tongue - K14.5 - Cannabidiol (CBD)
Ground Itch - B76.9 - Hybrid Cannabis
Grover's Disease or syndrome - L11.1 - Cannabidiol (CBD)
Growing Pains, children - R29.898 - Indicia Cannabis
Growth, fungoid, neoplastic, new - also neoplasm
Gruby's Disease - B35.0 - Hybrid Cannabis
Gubler-Millard Paralysis or syndrome - G46.3 - Hybrid Cannabis
Guerin-Stern Syndrome - Q74.3 - Hybrid Cannabis
Guidance, insufficient anterior, occlusal - M26.54 - Salvia Cannabis
Guillain-Barré Disease or syndrome - G61.0 - Hybrid Cannabis
Guinea Worms, infection, infestation - B72 - Cannabidiol (CBD)
Guinon's Disease, motor-verbal tic - F95.2 - Cannabidiol (CBD)
Gull's Disease - E03.4 - Indicia Cannabis
Gum - see condition
Gumboil - K04.7 - Indicia Cannabis
Gumma, syphilitic - A52.79 - Indicia Cannabis

Gunn's Syndrome - Q07.8 - Indicia - Cannabidiol (CBD)
Gunshot Wound - see also wound, open
Gynandrism - Q56.0 - Cannabidiol (CBD)
Gynandroblastoma
Gynecological examination, periodic, routine - Z01.419 - Indicia Cannabis
Gynecomastia - N62 - Tetrahydrocannabinol (THC)
Gynephobia - F40.291 - Indicia Cannabis
Gyrate scalp - Q82.8 - Salvia Cannabis

H

H (Hartnup's) - E72.02 - Indicia Cannabis
Haas' Disease or osteochondrosis also juvenile, head of a humerus - see osteochondrosis, juvenile, humerus
Habit, habituation
Haemophilus (H) - B96.3 - Indicia Cannabis
Haff Disease - also, poisoning, mercury
Hageman's Factor Defect, deficiency or disease - D68.2 - Salvia Cannabis
Haglund's Disease or osteochondrosis, juvenile, as tibial external - juvenile
Hailey-Hailey Disease - Q82.8 - Indicia Cannabis
Hair - see also condition
Hairball in Stomach - T18.2 - Salvia Cannabis
Hair-Pulling, pathological, compulsive - F63.3 - Cannabidiol (CBD)
Hairy Black Tongue - K14.3 - Cannabidiol (CBD)
Half Vertebra - Q76.49 - Indicia Cannabis
Halitosis - R19.6 - Hybrid Cannabis
Hallerman-Streiff Syndrome - Q87.0 - Hybrid Cannabis
Hallervorden-Spatz Disease - G23.0 - Hybrid Cannabis
Hallopeau's Acrodermatitis or disease - L40.2 - Cannabidiol (CBD)
Hallucination - R44.3 - Salvia Cannabis
Hallucinosis, chronic - F28 - Indicia Cannabis
Hallux
Halo, visual - H53.19 - Tetrahydrocannabinol (THC)
Hamartoma, hepatoblastoma - Q85.9 - Cannabidiol (CBD)
Hemarthrosis - Q85.9 - Salvia Cannabis
Hamman-Rich Syndrome - J84.114 - Cannabidiol (CBD)
Hammer Toe, acquired - also deformity, toe, hammer toe
Hand - see condition
Hand-Foot Syndrome - L27.1 - Indicia Cannabis
Handicap, handicapped

Hand-Schüller-Christian Disease or syndrome - C96.5 - Hybrid Cannabis
Hanging, asphyxia, strangulation, suffocation, Asphyxia, traumatic, due to mechanical threat
Hangnail - also cellulitis
Hangover, alcohol - F10.129 - Indicia Cannabis
Hanhart's Syndrome - Q87.0 - Hybrid Cannabis
Hanot-Chauffard, troisier - E83.19 - Salvia Cannabis
Hanot's Cirrhosis or disease - K74.3 - Cannabidiol (CBD)
Hansen's Disease - see leprosy
Hantaan Virus Disease, korean hemorrhagic fever - A98.5 - Hybrid Cannabis
Hantavirus Disease, with renal manifestations, dobrava, puumala - A98.5 - Salvia Cannabis
Happy Puppet Syndrome - Q93.5 - Indicia Cannabis
Harada's Disease or syndrome - H30.81 - Salvia Cannabis
Hardening
Harelip, complete, incomplete - see cleft, lip
Harlequin, newborn - Q80.4 - Cannabidiol (CBD)
Harley's Disease - D59.6 - Indicia Cannabis
Harmful use (of)
Harris' Lines - see arrest, epiphyseal
Hartnup's Disease - E72.02 - Hybrid Cannabis
Harvester's Lung - J67.0 - Cannabidiol (CBD)
Harvesting Ovum for in vitro fertilization - Z31.83 - Cannabidiol (CBD)
Hashimoto's Disease or thyroiditis - E06.3 - Indicia Cannabis
Hashitoxicosis, transient - E06.3 - Tetrahydrocannabinol (THC)
Hassal-Henle Bodies or warts, cornea - H18.49 - Hybrid Cannabis
Haut Mal - Epilepsy, generalized, specified NEC
Haverhill Fever - A25.1 - Hybrid Cannabis
Hay Fever - also fever, hay - J30.1 - Indicia Cannabis
Hayem-Widal Syndrome - D59.8 - Cannabidiol (CBD)
Haygarth's Nodes - M15.8 - Cannabidiol (CBD)
Haymaker's Lung - J67.0 - Indicia Cannabis
Hb (abnormal)
Head - see condition
Headache - R51 - Cannabidiol (CBD)
Healthy
Hearing Examination - Z01.10 - Indicia Cannabis
Heart - see condition

Heart Beat
Heartburn - R12 - Salvia Cannabis
Heat, effects - T67.9 - Cannabidiol (CBD)
Heavy for Dates (NEC), infant, (4000g to 4499g) - P08.1 - Salvia Cannabis
Hebephrenia, hebephrenic, schizophrenia - F20.1 - Tetrahydrocannabinol (THC)
Heberden's Disease or nodes, with arthropathy - M15.1 - Indicia Cannabis
Hebra's
Heel - see condition
Hereford's Disease - D86.89 - Cannabidiol (CBD)
Hegglin's Anomaly or syndrome - D72.0 - Indicia Cannabis
Heilmeyer-Schoner Disease - D45 - Cannabidiol (CBD)
Heine-Medin Disease - A80.9 - Hybrid Cannabis
Heinz Body Anemia, congenital - D58.2 - Indicia Cannabis
Heliophobia - F40.228 - Tetrahydrocannabinol (THC)
Heller's Disease or syndrome - F84.3 - Cannabidiol (CBD)
Hellp Syndrome - elevated liver enzymes and low platelet count - O14.2 - Cannabidiol (CBD)
Helminthiasis - see also Infestation, helminth
Heloma - L84 - Cannabidiol (CBD)
Hemangioblastoma - also neoplasm connective tissue, uncertain behavior
Hemangioendothelioma - see also neoplasm unpredictable behavior, by site
Hemangiofibroma - also neoplasm benign, by site
Hemangiolipoma - see lipoma
Hemangioma - D18.00 - Indicia Cannabis
Hemangiomatosis, systemic - I78.8 - Tetrahydrocannabinol (THC)
Hemangiopericytoma - also neoplasm connective tissue, uncertain behavior
Hemangiosarcoma - also neoplasm connective tissue, malignant
Hemarthrosis, nontraumatic - M25.00 -Salvia Cannabis
Hematemesis - K92.0 - Indicia Cannabis
Hematidrosis - L74.8 - Hybrid Cannabis
Hematinuria - see also hemoglobinuria
Hematobilia - K83.8 - Salvia Cannabis
Hematocele
Hematochezia - see also melena - K92.1 - Indicia Cannabis
Hematochyluria - see also infestation filarial
Hematocolpos, with hematosalpinx, hematometra or - N89.7 - Salvia Cannabis
Hematocornea - also cornea, stromal, pigmentation
Hematogenous - condition
Hematoma - skin surface intact, traumatic - see also contusion

Hematometra - N85.7 - Indicia Cannabis
Hematomyelia, central - G95.19 - Cannabidiol (CBD)
Hematomyelitis - G04.90 - Hybrid Cannabis
Hematoperitoneum - see hemoperitoneum
Hematophobia - F40.230 - Indicia Cannabis
Hemopneumothorax, see hemothorax
Hematopoiesis, cyclic - D70.4 - Salvia Cannabis
Hematoporphyria - see porphyria
Hematorachis, hem ator rhachis - G95.19 - Cannabidiol (CBD)
Hematosalpinx - N83.6 - Cannabidiol (CBD)
Hematospermia - R36.1 - Indicia Cannabis
Hematothorax, see hemothorax
Hematuria - R31.9 - Cannabidiol (CBD)
Hemeralopia, day blindness - H53.11 - Cannabidiol (CBD)
Hemi-akinesia - R41.4 - Salvia Cannabis
Hemianalgesia - R20.0 - Indicia Cannabis
Hemianencephaly - Q00.0 - Hybrid Cannabis
Hemianesthesia - R20.0 - Hybrid Cannabis
Hemianopia, hemianopsia, heteronymous - H53.47 - Cannabidiol (CBD)
Hemiathetosis - R25.8 - Salvia Cannabis
Hemiatrophy - R68.89 - Indicia Cannabis
Hemiballism (us) - G25.5 - Cannabidiol (CBD)
Hemicardia - Q24.8 - Salvia Cannabis
Hemicephalus, hemic ep Haly - Q00.0 - Indicia Cannabis
Hemichorea - G25.5 - Cannabidiol (CBD)
Hemicolitis Left - see colitis, left sided
Hemicrania
Hemidystrophy - see hemiatrophy
Hemiectromelia - Q73.8 - Indicia Cannabis
Hemihypalgesia - R20.8 - Hybrid Cannabis
Hemihypesthesia - R20.1 - Salvia Cannabis
Hemi-inattention - R41.4 - Cannabidiol (CBD)
Hemimelia - Q73.8 - Salvia Cannabis
Hemiparalysis - see hemiplegia
Hemiparesis - see hemiplegia
Hemiparesthesia - R20.2 - Cannabidiol (CBD)
Hemiparkinsonism - G20 - Hybrid Cannabis
Hemiplegia - G81.9 Indicia Cannabis
Hemisection, spinal cord - see Injury

Hemispasm - facial - R25.2 - Cannabidiol (CBD)
Hemiparesis - B48.8 - Salvia Cannabis
Hemitremor - R25.1 - Salvia Cannabis
Hemivertebra - Q76.49 - Cannabidiol (CBD)
Hemochromatosis - E83.119 - Indicia Cannabis
Hemoglobin - see also condition
Hemoglobinemia - D59.9 - Cannabidiol (CBD)
Hemoglobinopathy, mixed - D58.2 - Salvia Cannabis
Hemoglobinuria - R82.3 - Tetrahydrocannabinol (THC)
Hemolymphangioma - D18.1 - Indicia Cannabis
Hemolysis
Hemolytic - see condition
Hemopericardium - I31.2 - Cannabidiol (CBD)
Hemoperitoneum - K66.1 - Cannabidiol (CBD)
Hemophilia, classical, familial, hereditary - D66 - Indicia Cannabis
Hemophthalmos - H44.81- Salvia Cannabis
Hemopneumothorax - see also hemothorax
Hemoptysis - R04.2 - Salvia Cannabis
Hemorrhage, hemorrhagic, concealed - R58 - Hybrid Cannabis
Hemorrhoids, bleeding, without mention of degree - K64.9 - Hybrid Cannabis
Hemosalpinx - N83.6 - Hybrid Cannabis
Hemosiderosis, dietary - E83.19 - Indicia Cannabis
Hemothorax, bacterial, nontuberculous - J94.2 - Hybrid Cannabis
Henoch, - Schönlein Disease or syndrome purpura - D69.0 - Hybrid Cannabis
Henpue, Inouye - A66.6 - Tetrahydrocannabinol (THC)
Hepar, syphilitic - A52.74 - Indicia Cannabis
Hepatalgia - K76.89 - Hybrid Cannabis
Hepatitis - K75.9 - Hybrid Cannabis
Hepatization Lung, acute - see pneumonia, lobar
Hepatoblastoma - C22.2 - Salvia Cannabis
Hepatocarcinoma - C22.0 - Salvia Cannabis
Hepatocholangiocarcinoma - C22.0 - Tetrahydrocannabinol (THC)
Hepatocholangioma, benign - D13.4 - Cannabidiol (CBD)
Hepatocholangitis - K75.89 - Hybrid Cannabis
Hepatolenticular Degeneration - E83.01 - Cannabidiol (CBD)
Hepatoma, malignant - C22.0 - Hybrid Cannabis
Hepatomegaly - see also hypertrophy, liver
Hepatoptosis - K76.89 - Hybrid Cannabis
Hepatorenal Syndrome - following labor and delivery - O90.4 - Cannabidiol (CBD)

Hepatosis - K76.89 - Indicia Cannabis
Hepatosplenomegaly - R16.2 - Salvia Cannabis
Hereditary - see condition
Heredodegenerative, macular - see dystrophy, retina
Heredopathia Atactic Polyneuritiformis - G60.1 - Cannabidiol (CBD)
Heredosyphilis - see syphilis, congenital
Herlitz' Syndrome - Q81.1 - Indicia Cannabis
Hermansky-Pudlak Syndrome - E70.331 - Hybrid Cannabis
Hermaphrodite, hermaphroditism, actual - Q56.0 - Hybrid Cannabis
Hernia, hernia, acquired, recurrent - K46.9 - Cannabidiol (CBD)
Herniation - see also hernia
Herpangina - B08.5 - Indicia Cannabis
Herpes, herpes virus, herpetic - B00.9 - Hybrid Cannabis
Herpesvirus, human - see herpes
Herpetophobia - F40.218 - Cannabidiol (CBD)
Herrick's Anemia - see disease, sickle-cell
Hers' Disease - E74.09 - Cannabidiol (CBD)
Herter-Gee Syndrome - K90.0 - Indicia Cannabis
Herxheimer's Reaction - R68.89 - Salvia Cannabis
Hesitancy
Hesselbach's Hernia - see femoral, specified site NEC
Heterochromia, congenital - Q13.2 - Indicia Cannabis
Heterophoria - see strabismus, heterophoria
Heterophyes, heterophyids, small intestine - B66.8 - Hybrid Cannabis
Heterotopia, heterotopic - see also malposition, congenital
Heterotropia - see strabismus
Huebner-Herter Disease - K90.0 - Indicia Cannabis
Hexadactylism - Q69.9 - Hybrid Cannabis
Cytology Finding High Grade Squamous Intraepithelial Lesion on Cytologic (HGSIL)
Hibernoma - see Lipoma
Hiccup, hiccough - R06.6 - Salvia Cannabis
Hidden Penis, congenital - Q55.64 - Indicia Cannabis
Hidradenitis, axillary, suppurative - L73.2 - Salvia Cannabis
Hidradenoma, modular - also neoplasm, benign skin
Hidrocystoma - see neoplasm skin, benign
High
Hildenbrand's Disease - A75.0 - Indicia Cannabis
Hilum - see condition

Hip - see condition
Hippel's Disease - Q85.8 - Hybrid Cannabis
Hippophobia - F40.218 - Indicia Cannabis
Hippus - H57.09 - Hybrid Cannabis
Hirschsprung's Disease or megacolon - Q43.1 - Hybrid Cannabis
Hirsutism, hirsuties - L68.0 - Hybrid Cannabis
Hirudiniasis
Hiss-Russell Dysentery - A03.1 - Indicia Cannabis
Histidinemia, histidinuria - E70.41 - Hybrid Cannabis
Histiocytoma - see also neoplasm, skin, benign
Histiocytosis - D76.3 - Salvia Cannabis
Histoplasmosis - B39.9 - Hybrid Cannabis
History
His-Werner Disease - A79.0 - Hybrid Cannabis
Human Immunodeficiency Virus (HIV) - B20 - Hybrid Cannabis
Hives, bold - see urticaria
Hoarseness - R49.0 - Cannabidiol (CBD)
Hobo - Z59.0 - Hybrid Cannabis
Hodgkin Disease - see lymphoma, hodgkin
Hodgson's Disease - I71.2 - Hybrid Cannabis
Hoffa-Kastert Disease - E88.89 - Indicia Cannabis
Hoffa's Disease - E88.89 - Hybrid Cannabis
Hoffmann-Bouveret Syndrome - I47.9 - Tetrahydrocannabinol (THC)
Hoffmann's Syndrome - E03.9 - Salvia Cannabis
Hole (round)
Holiday Relief Care - Z75.5 - Indicia Cannabis
Hollenhorst's Plaque - see occlusion, artery, retina
Hollow Foot, congenital - Q66.7 - Salvia Cannabis
Holoprosencephaly - Q04.2 - Hybrid Cannabis
Holt-Oram Syndrome - Q87.2 - Salvia Cannabis
Homelessness - Z59.0 - Hybrid Cannabis
Homesickness - see disorder, adjustment
Homocysteinemia, homocystinuria - E72.11 - Hybrid Cannabis
Homogentisate 1,2-dioxygenase deficiency - E70.29 - Indicia Cannabis
Homologous Serum Hepatitis - prophylactic, therapeutic - see hepatitis
Honeycomb Lung - J98.4 - Cannabidiol (CBD)
Hooded
Hookworm, anemia, disease, infection, infestation - B76.9 - Salvia Cannabis
Hordeolum, eyelid, external, recurrent - H00.019 - Hybrid Cannabis

Horn
Horner, Claude Bernard - G90.2 - Hybrid Cannabis
Horseshoe Kidney, congenital - Q63.1 - Indicia Cannabis
Horton's Headache or neuralgia - G44.099 - Hybrid Cannabis
Hospital Hopper Syndrome - see disorder, fictitious
Hospitalism in Children - see disorder, adjustment
Hostility - R45.5 - Salvia Cannabis
Hot flashes
Hourglass, contracture - see also contraction, hourglass
Household, housing circumstance affecting care - Z59.9 - Indicia Cannabis
Housemaid's Knee - see bursitis, prepatellar
Hudson Stähli, line, cornea - see pigmentation, cornea, anterior
Human
Humidifier Lung or pneumonitis - J67.7 - Hybrid Cannabis
Humiliation, experience - Z62.898 - Indicia Cannabis
Humpback, acquired - see Kyphosis
Hunger - T73.0 - Hybrid Cannabis
Hungry Bone Syndrome - E83.81 - Salvia Cannabis
Hunner's Ulcer - see cystitis, chronic, interstitial
Hunter's
Huntington's Disease or chorea - G10 - Hybrid Cannabis
Hunt's
Hurler, Scheie - E76.02 - Hybrid Cannabis
Hurst's Disease - G36.1 - Indicia Cannabis
Hurthle Cell
Hutchinson-Boeck Disease or syndrome - see sarcoidosis
Hutchinson-Gilford Disease or syndrome - E34.8 - Hybrid Cannabis
Hutchinson's
Hyalin Plaque, sclera, senile - H15.89 - Indicia Cannabis
Hyaline Membrane - disease, lung, pulmonary - P22.0 - Hybrid Cannabis
Hyalinosis
Hyalitis, hypnosis, asteroid - also, crystalline
Hydatid, deposit
Hydatidiform Mole - benign, complicating pregnancy - O01.9 - Salvia Cannabis
Hydatidosis - see echinococcus
Hidradenitis, axillary, suppurative - L73.2 - Salvia Cannabis
Hidradenoma - see hidradenoma
Hydramnios - O40.- Hybrid Cannabis
Hydranencephaly, hydranencephaly - Q04.3 - Indicia Cannabis

Hydrargyrism (NEC) - see poisoning, mercury
Hydrarthrosis - see also effusion, joint
Hydremia - D64.89 - Salvia Cannabis
Hydrencephalocele, congenital - see encephalocele
Hydro Enephalalomeningocele, congenital - see encephalocele
Hydro - R23.8 - Salvia Cannabis
Hidradenitis, axillary, suppurative - L73.2 - Indicia Cannabis
Hydrocalycosis - see hydronephrosis
Hydrocele, spermatic cord, testis, tunica vaginal, - N43.3 - Hybrid Cannabis
Hydrocephalus - acquired, internal, malignant, recurrent - G91.9 - Indicia Cannabis
Hydrocolpos, congenital - N89.8 - Salvia Cannabis
Hydrocystoma - see neoplasm skin, benign
Hydroencephalocele, congenital - see encephalocele
Hydro encephalomeningocele, congenital - see encephalocele
Hydrohemato pneumothorax - see hemothorax
Hydromeningitis - see meningitis
Hydro Meningocele, spinal - see also spina bifida
Hydrometra - N85.8 p - Hybrid Cannabis
Hydrometrocolpos - N89.8 - Indicia Cannabis
Hydromicrocephaly - Q02 - Hybrid Cannabis
Hydrocepnalus, since birth - Q45.8 - Hybrid Cannabis
Hydromyelia - Q06.4 - Salvia Cannabis
Hydromyelocele - see spina bifida
Hydronephrosis, atrophic, early, intermittent, primary - N13.30 - Hybrid Cannabis
Hydropericarditis - see pericarditis
Hydropericardium - see pericarditis
Hydroperitoneum - R18.8 - Hybrid Cannabis
Hydrophobia - see rabies - Hybrid Cannabis
Hydro Phthalmos - Q15.0 - Salvia Cannabis
Hydro Pneumohemothorax - see hemothorax
Hydro Pneumopericarditis - see pericarditis
Hydro Pneumopericardium - see pericarditis
Hydro Pneumothorax - J94.8 - Salvia Cannabis
Hydrops - R60.9 - Hybrid Cannabis
Hydronephrosis - N13.6 - Tetrahydrocannabinol (THC)
Hydrorachis - Q06.4 - Hybrid Cannabis
Hydrorrhea, nasal - J34.89 - Cannabidiol (CBD)
Hidradenitis, axillary, suppurative - L73.2 - Indicia Cannabis
Hydrosalpinx, fallopian tube, follicular - N70.11 - Hybrid Cannabis

Hydrothorax, double, pleura - J94.8 - Salvia Cannabis
Hydroureter - see also hydronephrosis - N13.4 - Hybrid Cannabis
Hydroureteronephrosis - see hydronephrosis
Hydrourethra - N36.8 - Salvia Cannabis
Hydroxykynureninuria - E70.8 - Indicia Cannabis
Hydroxylysinemia - E72.3 - Hybrid Cannabis
Hydroxyprolinemia - E72.59 - Tetrahydrocannabinol (THC)
Hygiene, sleep
Hygroma, congenital, cystic - D18.1 - Hybrid Cannabis
Hymen - see condition
Hymenolepis, hymenolepiasis, diminutive, infection - B71.0 - Indicia Cannabis
Hypalgesia - R20.8 - Hybrid Cannabis
Hyperacidity, gastric - K31.89 - Hybrid Cannabis
Hyperactive, hyperactivity - F90.9 - Hybrid Cannabis
Hyperacusis - H93.23- Hybrid Cannabis
Hyperadrenalism - E27.5 - Indicia Cannabis
Hyperadrenocorticism - E24.9 - Tetrahydrocannabinol (THC)
Hyperaldosteronism - E26.9 - Hybrid Cannabis
Hyperalgesia - R20.8 - Salvia Cannabis
Hyperalimentation - R63.2 - Salvia Cannabis
Hyperaminoaciduria
Hyperammonemia, congenital - E72.20 - Hybrid Cannabis
Hyperazotemia - see uremia
Hyperbetalipoproteinemia, familial - E78.0 - Salvia Cannabis
Hyperbilirubinemia
Hypercalcemia, hypocalciuric, familial - E83.52 - Hybrid Cannabis
Hypercalciuria, idiopathic - E83.52 - Indicia Cannabis
Hypercapnia - R06.89 - Hybrid Cannabis
Hypercarotenemia, hypercarotenemia, dietary - E67.1 - Hybrid Cannabis
Hypercementosis - K03.4 - Hybrid Cannabis
Hyperchloremia - E87.8 - Hybrid Cannabis
Hyperchlorhydria - K31.89 - Hybrid Cannabis
Hypercholesterinemia - see hypercholesterolemia
Hypercholesterolemia - essential, familial, hereditary - E78.0 - Hybrid Cannabis
Hyperchylia Gastric, psychogenic - F45.8 - Salvia Cannabis
Hyperchylomicronemia, familial, primary - E78.3 - Cannabidiol (CBD)
Hypercoagulable, state - D68.59 - Indicia Cannabis
Hypercoagulation, state - D68.59 - Hybrid Cannabis

Hypercorticism, pituitary-dependent - E24.0 - Salvia Cannabis
Hypercortisolism - see cushing's, syndrome
Hypercorticosteronism - E24.2 - Hybrid Cannabis
Hypercortisolism - E24.2 - Hybrid Cannabis
Hyperekplexia - Q89.8 - Hybrid Cannabis
Hyperelectrolytemia - E87.8 - Indicia Cannabis
Hyperemesis - R11.10 - Hybrid Cannabis
Hyperemia, acute, passive - R68.89 - Tetrahydrocannabinol (THC)
Hyperesthesia, body surface - R20.3 - Salvia Cannabis
Hyperestrogenism, drug-induced, iatrogenic - E28.0 - Hybrid Cannabis
Hyperexplexia - Q89.8 - Hybrid Cannabis
Hyperfibrinolysis - see fibrinolysis
Hyperfructosemia - E74.19 - Indicia Cannabis
Hyperfunction
Hypergammaglobulinemia - D89.2 - Hybrid Cannabis
Hypergastrinemia - E16.4 - Hybrid Cannabis
Hyperglobulinemia - R77.1 - Salvia Cannabis
Hyperglycemia, hyperglycemic, transient - R73.9 - Hybrid Cannabis
Hyperglyceridemia, endogenous, hereditary, pure - E78.1 - Indicia Cannabis
Hyperglycinemia, non-ketotic - E72.51 - Hybrid Cannabis
Hypergonadism
Hyperheparinemia - D68.32 - Salvia Cannabis
Hyperhidrosis, hyperidrosis - R61 - Hybrid Cannabis
Hyperhistidinemia - E70.41 - Hybrid Cannabis
Hyperhomocysteinemia - E72.11 - Indicia Cannabis
Hyperhydroxyprolinemia - E72.59 - Hybrid Cannabis
Hyperinsulinism, functional - E16.1 - Tetrahydrocannabinol (THC)
Hyperkalemia - E87.5 - Salvia Cannabis
Hyperkeratosis - also keratosis - L85.9 - Hybrid Cannabis
Hyperkinesia, disease, reaction, syndrome, childhood, adolescence
Hyperleucine-Isoleucine Mia - E71.19 - Hybrid Cannabis
Hyperlipemia, hyperlipidemia - E78.5 - Indicia Cannabis
Hyperlipidosis - E75.6 - Hybrid Cannabis
Hyperlipoproteinemia - E78.5 - Hybrid Cannabis
Hyperlucent Lung, unilateral - J43.0 - Cannabidiol (CBD)
Hyperlysinemia - E72.3 - Salvia Cannabis
Hypermagnesemia - E83.41 - Hybrid Cannabis
Hypermenorrhea - N92.0 - Hybrid Cannabis
Hypermethioninemia - E72.19 - Indicia Cannabis

Hypermetropia, congenital - H52.0- Hybrid Cannabis
Hypermobility, hypermotility
Hypernasality - R49.21 - Tetrahydrocannabinol (THC)
Hypernatremia - E87.0 - Hybrid Cannabis
Hypernephroma - C64.- Indicia Cannabis
Hyperopia - see hypermetropia
Hyperoxia Nervosa - F50.2 - Salvia Cannabis
Hyperornithinemia - E72.4 - Hybrid Cannabis
Hyperosmia - R43.1 - Hybrid Cannabis
Hyperosmolality - E87.0 - Salvia Cannabis
Hyperostosis, mono melic - also disorder, bone, density and structure, specified
Hyperrealism - E28.8 - Hybrid Cannabis
Hyperoxaluria, primary - E72.53 - Hybrid Cannabis
Hyperparathyroidism - E21.3 - Salvia Cannabis
Hyperpathia - R20.8 - Hybrid Cannabis
Hyperperistalsis - R19.2 - Hybrid Cannabis
Hyperpermeability, capillary - I78.8 - Indicia Cannabis
Hyperphagia - R63.2 - Hybrid Cannabis
Hyperphenylalaninemia (NEC) - E70.1 - Salvia Cannabis
Hyperphoria, alternating - H50.53 - Hybrid Cannabis
Hyperphosphatemia - E83.39 - Hybrid Cannabis
Hyperpiesis, hyperpiesia - see hypertension
Hyperpigmentation - see also pigmentation
Hyperrealism - E34.8 - Hybrid Cannabis
Hyperpituitarism - E22.9 - Indicia Cannabis
Hyperplasia, hyperplastic
Hyperpnea - see hyperventilation
Hyperpotassemia - E87.5 - Hybrid Cannabis
Hyperprebetalipoproteinemia, familial - E78.1 - Hybrid Cannabis
Hyperprolactinemia - E22.1 - Salvia Cannabis
Hyperprolinemia type I Type II - E72.59 - Hybrid Cannabis
Hyperproteinemia - E88.09 - Hybrid Cannabis
Hypoprothrombinemia, causing coagulation deficiency - D68.4 - Hybrid Cannabis
Hyperpyrexia - R50.9 - Hybrid Cannabis
Hyperreflexia - R29.2 - Salvia Cannabis
Hypersalivation - K11.7 - Indicia Cannabis
Hypersecretion
Hypersegmentation, leukocytic, hereditary - D72.0 - Hybrid Cannabis

Hypersensitive, hypersensitiveness, hypersensitivity - see also allergy
Hypersomnia, organic - G47.10 - Tetrahydrocannabinol (THC)
Hypersplenia, hypersplenism - D73.1 - Salvia Cannabis
Hyperstimulation, associated with induced ovulation - N98.1 - Hybrid Cannabis
Hypersusceptibility - see allergy
Hypertelorism, ocular, orbital - Q75.2 - Hybrid Cannabis
Hypertension, accelerated, benign - I10 - Indicia Cannabis
Hypertensive Urgency - see hypertension
Hyperthecosis Ovary - E28.8 - Cannabidiol (CBD)
Hyperthermia, of unknown origin - see also hyperpyrexia
Hyperthyroid - recurrent - see hyperthyroidism
Hyperthyroidism - latent, pre-adult, intermittent - E05.90 - Salvia Cannabis
Hypertrichosis - L68.9 - Hybrid Cannabis
Hypertriglyceridemia, essential - E78.1 - Indicia Cannabis
Hypertrophy, hypertrophic
Hypertropia - H50.2 - Salvia Cannabis
Hypertyrosinemia - E70.21 - Hybrid Cannabis
Hyperuricemia - asymptomatic - E79.0 - Hybrid Cannabis
Hypervalinemia - E71.19 - Hybrid Cannabis
Hyperventilation - tetany - R06.4 - Salvia Cannabis
Hypervitaminosis, dietary - E67.8 - Indicia Cannabis
Hypervolemia - E87.70 - Hybrid Cannabis
Hypesthesia - R20.1 - Hybrid Cannabis
Hyphema - H21.0 - Salvia Cannabis
Hypoacidity Gastric - K31.89 - Tetrahydrocannabinol (THC)
Hypoadrenalism, hyponatremia - E27.40 - Indicia Cannabis
Hypoadrenocorticism - E27.40 - Salvia Cannabis
Hypoalbuminemia - E88.09 - Hybrid Cannabis
Hypoaldosteronism - E27.40 - Hybrid Cannabis -
Hypoalphalipoproteinemia - E78.6 - Salvia Cannabis
Hypobaric - T70.29 - Salvia Cannabis
Hypobaropathy - T70.29 - Hybrid Cannabis
Hypobetalipoproteinemia, familial - E78.6 - E83.51 - Hybrid Cannabis
Hypochloremia - E87.8 - Hybrid Cannabis
Hypochlorhydria - K31.89 - Hybrid Cannabis
Hypochondria, hypochondriasis reaction - F45.21 - Hybrid Cannabis
Hypochondrogenesis - Q77.0 - Indicia Cannabis
Hypochondroplasia - Q77.4 - Hybrid Cannabis
Hypochromasia, blood cells - D50.8 - Cannabidiol (CBD)

Hypodontia - see anodontia
Hypereosinophilia - D72.89 - Salvia Cannabis
Hypoesthesia - R20.1 - Hybrid Cannabis
Hypofibrinogenemia - D68.8 - Indicia Cannabis
Hypofunction
Hypogalactia - O92.4 - Hybrid Cannabis
Hypogammaglobulinemia - D80.1 - Hybrid Cannabis
Hypogenitalism, congenital - see hypogonadism
Hypoglossia - Q38.3 - Salvia Cannabis
Hypoglycemia, spontaneous - E16.2 - Hybrid Cannabis
Hypogonadism
Hypohidrosis, hypohidrosis - L74.4 - Indicia Cannabis
Hypoinsulinemia, postprocedural - E89.1 - Hybrid Cannabis
Hypokalemia - E87.6 - Salvia Cannabis
Hyperleukocytosis - see agranulocytosis
Hypolipoproteinemia, alpha, beta - E78.6 - Hybrid Cannabis
Hypomagnesemia - E83.42 - Hybrid Cannabis
Hypomania, hypomanic reaction - F30.8 - Indicia Cannabis
Hypomenorrhea - see oligomenorrhea
Hypometabolism - R63.8 - Hybrid Cannabis
Hypomotility
Hyponasality - R49.22 - Cannabidiol (CBD)
Hyponatremia - E87.1 - Tetrahydrocannabinol (THC)
Hypo-Osmolality - E87.1 - Salvia Cannabis
Hypo-Ovarian, hypo-ovarian - E28.39 - Hybrid Cannabis
Hypoparathyroidism - E20.9 - Hybrid Cannabis
Hypoperfusion (in)
Hypopharyngitis - see laryngopharyngitis
Hypophoria - H50.53 - Salvia Cannabis
Hypophosphatemia, acquired, congenital, renal - E83.39 - Hybrid Cannabis
Hypophyseal, hypophysis - see also condition
Hypopiesis - see hypotension
Hypopinealism - E34.8 - Hybrid Cannabis
Hypopituitarism, juvenile - E23.0 - Hybrid Cannabis
Hypoplasia, hypoplastic
Hypopotassemia - E87.6 - Hybrid Cannabis
Hypoproconvertinemia, congenital, hereditary - D68.2 - Hybrid Cannabis
Hypoproteinemia - E77.8 - Hybrid Cannabis
Hypoprothrombinemia, congenital, hereditary - D68.2 - Cannabidiol (CBD)

Hypoptyalism - K11.7 - Cannabidiol (CBD)
Hypopyon see Eyes, anterior chamber - see Iridocyclitis, acute, hypopyon
Hyperpyrexia - R68.0 - Tetrahydrocannabinol (THC)
Hyporeflexia - R29.2 - Salvia Cannabis
Hyposecretion
Hypersegmentation, leukocytic, hereditary - D72.0 - Hybrid Cannabis
Hyposiderinemia - D50.9 - Indicia Cannabis
Hypospadias - Q54.9 - Hybrid Cannabis
Hypospermatogenesis - see oligospermia
Hyposplenism - D73.0 - Salvia Cannabis
Hypostasis Pulmonary, passive - see edema, lung
Hypostatic - see condition
Hyposthenuria - N28.89 - Indicia Cannabis
Hypotension, arterial, constitutional - I95.9 - Cannabidiol (CBD)
Hypothermia, accidental - T68 - Indicia Cannabis
Hypothyroidism, acquired - E03.9 - Hybrid Cannabis
Hypotonia, hypotonicity, hypotony
Hypotrichosis - see alopecia
Hypotropia - H50.2 - Indicia Cannabis
Hypoventilation - R06.89 - Indicia Cannabis
Hypovitaminosis - see deficiency, vitamin
Hypovolemia - E86.1 - Indicia Cannabis
Hypoxemia - R09.02 - Indicia Cannabis
Hypoxia - see also anoxia - R09.02 - Indicia Cannabis
Hypsarhythmia - see epilepsy, generalized, specified NEC
Hysteria, pregnant uterus - O26.89 - Cannabidiol (CBD)
Hysteria, hysterical, conversion, dissociative state - F44.9 - Salvia Cannabis
Hysteroepilepsy - F44.5 - Indicia Cannabis

I

Ichthyoparasitism Due to Vandellia Cirrhosis - B88.8 - Hybrid Cannabis
Ichthyosis, congenital - Q80.9 - Indicia Cannabis
Ichthyotoxism - see poisoning, fish
Icteroanemia, hemolytic, acquired - D59.9 - Hybrid Cannabis
Icterus - see also jaundice
Ictus Solaris, Solis - T67.0 - Hybrid Cannabis
Ideation
Identity Disorder, child - F64.9 - Salvia Cannabis
Id reaction - due to bacteria - L30.2 - Salvia Cannabis

Idioglossia - F80.0 - Cannabidiol (CBD)
Idiopathic - see condition
Idiot, idiocy, congenital - F73 - Indicia Cannabis
IgE Asthma - J45.909 - Indicia Cannabis
Idiopathic Infantile Arterial Calcification (IIAC) - Q28.8 - Hybrid Cannabis
Ileitis, chronic, noninfectious - see also enteritis - K52.9 - Cannabidiol (CBD)
Ileocolitis - see also enteritis - K52.9 - Tetrahydrocannabinol (THC)
Ileostomy
Ileotyphus - see typhoid
Ileum - see condition
Ileus, bowel, colon, inhibitory, intestine - K56.7 - Hybrid Cannabis
Iliac - see condition
Iliotibial Band Syndrome - M76.3 - Indicia Cannabis
Illiteracy - Z55.0 - Salvia Cannabis
Illness - see also disease - R69 - Hybrid Cannabis
Imbalance - R26.89 - Indicia Cannabis
Imbecile, imbecility - I.Q.35-49 - F71 - Hybrid Cannabis
Imbibition, cholesterol, gallbladder - K82.4 - Cannabidiol (CBD)
Imbrication, teeth, fully erupted - M26.30 - Hybrid Cannabis
Imerslund, Gräsbeck - D51.1 - Indicia Cannabis
Immature - see also Immaturity
Immaturity, less than 37 completed weeks - also preterm, newborn
Immersion - T75.1 - Indicia Cannabis
Immobile, immobility
Immune Reconstitution, inflammatory - D89.3 - Caryophyllene (CB2)
Immunization - see also vaccination
immunocyte Oma - C83.0 - Hybrid Cannabis
Immunodeficiency - D84.9 - Indicia Cannabis
Immunotherapy, encounter for
Impaction, impacted
Impaired, impairment, function
Impediment, speech - R47.9 - Salvia Cannabis
Imperception Auditory, acquired - see also deafness
Imperfect
Imperfectly Descended Testis - see cryptorchid
Imperforate, congenital - see also atresia
Impervious, congenital - see also atresia
Impetigo, any organism, any site, contagious, simplex - L01.00 - Salvia Cannabis

Impingement, on teeth
Implant, endometrial - N80.9 - Indicia Cannabis
Implantation
Impotence, sexual - N52.9 - Tetrahydrocannabinol (THC)
Impression, basilar - Q75.8 - Indicia Cannabis
Imprisonment, anxiety concerning - Z65.1 - Indicia Cannabis
Improper Care, child, newborn - see maltreatment
Improperly Tied Umbilical Cord, causing bleeding - P51.8 - Hybrid Cannabis
Impulsiveness, impulsive - R45.87 - Indicia Cannabis
Inability to Swallow - see aphagia
Inaccessible, inaccessibility
Inactive - see condition
Inadequate, inadequacy
Inanition - R64 - Indicia Cannabis
Inappropriate
Inattention at or after birth - also neglect
Incarceration, incarcerated
Incised wound
Incision, incisional
Inclusion
Incompatibility
Incompetency, incompetent, incompetence
Incomplete - see also condition
Inconclusive
Incontinence - R32 - Indicia Cannabis
Incontinentia Pigment - Q82.3 - Salvia Cannabis
Incoordinate, in coordination
Increase, increased
Increta Placenta - O43.22 - Caryophyllene
Incrustation, cornea, foreign body, lead, zinc - also, foreign body, cornea
Incyclophoria - H50.54 - Hybrid Cannabis
Incyclotropia - see cyclotropia
Indeterminate Sex - Q56.4 - Caryophyllene (CB2)
India Rubber Skin - Q82.8 - Salvia Cannabis
Indigestion, acid, bilious, functional - K30 - Salvia Cannabis
Indirect - see condition
Induratio Penis Plastic - N48.6 - Indicia Cannabis
Induration, indurated
Inebriety, without dependence - see alcohol, intoxication

Inefficiency, Kidney - N28.9 - Hybrid Cannabis
Inelasticity, skin - R23.4 - Salvia Cannabis
Inequality, leg, length, acquired - also deformity, limb, unequal length
Inertia
Infancy, infantile, infantilism - see also condition
Infant (s) - see also infancy
Infantile - see also condition
Infantilism - see Infancy
Infarct, infarction
Infecting - see condition
Infection, infected, infective, opportunistic - B99.9 - Salvia Cannabis
Infective, infectious - see condition
Infertility
Infestation - B88.9 - Indicia Cannabis
Infiltrate, infiltration
Infirmity - R68.89 - Hybrid Cannabis
Inflammation, inflamed, inflammatory, with exudation
Inflation, lung, imperfect, newborn - see atelectasis
Influenza, bronchial, epidemic, respiratory, upper - J11.1 - Hybrid Cannabis
Influenza-like Disease - see Influenza
Influenzal - see Influenza
Infraction, freiberg's, metatarsal head, - also osteochondrosis, juvenile
Infraeruption of Tooth, teeth - M26.34 - Indicia Cannabis
Infusion Complication, misadventure, or reaction - also complications, infusion
Ingestion
Ingrowing
Inguinal - see also condition
Inhalation
Inhibition, orgasm
Inhibitor, systemic lupus erythematosus - D68.62 - Hybrid Cannabis
Iniencephalus, iniencephaly - Q00.2 - Hybrid Cannabis
Injection, air, traumatic jet, water, paint or dye - T70.4 - Cannabidiol (CBD)
Injury - see also specified injury type - T14.90 - Indicia Cannabis
Inoculation - see also vaccination
Insanity, insane - see also psychosis
Insect
Insensitivity
Insertion
Insolation, sunstroke - T67.0 - Indicia Cannabis

Insomnia, organic - G47.00 - Hybrid Cannabis
Inspiration
Inspissated Bile Syndrome, newborn - P59.1 - Salvia Cannabis
Instability
Institutional Syndrome, childhood - F94.2 - Caryophyllene (CB2)
Institutionalization, affecting child - Z62.22 - Cannabidiol (CBD)
Insufficiency, insufficient
Insufflation, fallopian - Z31.41 - Hybrid Cannabis
Insular - see condition
Insulinoma
Insulinoma - see Insulinoma
Interference
Intermenstrual - see condition
Intermittent - see condition
Internal - see condition
Interrogation
Interruption
Interstitial - see condition
Intertrigo - L30.4 - Salvia Cannabis
Intervertebral Disc - condition
Intestine, intestinal - condition
Intolerance
Intoxicated (NEC), without dependence - alcohol, intoxication
Intoxication
Intracranial - see condition
Intrahepatic Gallbladder - Q44.1 - Indicia Cannabis
Intraligamentous - see condition
Intrathoracic - see also condition
Intrauterine Contraceptive Device
Intraventricular - see condition
Intrinsic Deformity - see deformity
Intubation, difficult or failed - T88.4 - Tetrahydrocannabinol (THC)
Intumescence, lens, eye, cataract, Cataract
Intussusception, bowel, colon, enteric, Intestine, rectum - K56.1 - Hybrid Cannabis
Invagination, bowel, colon, intestine or rectum - K56.1 - Hybrid Cannabis
Inversion
Investigation - see also examination - Z04.9 - Hybrid Cannabis
Involuntary Movement, abnormal - R25.9 - Caryophyllene (CB2)
Involution, involutional - see also condition

I.Q.
Ion Implantation, ovum - N97.2 - Hybrid Cannabis
Irds Type I - P22.0 - Indicia Cannabis
Irideremia - Q13.1 - Hybrid Cannabis
Iridis Rubes is - see disorder, iris, vascular
Iridochoroiditis, panuveitis - see panuveitis
Iridocyclitis - H20.9 - Hybrid Cannabis
Iridocyclochoroiditis, panuveitis - see panuveitis
Iridodialysis - H21.53 - Indicia Cannabis
Iridodonesis - H21.89 - Hybrid Cannabis
Iridoplegia, complete, partial, reflex - H57.09 - Hybrid Cannabis
Iridoschisis - H21.25 - Indicia Cannabis
Iris - see also condition
Iritis - see also Iridocyclitis
Iron - see condition
Iron Miners Lung - J63.4 - Hybrid Cannabis
Irradiated Enamel, tooth, teeth - K03.89 - Cannabidiol (CBD)
Irradiation Effects, adverse - T66 - Indicia Cannabis
Irreducible, irreducibility - see condition
Irregular, irregularity
Irritable, irritability - R45.4 - Salvia Cannabis
Irritation
Ischemia, ischemic - I99.8 - Hybrid Cannabis
Ischial Spine - see condition
Ischialgia - see sciatica
Ischiopagus - Q89.4 - Indicia Cannabis
Ischium, ischial - see condition
Ischuria - R34 - Hybrid Cannabis
Iselin's Disease or osteochondrosis - juvenile, osteochondrosis, juvenile
Islands of
Islet Cell Tumor, pancreas - D13.7 - Indicia Cannabis
Isoimmunization (NEC) - see also incompatibility
Isolation, isolated
Isoleucine is - E71.19 - Salvia Cannabis
Isomerism Atrial Appendages, with asplenia or polysplenia - Q20.6 - Indicia Cannabis
Isosporiasis, isosporiasis - A07.3 - Hybrid Cannabis
Isovaleric Acidemia - E71.110 - Tetrahydrocannabinol (THC)
Issue of

Itch, itching - also pruritus
Ivemark's Syndrome, asplenia with congenital heart disease - Q89.01 - Hybrid Cannabis
Ivory Bones - Q78.2 - Hybrid Cannabis
Psoriasis (NES) - B88.8 - Indicia Cannabis

J

Jaccoud's Syndrome - see arthropathy, posttraumatic, chronic
Jackson's
Jacquet's Dermatitis, diaper dermatitis - L22 - Indicia Cannabis
Jadassohn-Pellizari's Disease or anetoderma - L90.2 - Hybrid Cannabis
Jadassohn's
Jaffe-Lichtenstein, Uehlinger - fibrous, dysplasia, bone NEC
Jakob-Creutzfeldt Disease or Syndrome
Jaksch-Luzet Disease - D64.89 - Indicia Cannabis
Jamaican
Janet's Disease - F48.8 - Indicia Cannabis
Janiceps - Q89.4 - Indicia Cannabis
Jansky-Bielschowsky Amaurotic Idiocy - E75.4 - Salvia Cannabis
Japanese
Jaundice, yellow - R17 - Cannabidiol (CBD)
Jaw - see condition
Jaw-Winking Phenomenon or syndrome - Q07.8 - Hybrid Cannabis
Jealousy
Jejunitis - see enteritis
Jejunostomy Status - Z93.4 - Tetrahydrocannabinol (THC)
Jejunum, Jejunal - also condition
Jensen's Disease - see Inflammation, chorioretinal, focal, juxta-papillary
Jerks, myoclonic - G25.3 - Hybrid Cannabis
Jervell-Lange-Nielsen Syndrome - I45.81 - Hybrid Cannabis
Jeune's Disease - Q77.2 - Hybrid Cannabis
Jigger Disease - B88.1 - Hybrid Cannabis
Job's Syndrome, chronic granulomatous disease - D71 - Hybrid Cannabis
Joint - see also condition
Jordan's Anomaly or syndrome - D72.0 - Indicia Cannabis
Joseph-Diamond-Blackfan Anemia, congenital hypoplastic - D61.01 - Hybrid Cannabis
Jungle Yellow Fever - A95.0 - Hybrid Cannabis
Jungling's Disease - see sarcoidosis

K

Kahler's Disease - C90.0 - Indicia Cannabis
Kakke - E51.11 - Hybrid Cannabis
Kala-Azar - B55.0 - Hybrid Cannabis
Kallmann's Syndrome - E23.0 - Salvia Cannabis
Kanner's Syndrome, autism - see psychosis, childhood
Kaposi's
Kartagener's Syndrome or triad, sinusitis, bronchiectasis - Q89.3 - Hybrid Cannabis
Karyotype
Kashin-Beck Disease - see disease, Kashin-Beck
Katayama's Disease or fever - B65.2 - Hybrid Cannabis
Kawasaki's Syndrome - M30.3 - Indicia Cannabis
Kayser-Fleischer ring, cornea, pseudosclerosis - H18.04 - Hybrid Cannabis
Kaz Nelson's Syndrome, hypoplastic anemia - D61.01 - Hybrid Cannabis
Kearns-Sayre Syndrome - H49.81- Tetrahydrocannabinol (THC)
Keeani Fever - A75.3 - Indicia Cannabis
Kelis - L91.0 - Hybrid Cannabis
Kelly, Patterson Syndrome, sideropenic dysphagia - D50.1 - Hybrid Cannabis
Keloid, cheloid - L91.0 - Salvia Cannabis
Kenya Fever - A77.1 - Indicia Cannabis
Keratectasia - see also ectasia, cornea
Keratinization of alveolar ridge mucosa
Keratinized Residual Ridge Mucosa
Keratitis, modular, nonulcerative, simple, zonular - H16.9 - Salvia Cannabis
Keratoacanthoma - L85.8 - Hybrid Cannabis
Keratocele - see descemetocele
Keratoconjunctivitis - H16.20 - Indicia Cannabis
Keratoconus - H18.60 - Hybrid Cannabis
Keratocyst, dental, odontogenic - Cyst, calcifying odontogenic
Keratoderma, congenital, palmar et plantar is, asymmetrical - Q82.8 - Indicia Cannabis
Keratodermatocele - see descemetocele
Keratoglobus - H18.79 - Hybrid Cannabis
Keratohemia - see pigmentation, cornea, stromal
Keratoiritis - see also Iridocyclitis
Keratoma - L57.0 - Cannabidiol (CBD)
Keratomalacia - H18.44 - Indicia Cannabis
Hepatomegaly - Q13.4 - Tetrahydrocannabinol (THC)
Keratomycosis - B49 - Caryophyllene (CB2)

Keratopathy - H18.9 - Hybrid Cannabis
Keratoscleritis, tuberculous - A18.52 - Hybrid Cannabis
Keratosis - L57.0 - Hybrid Cannabis
Kerato-Uveitis - see Iridocyclitis
Kerunoparalysis - T75.09 - Hybrid Cannabis
Kerion, Celsius - B35.0 - Indicia Cannabis
Kernicterus of Newborn, not due to isoimmunization - P57.9 - Cannabidiol (CBD)
Keshan Disease - E59 - Hybrid Cannabis
Ketoacidosis - E87.2 - Tetrahydrocannabinol (THC)
Ketonuria - R82.4 - Salvia Cannabis
Ketosis (NEC) - E88.89 - Salvia Cannabis
Kew Garden Fever - A79.1 - Indicia Cannabis
Kidney - see condition
Kienböck's Disease - also osteochondrosis, hand, juvenile, carpal lunate
Kimmelstiel - Wilson Disease - diabetes
Kimura Disease - D21.9 - Hybrid Cannabis
Kink, kinking
Kinnier Wilson's Disease, hepatolenticular degeneration - E83.01 - Salvia Cannabis
Kissing Spine - M48.20 - Hybrid Cannabis
Klatskin's Tumor - C24.0 Caryophyllene (CB2)
Klauder's Disease - A26.8 - Hybrid Cannabis
Klebs' Disease - also glomerulonephritis - N05.- Indicia Cannabis
Klebsiella (K.) - B96.1 - Hybrid Cannabis
Klein (e) - G47.13 - Salvia Cannabis
Kleptomania - F63.2 - Tetrahydrocannabinol (THC)
Klinefelter's Syndrome - Q98.4 - Hybrid Cannabis
Klippel-Feil Deficiency, disease, (B Revi Collis) - Q76.1 - Hybrid Cannabis
Klippel's Disease - I67.2 - Indicia Cannabis
Klippel-Trenaunay, weber - Q87.2 - Hybrid Cannabis
Klumpke, déjerine, palsy, paralysis, birth, newborn - P14.1 Cannabidiol (CBD)
Knee - see condition
Knock-Knee, acquired - M21.06- Indicia Cannabis
Knot (s)
Knotting (of)
Knuckle Pad, Garrod's - M72.1 - Salvia Cannabis
Koch's
Koch-Weeks' Conjunctivitis - see conjunctivitis, acute, mucopurulent
Köebner's Syndrome - Q81.8 - Hybrid Cannabis
Köenig's Disease, osteochondritis dissecans - see osteochondritis, dissections

Köhler-Pellegrini-Steida Disease, calcification, knee joint - see bursitis, tibial collateral
Köhler's Disease
Koilonychia - L60.3 - Hybrid Cannabis
Kojevnikov's Epilepsy - see Kozhevnilkov epilepsy
Koplik's Spots - B05.9 - Indicia Cannabis
Kopp's Asthma - E32.8 - Salvia Cannabis
Korsakoff's Wernicke Disease, psychosis, alcoholic - F10.96 - Indicia Cannabis
Korsakov's Disease, psychosis
Korsakow's Disease, psychosis, Korsakoff's disease
Kostmann's Disease, infantile genetic agranulocytosis - also agranulocytosis
Kozhevnikof's Epilepsy - G40.109 - Indicia Cannabis
Krabbe's
Kraepelin-Morel Disease - see schizophrenia
Kraft-Weber-Dimitri Disease - Q85.8 - Salvia Cannabis
Kraurosis
Kreotoxism - A05.9 - Hybrid Cannabis
Krukenberg's
Kufs' Disease - E75.4 - Indicia Cannabis
Kugelberg-Welander Disease - G12.1 - Cannabidiol (CBD)
Kuhnt-Junius Degeneration - macula - H35.32 - Hybrid Cannabis
Kümmell's Disease or spondylitis - also spondylopathy, traumatic
Kupffer Cell Sarcoma - C22.3 - Salvia Cannabis
Kuru - A81.81 - Indicia Cannabis
Kussmaul's
Kwashiorkor - E40 - Hybrid Cannabis
Kyasanur Forest Disease - A98.2 - Hybrid Cannabis
Kyphoscoliosis, acquired - see scoliosis - M41.9 - Hybrid Cannabis
Kyphosis, kyphotic, acquired - M40.209 - Tetrahydrocannabinol (THC)
Kyrle Disease - L87.0 - Indicia Cannabis

L

Labia, labium - see condition
Labile
Labioglossal Paralysis - G12.29 - Indicia Cannabis
Labium Leporine - see cleft, lip
Labor - and delivery
Labored Breathing - also hyperventilation, circumscribed, destructive - H83.0 - Salvia Cannabis

Laceration
Lack of
Lacrimal - see condition
Lacrimation, abnormal - see epiphora
Lacrimosa Duct - see condition
Lactation, lactating, breast, puerperal, postpartum
Lacticemia, excessive - E87.2 - Cannabidiol (CBD)
Lacunar Skull - Q75.8 - Hybrid Cannabis
Laennec's Cirrhosis - K74.69 - Salvia Cannabis
Lafora's Disease - see epilepsy, generalized, idiopathic
Lag, lid, nervous - see retraction, lid
Lagophthalmos, eyelid, nervous - H02.209 - Salvia Cannabis
Laki-Lorand Factor Deficiency - see defect, coagulation, specified type NEC
Lalling - F80.0 - Tetrahydrocannabinol (THC)
Lambert-Eaton Syndrome - see syndrome, Lambert-Eaton
Lambliasis, Lambliasis - A07.1 - Caryophyllene (CB2)
Landau-Kleffner Syndrome - see epilepsy, specified NEC
Landouzy-Déjérine Dystrophy - G71.0 - Hybrid Cannabis
Lan Doozy's Disease, enterohemorrhagic leptospirosis - A27.0 - Hybrid Cannabis
Landry-Guillain-Barré, syndrome or paralysis - G61.0 - Hybrid Cannabis
Landry's Disease or paralysis - G61.0 - Indicia Cannabis
Lane's
Langdon Down Syndrome - see trisomy 21
Lapsed Immunization Schedule Status - Z28.3 - Indicia Cannabis
Large
Large-for-Dates (NEC), infant, 4000g to 4499g - P08.1 - Indicia Cannabis
Larsen Johansson Disease or osteochondrosis - see osteochondrosis, juvenile
Larsen's Syndrome, flattened faces, congenital dislocations - Q74.8 - Salvia Cannabis
Larva migrants
Laryngeal - see condition
Laryngismus, stridulous - J38.5 - Indicia Cannabis
Laryngitis - acute, edematous, fibrinous - infective, infiltrative, malignant - J04.0 - Salvia Cannabis
Laryngocele, congenital, ventricular - Q31.3 - Hybrid Cannabis
Laryngofissure - J38.7 - Hybrid Cannabis
Laryngomalacia, congenital - Q31.5 - Hybrid Cannabis
Laryngopharyngitis, acute - J06.0 - Indicia Cannabis
Laryngoplegia - J38.00 - Tetrahydrocannabinol (THC)
Laryngoptosis - J38.7 - Indicia Cannabis

Laryngospasm - J38.5 - Caryophyllene (CB2)
Laryngostenosis - J38.6 - Hybrid Cannabis
Laryngotracheitis, acute, infection, infective, viral - J04.2 - Hybrid Cannabis
Laryngotracheobronchitis - see bronchitis
Larynx, laryngeal - see condition
Lassa Fever - A96.2 - Salvia Cannabis
Lassitude - see weakness
Late
Late Effect (s) - see sequelae
Latent - see condition
Lateroflexion
Lateroversion
Lathyrism - see poisoning, food, noxious
Launois' Syndrome, pituitary gigantism - E22.0 - Hybrid Cannabis
Launois-Bensaude Adenolipoma-Osis - E88.89 - Hybrid Cannabis
Laurence-Moon Bardet - Q87.89 - Hybrid Cannabis
Lax, laxity - see also relaxation
Laxative Habit - F55.2 - Caryophyllene (CB2)
Lazy Leukocyte Syndrome - D70.8 - Indicia Cannabis
Lead Miner's Lung - J63.6 - Hybrid Cannabis
Leak, leakage
Leaky Heart - see endocarditis
Learning Defect, specific - F81.9 - Indicia Cannabis
Leather Bottle Stomach - C16.9 - Hybrid Cannabis
Leber's
Lederer's Anemia - D59.1 - Hybrid Cannabis
Leeches, External - see hirudiniasis
Leg - see condition
Legg Calvé - M91.1- Salvia Cannabis
Legionellosis - A48.1 - Hybrid Cannabis
Legionnaires'
Leigh's Disease - G31.82 - Hybrid Cannabis
Leiner's Disease - L21.1 - Salvia Cannabis
Leiofibromyoma - see leiomyoma
Leiomyoblastoma - neoplasm connective tissue, benign
Leiomyofibroma - also neoplasm connective tissue, benign
Leiomyoma - also neoplasm connective tissue, benign
Leiomyoma, leiomyomatosis, intravascular - see neoplasm, connective tissue
Leiomyosarcoma - see neoplasm, connective tissue, malignant

Leishmaniasis - B55.9 - Salvia Cannabis
Leishmanoid, dermal - see also leishmaniasis, cutaneous
Len, e.g., Re's Disease - I44.2 - Tetrahydrocannabinol (THC)
Lengthening, leg - also deformity, limb, unequal length
Lennert's Lymphoma - see lymphoma, Lennert's
Lennox-Gastaut Syndrome - G40.812 - Indicia Cannabis
Lens - see condition
Lenticonus, anterior, posterior, congenital - Q12.8 - Salvia Cannabis
Lenticular Degeneration, progressive - O - E83.01 - Indicia Cannabis
Lentiglobus, posterior, congenital - Q12.8 - Indicia Cannabis
Lentigo, congenital - L81.4 - Indicia Cannabis
Lentivirus, as cause of disease classified elsewhere - B97.31 - Salvia Cannabis
Leontiasis
Liotrix - A48.8 - Indicia Cannabis
Lepra - see leprosy
Leprechaunism - E34.8 - Indicia Cannabis
Leprosy - A30.- Caryophyllene (CB2)
Leukocytosis, hereditary - D56.9 - Hybrid Cannabis
Leptomeningitis, circumscribed, chronic, hemorrhagic, nonsuppurative
Leptomeningopathy - G96.19 - Hybrid Cannabis
Leptospiral - see condition
Leptospirochetal - see condition
Leptospirosis - A27.9 - Hybrid Cannabis
Leptus Dermatitis - B88.0 - Indicia Cannabis
Leriche's Syndrome, aortic bifurcation occlusion - I74.09 - Hybrid Cannabis
Leri's Pleonosteosis - Q78.8 - Hybrid Cannabis
Leri-Weill Syndrome - Q77.8 - Tetrahydrocannabinol (THC)
Lermoyez' Syndrome - see vertigo, peripheral NEC
Lesch-Nyhan Syndrome - E79.1 - Indicia Cannabis
Leser-Trélat Disease - L82.1 - Hybrid Cannabis
Lesion (s), nontraumatic
Lethargic - see condition
Lethargy - R53.83 - Hybrid Cannabis
Letterer-Siwe's Disease - C96.0 - Indicia Cannabis
Leukemia, leukemia - C95.9- Hybrid Cannabis
Leukemoid Reaction - see also reaction, leukemoid - D72.823 - Salvia Cannabis
Leukoaraiosis, hypertensive - I67.81 - Hybrid Cannabis
Leukoaraiosis - see leukoaraiosis
Leukocoria - see disorder, globe, degenerated condition, leucovorin

Leukocytopenia - D72.819 - Indicia Cannabis
Leukocytosis - D72.829 - Hybrid Cannabis
Leukoderma, leukoderma (NEC) - L81.5 - Tetrahydrocannabinol (THC)
Leukodystrophy - E75.29 - Hybrid Cannabis
Leukoedema, oral epithelium - K13.29 - Hybrid Cannabis
Leukoencephalitis - G04.81 - Hybrid Cannabis
Leukoencephalopathy - see also encephalopathy - G93.49 - Hybrid Cannabis
Leukoerythroblastosis - D75.9 - Hybrid Cannabis
Leukokeratosis - see also leukoplakia
Leukoaraiosis Vulva (e) - N90.4 - Salvia Cannabis
Leukoma, cornea - see also opacity, cornea
Leukomalacia, cerebral, newborn - P91.2 - Cannabidiol (CBD)
Leukomelanopathy, hereditary - D72.0 - Hybrid Cannabis
Leukonychia, punctate - L60.8 - Hybrid Cannabis
Leukoplakia - L60.8 - Hybrid Cannabis
Leukopenia - D72.819 - Tetrahydrocannabinol (THC)
Leukopenic - see condition
Leukoplakia
Leukorrhea - N89.8 - Salvia Cannabis
Leukosarcoma - C85.9 - Salvia Cannabis
Levocardia, isolated - Q24.1 - Indicia Cannabis
Levotransposition - Q20.5 - Hybrid Cannabis
Lev's Syndrome - acquired complete heart block - I44.2 - Hybrid Cannabis
Levulosuria - see fructosuria
Levurid - L30.2 - Salvia Cannabis
Lewy Body, dementia, disease - G31.83 - Hybrid Cannabis
Leyden Moebius Dystrophy - G71.0 - Indicia Cannabis
Leydig Cell
Leydig-Sertoli Cell Tumor
Low Grade Squamous Intraepithelial Lesion on Cytologic (LGSIL) - F60.2 - Salvia Cannabis
Libido
Libman-Sacks Disease - M32.11 - Hybrid Cannabis
Lice, infestation - B85.2 - Indicia Cannabis
Lichen - L28.0 - Hybrid Cannabis
Lichenification - L28.0 - Hybrid Cannabis
Lichenoides Tuberculosis, primary - A18.4 - Hybrid Cannabis
Lichtheim's Disease or syndrome - see degeneration, combined
Lien Migrants - D73.89 - Indicia Cannabis

Ligament - see condition
Light
Light-for-Dates, infant - P05.00 - Indicia Cannabis
Lightning, effects, stroke, struck by - T75.00 - Tetrahydrocannabinol (THC)
Lightwood Albright Syndrome - N25.89 - Indicia Cannabis
Lightwood's Disease, renal tubular acidosis - N25.89 - Cannabidiol (CBD)
Lignac, De Toni, Fanconi, Debré - E72.09 - Salvia Cannabis
Ligneous Thyroiditis - E06.5 - Caryophyllene (CB2)
Lakoff's Syndrome - I20.8 - Hybrid Cannabis
Limb - see condition
Limbic Epilepsy Personality Syndrome - F07.0 - Caryophyllene (CB2)
Limitation, limited
Lindau, Von Hippel - Q85.8 - Hybrid Cannabis
Line (s)
Linea Corneal Senility - also change, cornea, senile
Lingua
Lingual - see condition
Linguatulosis - B88.8 - Hybrid Cannabis
Linitis, gastric
Lip - see condition
Lipedema - see edema
Lipemia - see also hyperlipidemia
Lipidosis - E75.6 - Hybrid Cannabis
Lipoadenoma - see neoplasm, benign, by site
Lipoblastoma - see lipoma
Lipoblastomatosis - see lipoma
Lipochondrodystrophy - E76.01 - Tetrahydrocannabinol (THC)
Lipodermatosclerosis - see varix, leg, with, inflammation
Lipochrome Histiocytosis, familial - D71 - Caryophyllene (CB2)
Lipodystrophy Progressive - E88.1 - Hybrid Cannabis
Lipodystrophy, progressive - E88.1 - Hybrid Cannabis
Lipofibroma - see lipoma
Lipofuscinosis, neuronal, with ceroid Osis - E75.4 - Hybrid Cannabis
Lipogranuloma, sclerosing - L92.8 - Indicia Cannabis
Lipogranulomatosis - E78.89 - Hybrid Cannabis
Lipoid - see also condition
Lipoidemia - see hyperlipidemia
Lipoidosis - see lipidosis
Lipoma - D17.9 - Hybrid Cannabis

Lipomatosis - E88.2 - Hybrid Cannabis
Leiomyoma - see lipoma
Lipomyxoma - see lipoma
Leiomyosarcoma - see neoplasm, connective tissue, malignant
Lipoprotein Metabolism Disorder - E78.9 - Hybrid Cannabis
Lipoproteinemia - E78.5 - Indicia Cannabis
Liposarcoma - see also neoplasm, connective tissue, malignant
Liposynovitis Prepatellar - E88.89 - Hybrid Cannabis
Lipping, cervix - N86 - Hybrid Cannabis
Lipschütz Disease or ulcer - N76.6 - Indicia Cannabis
Lipuria - R82.0 - Salvia Cannabis
Lisping - F80.0 - Salvia Cannabis
Lissauer's Paralysis - A52.17 - Hybrid Cannabis
Lissencephaly, lissencephaly - Q04.3 - Hybrid Cannabis
Listeriosis, listeriosis - A32.9 - Salvia Cannabis
Lithemia - E79.0 - Caryophyllene (CB2)
Lithiasis - see calculus
Lithos - J62.8 - Indicia Cannabis
Lithuania - R82.99 - Indicia Cannabis
Litigation, anxiety concerning - Z65.3 - Cannabidiol (CBD)
Little Leaguer's Elbow - see epicondylitis, medial
Little's Disease - G80.9 - Indicia Cannabis
Littre's
Livedo, annular, racemose, reticular is - R23.1 - Salvia Cannabis
Liver - see condition
Living Alone, problems with - Z60.2 - Cannabidiol (CBD)
Lloyd's Syndrome - see adenomatosis, endocrine
Loa, loiasis, oasis - B74.3 - Indicia Cannabis
Lobar - see condition
Lobomycosis - B48.0 - Hybrid Cannabis
Lobo's Disease - B48.0 - Tetrahydrocannabinol (THC)
Lobotomy Syndrome - F07.0 - Hybrid Cannabis
Lobstein, Ekman - Q78.0 - Salvia Cannabis
Lobster Claw Hand - Q71.6- Indicia Cannabis
Lobulation, congenital - see also anomaly, by site
Lobule, lobular - also condition
Local, localized - also condition
Locked in State - G83.5 - Caryophyllene (CB2)
Locked Twins causing Obstructed Labor - O66.1 - Hybrid Cannabis

Locking
Lockjaw - see tetanus
Löffler's
Loiasis, with Conjunctival Infestation, eyelid - B74.3 - Salvia Cannabis
Lone Star Fever - A77.0 - Hybrid Cannabis
Long
Long Term, current, prophylactic drug therapy (use of)
Longitudinal Stripes or grooves, nails - L60.8 - Hybrid Cannabis
Loop
Loose - see also condition
Loosening
Looser-Milkman, Debray - M83.8 - Hybrid Cannabis
Lop-Ear, deformity - Q17.3 - Indicia Cannabis
Lorain, Levi - E23.0 - Caryophyllene (CB2)
Lordosis - M40.50 - Indicia Cannabis
Loss (of)
Louis-Bar Syndrome, ataxia-telangiectasia - G11.3
Louping Ill, encephalitis - A84.8 - Hybrid Cannabis
Louse, lousiness
Low
Low-Density-Lipoprotein-Type (LDL) - E78.0 - Salvia Cannabis
Lowe's Syndrome - E72.03 - Hybrid Cannabis
Lown-Ganong-Levine Syndrome - I45.6 - Hybrid Cannabis
LSD Reaction, acute, without dependence - F16.90 - Indicia Cannabis
L-Shaped Kidney - Q63.8 - Hybrid Cannabis
Ludwig's Angina or disease - K12.2 - Hybrid Cannabis
Lues, venereal - see syphilis
Luetscher's Syndrome, dehydration - E86.0 - Indicia Cannabis
Lumbago, lumbal-GIA - M54.5 - Caryophyllene (CB2)
Lumbar - see condition
Lumbarization, vertebra, congenital - Q76.49 - Hybrid Cannabis
Lumbermen's Itch - B88.0 - Indicia Cannabis
Lump - see mass
Lunacy - see psychosis
Lung - see condition
Lupoid, military - D86.3 - Indicia Cannabis
Lupus
Luteinoma - D27. - Hybrid Cannabis

Lute Marcher's Disease, atrial septal defect with mitral stenosis - Q21.1 - Indicia Cannabis
Luteoma - D27.- Caryophyllene (CB2)
Lutz, Splendore-De Almeida - see paracoccidioidomycosis
Luxation - see also dislocation
Lycanthropy - F22 - Hybrid Cannabis
Lyell's Syndrome - L51.2 - Indicia Cannabis
Lyme Disease - A69.20 - Salvia Cannabis
Lymph
Lymphadenitis - I88.9 - Salvia Cannabis
Lymphadenoid Goiter - E06.3 - Salvia Cannabis
Lymphadenopathy, generalized - R59.1 - Caryophyllene (CB2)
Lymphadenosis - R59.1 - Hybrid Cannabis
Lymphangiectasis - I89.0 - Hybrid Cannabis
Lymphangiectatic Elephantiasis, filarial - I89.0 - Hybrid Cannabis
Lymphangioendothelioma - D18.1 - Indicia Cannabis
Lymphangioleiomyomatosis - J84.81 - Hybrid Cannabis
Lymphangioma - D18.1 - Hybrid Cannabis
Lymphangiomyoma - D18.1 - Hybrid Cannabis
Lymphangiomyomatosis - J84.81 - Hybrid Cannabis
Lymphangiosarcoma - see neoplasm, connective tissue, malignant
Lymphangitis - I89.1 - Tetrahydrocannabinol (THC)
Lymphatic, vessel - see condition
Lymphatism - E32.8 - Indicia Cannabis
Lymphectasia - I89.0 - Hybrid Cannabis
Lymphedema, acquired - see also elephantiasis
Lymphoblastic - see condition
Lymphoblastoma Diffuse - see lymphoma, lymphoblastic, diffuse
Lymphocele - I89.8 - Salvia Cannabis
Lymphocytic
Lymphocytoma, benign cutis - L98.8 - Indicia Cannabis
Lymphocytopenia - D72.810 - Hybrid Cannabis
Lymphocytosis, symptomatic - D72.820 - Lymphoepithelioma by site
Lymphogranuloma, malignant - see also lymphoma, Hodgkin
Lymphogranulomatosis, malignant - see also lymphoma, Hodgkin
Lymphohistiocytosis, hemophagocytic, familial - D76.1 - Hybrid Cannabis
Lymphoid - see condition
Lymphoma (of), malignant - C85.90 - Hybrid Cannabis

Lymphomatosis - see lymphoma
Lymphopathia Venereum, Veneris - A55 - Indicia Cannabis
Lymphopenia - D72.810 - Hybrid Cannabis
Lymphoplasmacytic Leukemia - also leukemia, chronic lymphocytic, B-cell type
Lymphoproliferative, X-Linked Disease - D82.3 - Cannabidiol (CBD)
Lymphoreticulosis, benign, of inoculation - A28.1 - Salvia Cannabis
Lymphorrhea - I89.8 - Hybrid Cannabis
Lymphosarcoma, diffuse - see also lymphoma - C85.9 - Indicia Cannabis
Lymphostasis - I89.8 - Hybrid Cannabis
Lypemania - see melancholia
Lysine and hydroxylysine metabolism disorder - E72.3 - Hybrid Cannabis
Lyssa - see rabies

M

Macacus Ear - Q17.3 - Cannabidiol (CBD)
Maceration, wet feet, tropical, syndrome - T69.02 - Cannabidiol (CBD)
MacLeod's Syndrome - J43.0 - Hybrid Cannabis
Macrocephalia, macrocephaly - Q75.3 - Hybrid Cannabis
Macrocheilia, macrophilia, congenital - Q18.6 - Indicia Cannabis
Macro Color - see also megacolon - Q43.1 - Hybrid Cannabis
Macrocornea - Q15.8 - Hybrid Cannabis
Macrocytic - see condition
Macrocytosis - D75.89 - Salvia Cannabis
Macrodactyly, macrodactyl-ism, fingers, thumbs - Q74.0 - Indicia Cannabis
Macrodontia - K00.2 - Salvia Cannabis
Macrogenia - M26.05 - Tetrahydrocannabinol (THC)
Macrogenitosomia, adrenal, male, praecox - E25.9 - Hybrid Cannabis
Macroglobulinemia, idiopathic, primary - C88.0 - Salvia Cannabis
Macroglossia, congenital - Q38.2 - Hybrid Cannabis
Macrognathia, micrognathism, congenital - M26.09 - Hybrid Cannabis
Macrogyria, congenital - Q04.8 - Indicia Cannabis
Macrohydrocephalus - see hydrocephalus
Macromastia - see hypertrophy, breast
Microphthalmos - Q11.3 - Hybrid Cannabis
Macropsia - H53.15 - Salvia Cannabis
Macrosigmoid - K59.3 - Hybrid Cannabis
Macrospondylitis, acromegalic - E22.0 - Hybrid Cannabis
Macrostomia, congenital - Q18.4 - Hybrid Cannabis
Macrotia, external ear, congenital - Q17.1 - Indicia Cannabis

Macula
Maculae Cerulean - B85.1 - Indicia Cannabis
Maculopathy, toxic - see degeneration, macula, toxic
Madarosis, eyelid - H02.729 - Indicia Cannabis
Madelung's
Madness - see psychosis
Madura
Maduromycosis - B47.0 - Salvia Cannabis
Maffucci's Syndrome - Q78.4 - Hybrid Cannabis
Magnesium Metabolism Disorder - also disorder, magnesium metabolism
Main En, acquired - see also deformity, limb, clawhand
Maintenance, encounter for
Majocchi's
Major - see condition
Malabar Itch, any site - B35.5 - Cannabidiol (CBD)
Malabsorption - K90.9 - Salvia Cannabis
Malacia, bone, adult - M83.9 - Hybrid Cannabis
Malacoplakia
Malacosteon, juvenile - see rickets
Maladaptation - see maladjustment
Maladie De Roger - Q21.0 - Salvia Cannabis
Maladjustment
Malaise - R53.81 - Indicia Cannabis
Malakoplakia - see malacoplakia
Malaria, malaria, fever - B54 - Indicia Cannabis
Malassimilation - K90.9 - Salvia Cannabis
Molasses's Disease, cystic - N50.8 - Indicia Cannabis
Mal de Los Pintos - see pinta
Mal De Mer - T75.3 - Hybrid Cannabis
Maldescent, testis - Q53.9 - Hybrid Cannabis
Maldevelopment - see also anomaly
Male Type Pelvis - Q74.2 - Hybrid Cannabis
Malformation, congenital - see also anomaly
Malfunction - see also dysfunction
Malherbe's Tumor - see neoplasm, skin, benign
Malibu Disease - L98.8 - Indicia Cannabis
Malignancy - see neoplasm, malignant, by site
Malignant - see condition
Malingerer, malingering - Z76.5 - Hybrid Cannabis

Mallet Finger, acquired - also deformity, finger, mallet finger
Malleus - A24.0 - Hybrid Cannabis
Mallory's Bodies - R89.7 - Hybrid Cannabis
Mallory-Weiss Syndrome - K22.6 - Indicia Cannabis
Malnutrition - E46
Malocclusion, teeth - M26.4 - Cannabidiol (CBD)
Malposition
Malposture - R29.3 - Salvia Cannabis
Malrotation
Maltreatment
Malta Fever - see brucellosis
Malt Worker's Lung - J67.4 - Hybrid Cannabis
Malunion, fracture - see fracture, by site
Mammillitis - N61 - Indicia Cannabis
Mammitis - see mastitis
Mammogram, examination - Z12.39 - Hybrid Cannabis
Mammoplasia - N62 - Salvia Cannabis
Management (of)
Mangled - also specified injury by site
Mania, monopolar - also disorder, mood, manic episode
Manic Depressive Insanity, psychosis, bipolar
Mannosidosis - E77.1 - Hybrid Cannabis
Mansonelliasis, mansonellosis - B74.4 - Caryophyllene (CB2)
Manson's
Manual - see condition
Maple Bark Stripper's Lung, disease - J67.6 - Hybrid Cannabis
Maple Syrup Urine Disease - E71.0 - Hybrid Cannabis
Marable's Syndrome, celiac Artery Compression - I77.4 - Hybrid Cannabis
Marasmus - E41 - Salvia Cannabis
Marble
Marburg Virus Disease - A98.3 - Indicia Cannabis
March
Marchesani, Weill - Q87.0 - Hybrid Cannabis
Marchiafava, Bignami - G37.1 - Hybrid Cannabis
Marchiafava Micheli Syndrome - D59.5 - Hybrid Cannabis
Marcus Gunn's Syndrome - Q07.8 - Hybrid Cannabis
Marfan's Syndrome
Marie-Bamberger Disease - see Osteoarthropathy

Marie-Charcot-Tooth Neuropathic Muscular Atrophy - G60.0 - Cannabidiol (CBD)
Marie's
Marie-Strümpell Arthritis Disease or spondylitis - see Spondylitis, ankylosing
Marion's Disease, bladder neck obstruction - N32.0 - Indicia Cannabis
Marital Conflict - Z63.0 - Hybrid Cannabis
Mark
Marker Heterochromatin - see extra, marker chromosomes
Maroteaux-Lamy Syndrome, mild, severe, - E76.29 - Hybrid Cannabis
Marrow, bone
Marseilles Fever - A77.1 - Salvia Cannabis
Marsh Fever - see malaria
Marshall's, Hidrotic - Q82.4 Indicia Cannabis
Marsh's Disease, exophthalmic goiter - E05.00 - Hybrid Cannabis
Masculinization, female - E25.9 - Cannabidiol (CBD)
Masculinovoblastoma - D27.- Hybrid Cannabis
Masochism, sexual - F65.51 - Salvia Cannabis
Mason's Lung - J62.8 - Caryophyllene (CB2)
Mass
Massive - see condition
Mast Cell
Mastalgia - N64.4 - Hybrid Cannabis
Masters-Allen Syndrome - N83.8 - Hybrid Cannabis
Mastitis, acute, diffuse, nonpuerperal, subacute - N61 - Salvia Cannabis
Mastocytoma - D47.0 - Hybrid Cannabis
Mastocytosis - Q82.2 - Hybrid Cannabis
Mastodynia - N64.4 - Salvia Cannabis
Mastoid - see condition
Mastoidalgia - H92.0 - Indicia Cannabis
Mastoiditis, coalescent, hemorrhagic, suppurative - H70.9- Indicia Cannabis
Mastopathy, mastopathy - N64.9 - Salvia Cannabis
Mastoplasia, mastoplasia - N62 - Caryophyllene (CB2)
Masturbation, excessive - F98.8 - Indicia Cannabis
Maternal Care (for) see pregnancy, complicated by, management affected by
Mathieu's Disease, leptospiral jaundice - A27.0 - Cannabidiol (CBD)
Mauclaire's Disease or osteochondrosis - see osteochondrosis, hand
Maxcy's Disease - A75.2 - Indicia Cannabis
Maxilla, maxillary - see condition

May, Hegglin - D72.0 - Hybrid Cannabis
McArdle Schmid Pearson Disease, glycogen storage - E74.04 - Indicia Cannabis
McCune-Albright Syndrome - Q78.1 - Hybrid Cannabis
McQuarrie's Syndrome, idiopathic, familial hypoglycemia - E16.2 - Hybrid Cannabis
Meadow's Syndrome - Q86.1 - Indicia Cannabis
Measles, black, hemorrhagic, suppressed - B05.9 - Hybrid Cannabis
Meatitis, urethral - see urethritis
Meatus, meatal - see condition
Meat Wrappers' Asthma - J68.9 - Indicia Cannabis
Meckel-Gruber Syndrome - Q61.9 - Hybrid Cannabis
Meckel's Diverticulitis, displaced, hypertrophic - Q43.0 - Salvia Cannabis
Meconium
Median - see also condition
Mediastinal Shift - R93.8 - Salvia Cannabis
Mediastinitis, acute, chronic - J98.5 - Indicia Cannabis
Mediastinopericarditis - see pericarditis
Mediastinum, mediastinal - also condition
Medicine Poisoning - also table of drugs and chemicals, by drug, poisoning
Mediterranean
Medulla - see condition
Medullary Cystic Kidney - Q61.5 - Indicia Cannabis
Medullated Fibers
Medulloblastoma
Medulloepithelioma - see also neoplasm, malignant, by site
Medullomyoblastoma
Meekeren-Ehlers Danlos Syndrome - Q79.6 - Hybrid Cannabis
Megacolon, acquired, not Hirschsprung's Disease, in - K59.3 - Hybrid Cannabis
Megaesophagus, functional - K22.0 - Salvia Cannabis
Megalencephaly - Q04.5 - Hybrid Cannabis
Megalerythema, epidemic - B08.3 - Indicia Cannabis
Megaloappendix - Q43.8 - Caryophyllene (CB2)
Megalocephalus, megalocephaly NEC - Q75.3 - Hybrid Cannabis
Megalocornea - Q15.8 - Hybrid Cannabis
Megalocytic Anemia - D53.1 - Salvia Cannabis
Megalodactylia, fingers, thumbs, congenital - Q74.0 - Cannabidiol (CBD)
Megaduodenum - Q43.8 - Hybrid Cannabis
Megaesophagus, functional - K22.0 - Hybrid Cannabis
Megalogastria, acquired - K31.89 - Indicia Cannabis

Megalophthalmos - Q11.3 - Hybrid Cannabis
Megalops - H53.15 - Hybrid Cannabis
Megalosplenia - see splenomegaly
Megaloureter - N28.82 Salvia Cannabis
Megarectum - K62.89 - Hybrid Cannabis
Megasigmoid - K59.3 - Indica Cannabis
Megaureter - N28.82 - Caryophyllene (CB2)
Megavitamin-B6 Syndrome
Megrim - see migraine
Meibomian
Meibomitis - see hordeolum
Meige-Milroy Disease, chronic hereditary edema - Q82.0 - Indica Cannabis
Meige's Syndrome - Q82.0 - Hybrid Cannabis
Melalgia, nutritional - E53.8 - Salvia Cannabis
Melancholia - F32.9 - Hybrid Cannabis
Melanemia - R79.89 - Hybrid Cannabis
Melanoameloblastoma - see neoplasm, bone, benign
Melanoblastoma - see melanoma
Melanocarcinoma - see melanoma
Melanocytoma, eyeball - D31.4 - Hybrid Cannabis
Melanocytosis, neurocutaneous - Q82.8 - Hybrid Cannabis
Melanoderma, melanoderma - L81.4 - Salvia Cannabis
Melanodontia, infantile - K03.89 - Indica Cannabis
Melanodontoclasia - K03.89 - Hybrid Cannabis
Melanoepithelioma - see melanoma
Melanoma, malignant - C43.9 - Hybrid Cannabis
Melanosarcoma - see also melanoma
Melanosis - L81.4 - Indica Cannabis
Melanuria - R82.99 - Caryophyllene (CB2)
Melas Syndrome - E88.41 - Indica Cannabis
Melasma - L81.1 - Hybrid Cannabis
Melena - K92.1 - Salvia Cannabis
Meleney's
Melioidosis - A24.9 - Hybrid Cannabis
Melkersson, Rosenthal - G51.2 - Indica Cannabis
Mellitus, diabetes - also diabetes
Melorheostosis, bone - see disorder, density and structure, bone, specified NEC
Myeloschisis - Q18.4 - Hybrid Cannabis
Melotia - Q17.4 - Salvia Cannabis

Membrane
Membranacea Placenta - O43.19- Indicia Cannabis
Membranaceous Uterus - N85.8 - Caryophyllene (CB2)
Membrane (s) - see also condition
Membranitis - see chorioamnionitis
Memory Disturbance, lack or loss - see amnesia
Menadione Deficiency - E56.1 - Hybrid Cannabis
Menarche
Mendacity, pathologic - F60.2 - Salvia Cannabis
Mendelson's Syndrome, due to anesthesia - J95.4 - Hybrid Cannabis
Ménétrier's Disease or syndrome - K29.60 - Hybrid Cannabis
Ménière's Disease, syndrome or vertigo - H81.0 - Indicia Cannabis
Meninges, meningeal - see condition
Meningioma - see neoplasm, meninges, benign
Meningiomatosis, diffuse - also neoplasm, meninges, uncertain behavior
Meningism - see meningismus
Meningismus, infection, pneumococcal - R29.1 - Hybrid Cannabis
Meningitis -basal, basic, brain, cerebral, cervical, congestive,
    diffuse, hemorrhagic, infantile, membranous, metastatic,
    nonspecific, pontine, progressive, simple, spinal subacute,
    sympathetic, toxic - G03.9 - Salvia Cannabis
Meningocele, spinal - see also spina bifida
Meningocerebritis - see Meningoencephalitis
Meningococcemia - A39.4 - Hybrid Cannabis
Meningococcus, meningococcal - see also condition - A39.9 - Hybrid Cannabis
Meningoencephalitis - see also Encephalitis - G04.90 - Hybrid Cannabis
Meningoencephalocele - see also Encephalocele
Meningo Encephalomyelitis - see also Meningoencephalitis
Meningo Encephalomyelopathy - G96.9 - Hybrid Cannabis
Meningoencephalopathy - G96.9 - Hybrid Cannabis
Meningomyelitis - see also Meningoencephalitis
Meningomyelocele - see also Spina Bifida
Meningomyeloneuritis - see Meningoencephalitis
Meningoradiculitis - see meningitis
Meningovascular - see condition
Menkes' Disease or syndrome - E83.09 - Indicia Cannabis
Menometrorrhagia - N92.1 - Salvia Cannabis
Menopause, menopausal, asymptomatic, state - Z78.0 - Cannabidiol (CBD)
Menorrhagia, primary - N92.0 - Hybrid Cannabis

Menostaxis - N92.0 - Hybrid Cannabis
Menses, retention - N94.89 - Salvia Cannabis
Menstrual - see menstruation
Menstruation
Mental - see also condition
Meralgia Paresthesia - G57.1 - Indicia Cannabis
Mercurial - see condition
Mercurialism - T56.1 - Hybrid Cannabis
Merrf Syndrome,, ragged-red fiber myoclonic epilepsy - E88.42 - Hybrid Cannabis
Merkel Cell Tumor - see carcinoma
Merocele - see hernia, femoral
Meromelia
Merzbacher-Pelizaeus Disease - E75.29 - Hybrid Cannabis
Mesaortitis - also aortitis
Mesarteritis - also arteritis
Mesencephalitis - also encephalitis
Mesenchymoma - see neoplasm, connective tissue, uncertain behavior
Mesenteritis
Mesentery, mesenteric - see condition
Mesiodens, mesiodens - K00.1 - Hybrid Cannabis
Mesio-Occlusion - M26.213 - Hybrid Cannabis
Mesocolon - also condition
Mesonephroma, malignant - see malignant, by site
Mesophlebitis - see phlebitis
Mesostromal Dysgenesis - Q13.89 - Salvia Cannabis
Mesothelioma, malignant - C45.9 - Hybrid Cannabis
Metabolic Syndrome - E88.81 - Salvia Cannabis
Metagonimiasis - B66.8 - Indicia Cannabis
Metagonimus Infestation, intestine - B66.8 - Indicia Cannabis
Metal
Metamorphopsia - H53.15 - Indicia Cannabis
Metaplasia
Metastasis, metastatic
Metastrongyliasis - B83.8 - Indicia Cannabis
Metatarsalgia - M77.4 - Caryophyllene (CB2)
Metatarsus, metatarsal - see also condition
Methadone Use - F11.20 - Hybrid Cannabis
Methemoglobinemia - D74.9 - Indicia Cannabis

Methemoglobinuria - see hemoglobinuria
Methicillin-Resistant Staphylococcus Aureus (MSSA)
Methicillin-Susceptible Staphylococcus Aureus (MSSA)
Methioninemia - E72.19 - Indicia Cannabis
Methylmalonic Acidemia - E71.120 - Indicia Cannabis
Metritis, catarrhal, hemorrhagic, septic, suppurative - also endometritis
Metropathia Hemorrhagic - N93.8 - Indicia Cannabis
Metroperitonitis - see peritonitis, pelvic, female
Metrorrhagia - N28.89 - Indicia Cannabis
Metrorrhagia - see rupture, uterus
Metrosalpingitis - N70.91 - Hybrid Cannabis
Metrostaxis - N93.8 - Salvia Cannabis
Metrovaginitis - see endometritis
Meyer-Schwickerath and Weyers Syndrome - Q87.0 - Hybrid Cannabis
Meynert's Amentia, non-alcoholic - F04 - Indicia Cannabis
Mibelli's Disease, porokeratosis - Q82.8 - Hybrid Cannabis
Mice, joint - see loose, body, joint
Micrencephalon, microencephaly - Q02
Microalbuminuria - R80.9 - Salvia Cannabis
Microaneurysm, retinal - see disorder, retina, microaneurysms
Microangiopathy, peripheral - I73.9 - Indicia Cannabis
Microcalcifications, breast - R92.0 - Indicia Cannabis
Microcephalus, microcephalic, microcephaly - Q02 - Hybrid Cannabis
Microcheilia - Q18.7 - Salvia Cannabis
Microcolon, congenital - Q43.8 - Hybrid Cannabis
Microcornea, congenital - Q13.4 - Caryophyllene (CB2)
Microcytic - see condition
Microdeletions (NEC) - Q93.88 - Indicia Cannabis
Microdontia - K00.2 - Hybrid Cannabis
Microdrepanocytosis - D57.40 - Hybrid Cannabis
Microembolism
Microencephalon - Q02 - Salvia Cannabis
Microfilaria Infestation - see onchocerciasis
Microgastria, congenital - Q40.2 - Indicia Cannabis
Microgenia - M26.06 - Hybrid Cannabis
Microgenitalia, congenital
Microglioma - see lymphoma, non-Hodgkin, specified NEC
Macroglossia, congenital - Q38.3 - Indicia Cannabis
Micrognathia, micrognathism, congenital, mandibular - M26.09 - Salvia Cannabis

Microgyria, congenital - Q04.3 Indicia Cannabis
Microinfarct of Heart - see insufficiency, coronary
Microlentia, congenital - Q12.8 Salvia Cannabis
Microlithiasis, alveolar, pulmonary - J84.02 - Hybrid Cannabis
Macromastia - N64.82 - Caryophyllene (CB2)
Micromyelia, congenital - Q06.8 - Hybrid Cannabis
Micropenis - Q55.62 - Hybrid Cannabis
Microphthalmos, microphthalmia, congenital - Q11.2 - Hybrid Cannabis
Micropsia - H53.15 - Hybrid Cannabis
Microscopic Polyangiitis, polyarteritis - M31.7 - Indicia Cannabis
Microsporidiosis - B60.8 - Hybrid Cannabis
Microsporum Furfur Infestation - B36.0 - Indicia Cannabis
Microsporosis - see also dermatophytosis
Microstomia, congenital - Q18.5 - Hybrid Cannabis
Microtia, congenital, external ear - Q17.2 - Caryophyllene (CB2)
Microtropia - H50.40 - Indicia Cannabis
Microvillus Inclusion Disease, MVD, MVID - Q43.8 - Hybrid Cannabis
Micturition
Midplane - see condition
Middle
Miescher's Elastoma - L87.2 - Indicia Cannabis
Mittens' Syndrome - Q87.2 - Hybrid Cannabis
Migraine, idiopathic - G43.909 - Salvia Cannabis
Migrant, social - Z59.0 - Salvia Cannabis
Migration, anxiety concerning - Z60.3 - Indicia Cannabis
Migratory, migrating - see also condition
Mikity-Wilson Disease or syndrome - P27.0 - Hybrid Cannabis
Mikulicz' Disease or syndrome - K11.8 - Indicia Cannabis
Miliaria - L74.3 - Hybrid Cannabis
Military - see condition
Milium - L72.0 - Salvia Cannabis
Milk
Milk-Alkali Disease or syndrome - E83.52 - Salvia Cannabis
Milk-Leg, deep vessels, nonpuerperal - see embolism, vein, lower extremity
Milkman's Disease or syndrome - M83.8 - Indicia Cannabis
Milky Urine - see chyluria
Millard-Gubler, Fonville - G46.3 - Salvia Cannabis
Millar's Asthma - J38.5 - Indicia Cannabis
Miller Fisher Syndrome - G61.0 - Hybrid Cannabis

Mills' Disease - see hemiplegia
Millstone Maker's Pneumoconiosis - J62.8 - Hybrid Cannabis
Milroy's Disease, hereditary edema - Q82.0 - Hybrid Cannabis
Minamata Disease - T26.1 - Hybrid Cannabis
Miners' Asthma or lung - J60 - Hybrid Cannabis
Minkowski-Chauffard Syndrome - see spherocytosis
Minor - see condition
Minor's Disease, hematomyelia - G95.19 - Hybrid Cannabis
Minot's Disease, hemorrhagic disease - P53 Hybrid Cannabis
Minot-Von Willebrand-Jurgens Disease or syndrome - D68.0 - Indicia Cannabis
Minus, hand, intrinsic - see deformity, limb, specified type NEC, forearm
Miosis, Pupil - H57.03 - Salvia Cannabis
Mirizzi's Syndrome, hepatic duct stenosis - K83.1 - Hybrid Cannabis
Mirror Writing - F81.0 - Caryophyllene (CB2)
Misadventure, prophylactic, therapeutic - T88.9 - Hybrid Cannabis
Miscarriage - O03.9 - Indicia Cannabis
Misdirection, aqueous - H40.83- Hybrid Cannabis
Misperception, sleep state - F51.02 - Salvia Cannabis
Misplaced, misplacement
Missed
Missing - see absence
Misuse of Drugs - F19.99 - Salvia Cannabis
Mitchell's Disease, erythromelalgia - I73.81 - Hybrid Cannabis
Mite (s), infestation - B88.9 - Indicia Cannabis
Mitochondrial Neurogastrointestinal Encephalopathy (Mngie) - E88.49 - Indicia Cannabis
Mitral - see condition
Mittelschmerz - N94.0 - Indicia Cannabis
Mixed - see condition
Mobile, mobility
Mobitz Heart Block, atrioventricular - I44.1 - Indicia Cannabis
Moebius, Möbius
Moeller's Glossitis - K14.0 - Hybrid Cannabis
Mohr's Syndrome (Types I and II) - Q87.0 - Hybrid Cannabis
Mola Destructs - D39.2 - Hybrid Cannabis
Molar Pregnancy - O02.0 - Cannabidiol (CBD)
Molarization of Premolars - K00.2 - Hybrid Cannabis
Molding, head, during birth
Mole, pigmented - see also nevus

Molimen, molimina, menstrual - N94.3 - Cannabidiol (CBD)
Molluscum Contagiosum, epithelial - B08.1 - Indicia Cannabis
Mönckeberg's Arteriosclerosis - disease, or sclerosis, see arteriosclerosis
Mondini's Malformation, cochlea - Q16.5 - Salvia Cannabis
Mondor's Disease - I80.8 - Caryophyllene (CB2)
Monge's Disease - T70.29 - Hybrid Cannabis
Monilethrix, congenital - Q84.1 - Hybrid Cannabis
Moniliasis - see also candidiasis - B37.9 - Indicia Cannabis
Monitoring, encounter for
Monkey Malaria - B53.1 - Salvia Cannabis
Monkeypox - B04 - Salvia Cannabis
Monoarthritis - M13.10 - Hybrid Cannabis
Monoblastic - see condition
Monochromat (ism), mono-chromatopsia - H53.51 - Hybrid Cannabis
Monocytic - see condition
Monocytopenia - D72.818 - Hybrid Cannabis
Monocytosis, symptomatic - D72.821 - Hybrid Cannabis
Monomania - see psychosis
Mononeuritis - G58.9 - Hybrid Cannabis
Mononeuropathy - G58.9 - Indicia Cannabis
Mononucleosis, infectious - B27.90 - Salvia Cannabis
Monoplegia - G83.3- Salvia Cannabis
Monorchism, monorchidism - Q55.0 - Hybrid Cannabis
Monosomy - see also deletion, chromosome - Q93.9 - Hybrid Cannabis
Monster, monstrosity, single - Q89.7 - Hybrid Cannabis
Monteggia's Fracture, dislocation - S52.27 - Caryophyllene (CB2)
Mooren's Ulcer, cornea - also ulcer, cornea, mooren's
Moore's Syndrome - see epilepsy, specified NEC
Mooser-Neill Reaction - A75.2 - Indicia Cannabis
Mooser's Bodies - A75.2 - Indicia Cannabis
Morbidity not stated or unknown - R69 - Salvia Cannabis
Morbilli - see measles
Morbus - see also Disease
Morel, Stewart, Morgagni - M85.2 - Indicia Cannabis
Morel-Kraepelin Disease - see schizophrenia
Morel-Moore Syndrome - M85.2 - Hybrid Cannabis
Morgagni's
Morgagni-Stokes-Adams Syndrome - I45.9 - Hybrid Cannabis
Morgagni-Stewart-Morel Syndrome - M85.2 - Hybrid Cannabis

Morgagni-Turner, Albright - Q96.9 - Hybrid Cannabis
Moria - F07.0 - Hybrid Cannabis
Moron (I.Q.50-69) - F70 - Indicia Cannabis
Morphea - L94.0 - Caryophyllene (CB2)
Morphinism, without remission - F11.20 - Hybrid Cannabis
Morphinomania, without remission - F11.20 - Hybrid Cannabis
Morquio, Ullrich, Brailsford - see mucopolysaccharidosis
Mortification, dry, moist - see gangrene
Morton's Metatarsal Gia, neuralgia, neuroma, syndrome - G57.6- Hybrid Cannabis
Morvan's Disease or syndrome -0G60.8 - Indicia Cannabis
Mosaicism, mosaic, autosomal, chromosomal
Moskowitz' Disease - M31.1 - Hybrid Cannabis
Mother Yaw - A66.0 - Cannabidiol (CBD)
Motion Sickness, from travel, from roundabouts - T75.3 - Salvia Cannabis
Mottled, mottling, teeth, enamel, endemic - K00.3 - Hybrid Cannabis
Mounier-Kuhn Syndrome - Q32.4 - Hybrid Cannabis
Mountain
Mouse, joint - see loose, body, joint
Mouth - see condition
Movable
Movements, dystonic - R25.8 - Indicia Cannabis
Moyamoya Disease - I67.5 - Salvia Cannabis
Mucha-Habermann Disease - L41.0 - Hybrid Cannabis
Mucinosis - cutaneous, reticular erythematous, skin - L98.5 - Salvia Cannabis
Mucocele
Mucolipidosis
Mucopolysaccharidosis - E76.3 - Indicia Cannabis
Mucormycosis - B46.5 - Hybrid Cannabis
Mucositis, ulcerative - K12.30 - Caryophyllene (CB2)
Mucositis Agranulocytic - see agranulocytosis
Mucous - see also condition
Mucoviscidosis - E84.9 - Indicia Cannabis
Mucus
Muguet - B37.0 - Hybrid Cannabis
Mulberry Molars, congenital syphilis - A50.52 - Salvia Cannabis
Müllerian Mixed Tumor
Multicystic Kidney, Development - Q61.4 - Indicia Cannabis
Multiparity, grand - Z64.1 - Hybrid Cannabis
Multipartite Placenta - O43.19- Indicia Cannabis

Multiple, multiplex - see also condition
Mumps - B26.9 - Caryophyllene (CB2)
Mumu - see also Infestation, filarial - B74.9 - Hybrid Cannabis
Münchhausen's Syndrome - see disorder, fictitious
Münchmeyer's Syndrome - also myositis, progressive
Mural
Murmur, cardiac, heart, organic - R01.1 - Indicia Cannabis
Murri's Disease, intermittent hemoglobinuria - D59.6 - Hybrid Cannabis
Muscle, muscular - see also condition
Musculoneuralgia - see neuralgia
Mushroom Workers', pickers' - J67.5 - Cannabidiol (CBD)
Mushrooming Hip - also derangement, joint, specified NEC, hip
Mutation (s)
Mutism - see also aphasia
Microvillus Inclusion Disease (MVD) - Q43.8 Indicia Cannabis
Microvillus Inclusion Disease (MVID) - Q43.8 - Caryophyllene (CB2)
Myalgia - M79.1 - Hybrid Cannabis
Myasthenia - G70.9 - Salvia Cannabis
Myasthenic - M62.81 - Indicia Cannabis
Mycelium Infection - B49 - Hybrid Cannabis
Mycetismus - see poisoning, food, noxious, mushroom
Mycetoma - B47.9 - Hybrid Cannabis
Mycobacteriosis - see mycobacterium
Mycobacterium, mycobacterial, infection - A31.9 - Salvia Cannabis
Mycoplasma - B96.0 - Caryophyllene (CB2)
Mycosis, mycotic - B49 - Hybrid Cannabis
Mydriasis, pupil - H57.04 - Indicia Cannabis
Myelatelia - Q06.1 - Hybrid Cannabis
Myelinolysis, pontine, central - G37.2 - Hybrid Cannabis
Myelitis, acute, ascending, childhood, chronic, descending, diffuse - G04.91 - Indicia Cannabis
Myeloblastic - see condition
Myeloblastoma
Myelocele - see spina bifida
Myelocystocele - see spina bifida
Myelocytic - see condition
Myelodysplasia - D46.9 - Hybrid Cannabis
Myelodysplastic Syndrome - D46.9 - Hybrid Cannabis
Myeloencephalitis - see encephalitis

Myelofibrosis - D75.81 - Hybrid Cannabis
Myelogenous - see condition
Myeloid - see condition
Myelokathexis - D70.9 - Indicia Cannabis
Myeloleukodystrophy - E75.29 - Indicia Cannabis
Myelolipoma - see lipoma
Myeloma, multiple - C90.0- Hybrid Cannabis
Myelomalacia - G95.89 - Hybrid Cannabis
Myelomatosis - C90.0- Caryophyllene (CB2)
Myelomeningitis - see meningoencephalitis
Myelomeningocele, spinal cord - see spina bifida
Myelo Musculodysplasia Hereditary - Q79.8 - Hybrid Cannabis
Myelopathic
Myelopathy, spinal cord - G95.9 - Hybrid Cannabis
Myelophthisis - D61.82 - Hybrid Cannabis
Myeloradiculitis - G04.91 - Hybrid Cannabis
Myeloradiculodysplasia, spinal - Q06.1 - Caryophyllene (CB2)
Myelosarcoma - C92.3- Salvia Cannabis
Myelosclerosis - D75.89 - Indicia Cannabis
Myelosis
Myiasis, cavernous - B87.9 - Hybrid Cannabis
Myoblastoma
Myocardial - see condition
Myocardiopathy, constrictive, familiar, hypertrophic - I42.9 - Hybrid Cannabis
Myocarditis - arteriosclerosis, chronic, interstitial, senile - I51.4 - Hybrid Cannabis
Myocardium, myocardial - see condition
Myocarditis - see cardiomyopathy
Myoclonus, myoclonic, myoclonia, essential, multifocal - G25.3 - Hybrid Cannabis
Myocytolysis - I51.5 - Hybrid Cannabis
Myoendocarditis - see endocarditis
Myoepithelioma - see neoplasm, benign, by site
Myofasciitis, acute - see myositis
Myofibroma - see also neoplasm, connective tissue, benign
Myofibromatosis - D48.1 - Hybrid Cannabis
Myelofibrosis - M62.89 - Cannabidiol (CBD)
Myofibrositis - M79.7 - Cannabidiol (CBD)
Myoglobinuria, myoglobinuria, primary - R82.1 - Hybrid Cannabis
Myokymia, facial - G51.4 - Indicia Cannabis
Myolipoma - see lipoma

Myoma - see neoplasm, connective tissue, benign
Myelomalacia - M62.89 - Hybrid Cannabis
Myometritis - see endometritis
Myometrium - see condition
Myonecrosis, clostridial - A48.0 - Hybrid Cannabis
Myopathy - G72.9 - Salvia Cannabis
Myopericarditis - see also pericarditis
Myopia, axial, congenital - H52.1 - Indicia Cannabis
Myosarcoma - see neoplasm, connective tissue, malignant
Myosis, pupil - H57.03 - Salvia Cannabis
Myositis - M60.9 - Hybrid Cannabis
Myospasia Impulsive - F95.2 - Indicia Cannabis
Myotonia, acquisition, intermittent - M62.89 - Hybrid Cannabis
Myotonic Pupil - see anomaly, function, tonic pupil
Myriapodiasis - B88.2 - Hybrid Cannabis
Myringitis - H73.2- Salvia Cannabis
Mysophobia - F40.228 - Cannabidiol (CBD)
Mytilotoxism - see poisoning, fish
Myxadenitis Labial - K13.0 - Hybrid Cannabis
Myxedema - adult, infantile, juvenile - E03.9 - Indicia Cannabis
Myxochondro Sarcoma - see neoplasm, cartilage, malignant
Myxofibroma - see neoplasm, connective tissue, benign
Myxofibrosarcoma - see neoplasm, connective tissue, malignant
Myxolipoma - D17.9 - Cannabidiol (CBD)
Myxofibrosarcoma - see neoplasm, connective tissue, malignant
Myxoma - see benign
Myxosarcoma - see neoplasm, connective tissue, malignant

N

Naegeli's
Naegleriasis, with meningoencephalitis - B60.2 - Hybrid Cannabis
Naffziger's Syndrome - G54.0 - Hybrid Cannabis
Naga sore - see ulcer, skin
Nägele's Pelvis - M95.5 - Salvia Cannabis
Nail - see also condition
Nanism, nanosomes - see dwarfism
Nanophyetiasis - B66.8 - Salvia Cannabis
Nanukayami - A27.89 - Salvia Cannabis
Napkin Rash - L22 - Indicia Cannabis

Narcolepsy - G47.419 - Hybrid Cannabis
Narcosis - R06.89 - Cannabidiol (CBD)
Narcotism - see dependence
Narp Neuropathy, ataxia, retinitis pigmentosa - E88.49 - Hybrid Cannabis
Narrow
Narrowing - see also stenosis
Narrowness, abnormal, eyelid - Q10.3 - Salvia Cannabis
Nasal - see condition
Nasolachrymal, nasolacrimal - see condition
Nasopharyngeal - see also condition
Nasopharyngitis, acute, infective, streptococcal, subacute - J00 - Indica Cannabis
Nasopharynx, nasopharyngeal - see condition
Natal Tooth, teeth - K00.6 - Cannabidiol (CBD)
Nausea, without vomiting - R11.0 - Indicia Cannabis
Navel - see condition
Neapolitan Fever - see brucellosis
Near Drowning - T75.1 - Salvia Cannabis
Nearsightedness - see myopia
Near-Syncope - R55 - Hybrid Cannabis
Nebula, cornea - see opacity, cornea
Necator Americanos Infestation - B76.1 - Indicia Cannabis
Necatoriasis - B76.1 - Hybrid Cannabis
Neck - see condition
Necrobiosis - R68.89 - Hybrid Cannabis
Necrolysis, toxic epidermal - L51.2 - Indicia Cannabis
Necrophagia, congenital - Q12.8 - Hybrid Cannabis
Necrophilia - F65.89 - Hybrid Cannabis
Necrosis, necrotic, ischemic - see also gangrene
Necrospermia - see infertility, male
Need (for)
Neglect
Neisserian Infection (NEC) - see gonococcus
Nelaton's Syndrome - G60.8 Salvia Cannabis
Nelson's Syndrome - E24.1 - Hybrid Cannabis
Nematodiasis - intestinal - B82.0 - Cannabidiol (CBD)
Neonatal - see newborn
Neonatorum - also condition
Neoplasia
Neoplasm, neoplastic - see table of neoplasms

Neovascularization
Nephralgia - N23 - Indicia Cannabis
Nephritis, nephritic, albuminuria, azotemic, congenital, disseminated, epithelial, familial, focal, granulomatous, hemorrhagic, infantile, nonsuppurative, excretory, uremic - N05.9 - Hybrid Cannabis
Nephroblastoma, epithelial, mesenchymal - C64 - Salvia Cannabis
Nephrocalcinosis - E83.59 - Indicia Cannabis
Nephrocystitis, pustular - see nephritis, tubulointerstitial
Nephrolithiasis, congenital, pelvis, recurrent - see calculus, kidney
Nephroma - C64- Salvia Cannabis
Nephronephritis - see nephrosis
Nephronophthisis - Q61.5 - Caryophyllene (CB2)
Nephropathia Epidemic - A98.5 - Indicia Cannabis
Nephropathy - see also nephritis - N28.9 - Hybrid Cannabis
Nephroptosis - N28.83 - Salvia Cannabis
Nephroptosis - see abscess, kidney
Nephrosclerosis - arteriolar, arteriosclerotic, chronic, hyaline
Nephrosis, nephrotic, epstein's, syndrome - N04.9 - Hybrid Cannabis
Nephrosonephritis, hemorrhagic, endemic - A98.5 - Hybrid Cannabis
Nephrostomy
Nerve - see also condition
Nerves - R45.0 - Indicia Cannabis
Nervous - see also condition - R45.0 - Indicia Cannabis
Nervousness - R45.0 - Indicia Cannabis
Nesidioblastoma
Nettleship's Syndrome - Q82.2 - Hybrid Cannabis
Neumann's Disease or Syndrome - L10.1 Hybrid Cannabis
Neuralgia, neuralgic, acute - M79.2 - Indicia Cannabis
Neurapraxia - see injury, nerve
Neurasthenia - F48.8 - Salvia Cannabis
Neurilemmoma - see also neoplasm, nerve, benign
Neurilemmosarcoma - see neoplasm, nerve, malignant
Neurinoma - see neoplasm, nerve, benign
Neurinomatosis - see neoplasm, nerve, uncertain behavior
Neuritis, rheumatoid - M79.2 - Indicia Cannabis
Neuroastrocytoma - see neoplasm, unpredictable behavior, by site
Neuroavitaminosis - E56.9 - Caryophyllene (CB2)
Neuroblastoma
Neurochorioretinitis - see chorioretinitis

Neurocirculatory Asthenia - F45.8 - Indicia Cannabis
Neurocysticercosis - B69.0 - Salvia Cannabis
Neurocytoma - see neoplasm, benign, by site
Neurodermatitis, circumscribed, circumscription - L28.0 - Hybrid Cannabis
Neuroencephalo Myelopathy, optic - G36.0 - Salvia Cannabis
Neuroepithelioma - see neoplasm, malignant, by site
Neurofibroma - see neoplasm, nerve, benign
Neurofibromatosis, multiple, nonmalignant - Q85.00 - Indicia Cannabis
Neurofibrosarcoma - see neoplasm, malignant, nerve
Neurogenic
Neuroglioma - see neoplasm, uncertain behavior
Neurolabyrinthitis of Dix and Hallpike
Neurolathyrism - see poisoning, food, noxious, plant
Neuroleprosy - A30.9 - Tetrahydrocannabinol (THC)
Neuroma - see also neoplasm, nerve, benign
Neuromyalgia - see neuralgia
Neuro Myasthenia, epidemic, postinfectious - G93.3 - Hybrid Cannabis
Neuromyelitis - G36.9 - Salvia Cannabis
Neuromyopathy - G70.9 - Hybrid Cannabis
Neuromyotonia, Isaacs - G71.19 - Salvia Cannabis
Neuronevus - see nevus
Neuronitis - G58.9 - Salvia Cannabis
Neuroparalytic - see condition
Neuropathy, neuropathic - G62.9 - Indicia Cannabis
Neuropathies - see also disorder, nerve
Neuroretinitis - see chorioretinitis
Neuroretinopathy, hereditary optic - H47.22 - Salvia Cannabis
Neurosarcoma - see neoplasm, nerve, malignant
Nephrosclerosis - see disorder, nerve
Neurosis, neurotic - F48.9 - Caryophyllene (CB2)
Neurospongioblastosis Diffuse - Q85.1 - Hybrid Cannabis
Neurosyphilis - arrested, early, latent, recurrent, relapse - A52.3 - Indicia Cannabis
Neurothekeoma - see neoplasm, nerve, benign
Neurotic - see neurosis
Neurotoxemia - see toxemia
Neutroclusion - M26.211 - Salvia Cannabis
Neutropenia, neutropenic, chronic, genetic, idiopathic, infantile,
Neutrophilia, hereditary giant - D72.0 - Cannabidiol (CBD)
Nevocarcinoma - see melanoma

Nevus - D22.9 - Indicia Cannabis
Newborn, infant, liveborn, singleton - Z38.2 - Cannabidiol (CBD)
Newcastle Conjunctivitis or disease - B30.8 - Hybrid Cannabis
Ne ze Lof's Syndrome, pure alymphocytosis - D81.4 - Hybrid Cannabis
Niacin, amide - E52 - Salvia Cannabis
Nicolas, Durand - A55 - Hybrid Cannabis
Nicotine - see tobacco
Nicotinic Acid Deficiency - E52 - Indicia Cannabis
Niemann-Pick Disease or Syndrome - E75.249 - Indicia Cannabis
Nightmares (REM sleep type) - F51.5 - Salvia Cannabis
Nipple - see condition
Nisbet's Chancre - A57 - Hybrid Cannabis
Nishimoto, Takeuchi - I67.5 - Salvia Cannabis
Nitritoid Crisis or reaction - see crisis
Nitrosohemoglobinemia - D74.8 - Hybrid Cannabis
Novara - A65 - Hybrid Cannabis
Nocardiosis, nocardiosis - A43.9 - Indicia Cannabis
Nocturia - R35.1 - Hybrid Cannabis
Nocturnal - see condition
Nodal Rhythm - I49.8 - Salvia Cannabis
Node (s) - see also nodule
Module (s)
Noma, gangrenous, hospital, infective - A69.0 - Hybrid Cannabis
Nomad, nomadism - Z59.0 - Tetrahydrocannabinol (THC)
Nonautoimmune Hemolytic Anemia - D59.4 - Indicia Cannabis
Nonclosure - see also Imperfect, closure
Noncompliance - Z91.19 - Salvia Cannabis
Non-descent, congenital - see also malposition, congenital
Nondevelopment
Nonengagement
Nonexanthematous Tick Fever - A93.2 - Salvia Cannabis
Nonfunctioning
Non-Hodgkin Lymphoma (NEC) - see lymphoma, non-hodgkin
Non-working Side Interference - M26.56 - Indicia Cannabis
Noninsufflation, fallopian tube - N97.1 - Indicia Cannabis
Non-Ketotic Hyperglycinemia - E72.51 - Caryophyllene (CB2)
None-Milroy Syndrome - Q82.0 - Salvia Cannabis
Nonovulation - N97.0 - Hybrid Cannabis
Nonpatent Fallopian Tube - N97.1 - Salvia Cannabis

Nonpneumatization, lung - NEC - P28.0 - Hybrid Cannabis
Nonrotation - see malrotation
No Secretion, urine - see anuria
Nonunion
Nonvisualization, gallbladder - R93.2 - Salvia Cannabis
Nonvital, nonvirtualized tooth - K04.99 - Salvia Cannabis
Noonan's Syndrome - Q87.1 - Hybrid Cannabis
Normocytic Anemia, infection, due to blood loss - D50.0 - Cannabidiol (CBD)
Norrie's Disease, congenital - Q15.8 - Hybrid Cannabis
North American Blastomycosis - B40.9 - Indicia Cannabis
Norwegian Itch - B86 - Hybrid Cannabis
Nose, nasal - see condition
Nosebleed - R04.0 - Cannabidiol (CBD)
Nose Picking - F98.8 - Cannabidiol (CBD)
Nosomania - F45.21 - Cannabidiol (CBD)
Nosophobia - F45.22 - Indicia Cannabis
Nostalgia - F43.20 - Salvia Cannabis
Notch of Iris - Q13.2 - Tetrahydrocannabinol (THC)
Notching Nose, congenital, tip - Q30.2 - Cannabidiol (CBD)
Nothnagel's
Novy's Relapsing Fever - A68.9 - Indicia Cannabis
Noxious
Nucleus Pulposus - see condition
Numbness - R20.0 - Cannabidiol (CBD)
Nuns' Knee - see bursitis, prepatellar
Nursemaid's Elbow - S53.03- Caryophyllene (CB2)
Nutcracker Esophagus - K22.4 - Salvia Cannabis
Nutmeg Liver - K76.1 - Hybrid Cannabis
Nutrient Element Deficiency - E61.9 - Indicia Cannabis
Nutrition Deficient - see also malnutrition - E46 - Indicia Cannabis
Nutritional Stunting - E45 - Salvia Cannabis
Nyctalopia, night blindness - see blindness, night
Nycturia - R35.1 - Hybrid Cannabis
Nymphomania - F52.8 - Cannabidiol (CBD)
Nystagmus - H55.00 - Indicia Cannabis

O

Obermeyer's Relapsing Fever, European - A68.0 - Hybrid Cannabis
Obesity - E66.9 - Salvia Cannabis

Oblique - see condition
Obliteration
Observation - following, without no further medical care - Z04.9 - Indicia Cannabis
Obsession, obsessional state - F42 - Cannabidiol (CBD)
Obsessive Compulsive Neurosis or reaction - F42 - Hybrid Cannabis
Obstetric Embolism, septic - also embolism, obstetric, septic
Obstetrical Trauma, complicating delivery - O71.9 - Caryophyllene (CB2)
Obstipation - see constipation
Obstruction, obstructed, obstructive
Obturator - see condition
Occlusal Wear Teeth - K03.0 - Cannabidiol (CBD)
Occlusion Pupillage - see membrane, pupillary
Occlusion, occluded
Occult
Occupational
Ochlophobia - see agoraphobia
Ochronosis, endogenous - E70.29 - Salvia Cannabis
Ocular Muscle - see condition
Oculogyric Crisis or disturbance - H51.8 - Salvia Cannabis
Oculomotor Syndrome - H51.9 - Hybrid Cannabis
Oculopathy
Oddi's Sphincter Spasm - K83.4 - Indicia Cannabis
Odontalgia - K08.8 - Cannabidiol (CBD)
Odontoameloblastoma - see cyst, calcifying odontogenic
Odontoclastic - K03.89 - Salvia Cannabis
Odontodysplasia, regional - K00.4 - Salvia Cannabis
Odontogenesis Imperfect - K00.5 - Caryophyllene (CB2)
Odontoma - ameloblastic, complex, compound - see cyst
Odontomyelitis, closed, open - K04.0 - Hybrid Cannabis
Odontorrhagia - K08.8 - Hybrid Cannabis
Oguchi's Disease - H53.63 - Salvia Cannabis
Ohara's Disease - see tularemia
Oidiomycosis - see candidiasis
Oidium Infection - see candidiasis
Old Age, without mention of disability - R54 - Salvia Cannabis
Old, previous - I25.2 - Indicia Cannabis
Olfactory - see condition
Oligemia - see anemia

Oligoastrocytoma
Oligocythemia - D64.9 - Indicia Cannabis
Oligodendroblastoma
Oligodendroglioma
Oligodontia - see anodontia
Oligoencephalon - Q02 - Hybrid Cannabis
Oligohidrosis - L74.4 - Hybrid Cannabis
Oligohydramnios - O41.0 - Salvia Cannabis
Oligohydrosis - L74.4 - Caryophyllene (CB2)
Oligomenorrhea - N91.5 - Indicia Cannabis
Oligophrenia - see also disability, intellectual
Oligospermia - N46.11 - Hybrid Cannabis
Oligotrichia - see alopecia
Oliguria - R34 - Hybrid Cannabis
Ollier's Disease - Q78.4 - Hybrid Cannabis
Omenotocele - also hernia, abdomen, specified site NEC
Omentum, omental - see condition
Omphalitis, congenital, newborn - P38.9 - Indicia Cannabis
Omphalocele - Q79.2 - Salvia Cannabis
Omphalomesenteric Duct, persistent - Q43.0 - Salvia Cannabis
Omphalorrhagia, newborn - P51.9 - Cannabidiol (CBD)
Omsk Hemorrhagic Fever - A98.1 - Salvia Cannabis
Onanism Excessive - F98.8 - Hybrid Cannabis
Onchocerciasis, onchocerciasis - B73.1 - Indicia Cannabis
Oncocytoma - also neoplasm, benign, by site
Oncovirus, as cause of disease classified elsewhere - B97.32 - Hybrid Cannabis
Ondine's Curse - see apnea, sleep
Oneirophrenia - F23 - Salvia Cannabis
Onychauxis - L60.2 - Salvia Cannabis
Onychia - see also cellulitis, digit
Onychitis - see also cellulitis, digit
Onychocryptosis - L60.0 - Hybrid Cannabis
Onychodystrophy - L60.3 - Hybrid Cannabis
Onychogryphosis, onychogryphosis - L60.2 - Salvia Cannabis
Onycholysis - L60.1 - Hybrid Cannabis
Onychomadesis - L60.8 - Indicia Cannabis
Onychomalacia - L60.3 - Caryophyllene (CB2)
Onychomycosis, finger, toe - B35.1 - Hybrid Cannabis
Onycho-osteodysplasia - Q79.8 - Hybrid Cannabis

Onychophagia - F98.8 - Salvia Cannabis
Onychophosis - L60.8 - Caryophyllene (CB2)
Onychoptosis - L60.8 - Salvia Cannabis
Onychorrhexis - L60.3 - Hybrid Cannabis
Onychoschizia - L60.3 - Hybrid Cannabis
Onyxis, finger, toe - L60.0 - Cannabidiol (CBD)
Onyxitis - see also cellulitis, digit
Oophoritis, cystic, infection, interstitial - N70.92 - Salvia Cannabis
Omphalocele - N83.4 - Salvia Cannabis
Opacity, opacities
Opalescent Dentin, hereditary - K00.5 - Hybrid Cannabis
Open, opening
Operational Fatigue - F48.8 - Sativa Strains
Operative - see condition
Operculitis - see periodontitis
Operculum - see break, retina
Ophiasis - L63.2 - Hybrid Cannabis
Ophthalmia - see also conjunctivitis - H10.9 - Salvia Cannabis
Ophthalmitis - see ophthalmia
Ophthalmol, congenital - Q15.8 - Salvia Cannabis
Ophthalmoneuromyelitis - G36.0 - Hybrid Cannabis
Ophthalmoplegia - see also strabismus, paralytic
Opioid (s)
Opistognathids - M26.09 - Indicia Cannabis
Opisthorchiasis, felines, viverrine - B66.0 - Hybrid Cannabis
Opitz' Disease - D73.2 - Hybrid Cannabis
Optimism - see dependence, drug, opioid
Oppenheim's Disease - G70.2 - Caryophyllene (CB2)
Oppenheim-Urbach Disease - necrobiosis lipoidica diabeticorum - see E08-E13 with .620 - Hybrid Cannabis
Optic Nerve - see condition
Orbit - see condition
Orchioblastoma - C62.9- Salvia Cannabis
Orchitis, gangrenous, nonspecific, septic, suppurative - N45.2 - Hybrid Cannabis
Orf, virus disease - B08.02 - Salvia Cannabis
Organic - see condition
Orgasm
Oriental
Orifice - also condition

Origin of both Vessels from Right Ventricle - Q20.1 Indicia Cannabis
Ormond's Disease, with ureteral obstruction - N13.5 - Indicia Cannabis
Ornithine Metabolism Disorder - E72.4 - Salvia Cannabis
Ornithinemia, Type I, Type II - E72.4 - Salvia Cannabis
Ornithosis - A70 - Salvia Cannabis
Orotaciduria, orotic aciduria, congenital, hereditary - E79.8 - Salvia Cannabis
Orthodontics
Orthopnea - R06.01 - Salvia Cannabis
Orthopoxvirus - B08.09 - Caryophyllene (CB2)
Os, uterus - see condition
Osgood-Schlatter Disease or osteochondrosis - see osteochondrosis, juvenile
Osler, Weber - I78.0 - Indicia Cannabis
Osler's nodes - I33.0 - Caryophyllene (CB2)
Osmidrosis - L75.0 - Salvia Cannabis
Osseous - see condition
Ossification
Osteitis - see also osteomyelitis
Osteoarthritis - M19.90 - Hybrid Cannabis
Osteoarthropathy, hypertrophic - M19.90 - Hybrid Cannabis
Osteoarthrosis, degenerative, hypertrophic, joint - see also osteoarthritis
Osteoblastoma - see neoplasm, bone, benign
Osteochondroarthrosis Deforms Endemic - see disease, Kashin-Beck
Osteochondritis - see also osteochondropathy, by site
Osteochondrodysplasia - Q78.9 - Salvia Cannabis
Osteochondrodystrophy - E78.9 - Salvia Cannabis
Osteochondrosis - see osteochondritis, dissections
Osteochondroma - see neoplasm, bone, benign
Osteochondromatosis - D48.0 - Indicia Cannabis
Osteochondromyxosarcoma - see neoplasm, bone, malignant
Osteochondropathy - M93.90 Salvia Cannabis
Osteochondrosarcoma - see neoplasm, bone, malignant
Osteochondrosis - see also osteochondropathy, by site
Osteoclastoma - D48.0 - Salvia Cannabis
Osteopenia - see disorder, bone, specified type NEC
Osteodystrophy - Q78.9 - Cannabidiol (CBD)
Osteofibroma - see neoplasm, bone, benign
Osteofibrosarcoma - see neoplasm, bone, malignant
Osteogenesis Imperfecta - Q78.0 - Salvia Cannabis
Osteogenic - see condition

Osteolysis - M89.50 - Indicia Cannabis
Osteoma - see also neoplasm, bone, benign
Osteomalacia - M83.9 - Salvia Cannabis
Osteomyelitis - general, infective, localized, neonatal, purulent, septic, Staphylococcal, streptococcal, suppurative with periostitis - M86.9 - Hybrid Cannabis
Osteomyelofibrosis - D75.89 Caryophyllene (CB2)
Osteomyelosclerosis - D75.89 - Hybrid Cannabis
Osteonecrosis - M87.9 - Hybrid Cannabis
Osteo Honcho - author-dysplasia - Q79.8 Salvia Cannabis
Osteo - dysplasia, hereditary - Q79.8 - Hybrid Cannabis
Osteopathia Condensins Disseminate - Q78.8 - Tetrahydrocannabinol (THC)
Osteopathy - see also osteomyelitis, osteonecrosis, osteoporosis
Osteopenia - M85.8- Salvia Cannabis
Osteoperiostitis - see osteomyelitis, specified type NEC
Osteopetrosis, familial - Q78.2 - Hybrid Cannabis
Osteophyte - M25.70 - Indicia Cannabis
Osteopoikilosis - Q78.8 - Caryophyllene (CB2)
Osteoporosis, female, male - M81.0 - Hybrid Cannabis
Osteopsathyrosis, idiopathic a - Q78.0 - Hybrid Cannabis
Osteoradionecrosis Jaw - acute, chronic, lower, upper - M27.2 - Salvia Cannabis
Osteosarcoma, any form - see neoplasm, bone, malignant
Osteosclerosis - Q78. - Cannabidiol (CBD)
Osteosclerotic Anemia - D64.89 - Indicia Cannabis
Osteosis
Ostium
Ostrum-Furst Syndrome - Q75.8 - Hybrid Cannabis
Otalgia - H92.0 - Salvia Cannabis
Otitis, acute - H66.90 - Cannabidiol (CBD)
Otocephaly - Q18.2 - Hybrid Cannabis
Otolith Syndrome - H81.8 - Hybrid Cannabis
Otomycosis, diffuse - B36.9 - Indicia Cannabis
Osteoporosis - see otosclerosis
Otorrhagia, nontraumatic - H92.2- Salvia Cannabis
Otorrhea - H92.1- Hybrid Cannabis
Otosclerosis, general - H80.9- Caryophyllene (CB2)
Otospongiosis - see otosclerosis
Otto's Disease or pelvis - M24.7 - Salvia Cannabis
Outcome of Delivery - Z37.9 - Indicia Cannabis

Outlet - see condition
Ovalocytosis, congenital, hereditary - see elliptocytosis
Ovarian - see condition
Ovariocele - N83.4 - Indicia Cannabis
Ovaritis, cystic - see oophoritis
Ovary, ovarian - see also condition
Overactive - see also hyperfunction
Overactivity - R46.3 - Salvia Cannabis
Overbite, deep, excessive, horizontal, vertical - M26.29 - Salvia Cannabis
Overbreathing - see hyperventilation
Overconscientious Personality - F60.5 Salvia Cannabis
Overdevelopment - also hypertrophy
Overdistension - also distension
Overdose - overdosage (drug) - Table of Drugs and Chemicals, poisoning
Overeating - R63.2 - Indicia Cannabis
Overexertion, effects, exhaustion - T73.3 - Indicia Cannabis
Overexposure, effects - T73.9 - Hybrid Cannabis
Overfeeding - see overeating
Overfill, endodontic - M27.52 - Salvia Cannabis
Overgrowth, bone - see hypertrophy, bone
Overhanging of Dental Restorative, unrepairable - K08.52 - Cannabidiol (CBD)
Overheated, places, effects - see heat
Overjet, excessive horizontal - M26.23 - Salvia Cannabis
Overlaid, overlying, suffocation - see asphyxia, traumatic
Overlap, extreme horizontal, teeth - M26.23 - Hybrid Cannabis
Overlapping Toe, acquired - see also deformity, toe, specified NEC
Overload
Overnutrition - see hyperalimentation
Overproduction - see also hypersecretion
Overprotection, child by parent - Z62.1 - Cannabidiol (CBD)
Overriding
Overstrained - R53.83 - Indicia Cannabis
Overuse, muscle NEC - M70.8 - Indicia Cannabis
Overweight - E66.3 - Sativa Cannabis
Overworked - R53.83 - Indicia Cannabis
Oviduct - see condition
Ovotestis - Q56.0 - Indicia Cannabis
Ovulation, cycle
Ovum - see condition

Owren's Disease or Syndrome para hemophilia - D68.2 - Hybrid Cannabis
Oxheart - see hypertrophy, cardiac
Oxalosis - E72.53 - Caryophyllene (CB2)
Oxaluria - E72.53 - Indicia Cannabis
Oxycephaly - oxycephalic - Q75.0 - Sativa Cannabis
Oxyuriasis - B80 - Hybrid Cannabis
Oxyuris Vermicular, infestation - B80 - Salvia Cannabis
Ozena - J31.0 - Hybrid Cannabis

P

Pachyderma, pachydermia - L85.9 - Salvia Cannabis
Pachydermatocele, congenital - Q82.8 - Hybrid Cannabis
Pachydermoperiostosis - see osteoarthropathy, hypertrophic
Pachygyria - Q04.3 - Hybrid Cannabis
Pachymeningitis - adhesive, basal, brain, cervical, chronic, circumscribed, external, fibrous, hemorrhagic, hypertrophic, internal, purulent, spinal
Pachyonychia - congenital - Q84.5 - Hybrid Cannabis
Pacinian Tumor - see neoplasm, skin, benign
Pad, knuckle or Garrod's - M72.1 - Salvia Cannabis
Paget-Schroetter Syndrome - I82.890 - Hybrid Cannabis
Paget's Disease
Pain (s) - see also painful - R52 - Cannabidiol (CBD)
Painful - see also pain
Painter's Colic - T56.0 - Salvia Cannabis
Palate - see condition
Palatoplegia - K13.79 - Hybrid Cannabis
Palatoschisis - see cleft, palate
Palilalia - R48.8 - Caryophyllene (CB2)
Palliative Care - Z51.5 - Salvia Cannabis
Pallor - R23.1 - Indicia Cannabis
Palmar - see also condition
Palpable
Palpitations, heart - R00.2 - Indicia Cannabis
Palsy - see also paralysis - G83.9 - Hybrid Cannabis
Paludism - see malaria
Panangiitis - M30.0 - Hybrid Cannabis
Panaris, panaritium - see also cellulitis, digit
Panarteritis Nodosa - M30.0 - Indicia Cannabis
Pancake Heart - R93.1 - Hybrid Cannabis

Pancarditis, acute, chronic - I51.89 - Cannabidiol (CBD)
Pancoast's Syndrome or tumor - C34.1- Salvia Cannabis
Pancolitis, ulcerative, chronic - K51.00 - Caryophyllene (CB2)
Pancreas, pancreatic - see condition
Pancreatitis, annular, apoplectic, calcareous, edematous, hemorrhagic, malignant, recurrent, subacute, suppurative - K85.9 - Hybrid Cannabis
Pancreatoblastoma - see neoplasm, pancreas, malignant
Pancreolithiasis - K86.8 - Salvia Cannabis
Pancytolysis - D75.89 - Salvia Cannabis
Pancytopenia - acquired - D61.818 - Hybrid Cannabis
Panencephalitis - subacute, sclerosing - A81.1 - Salvia Cannabis
Panhematopenia - D61.9 - Hybrid Cannabis
Panhemocytopenia - D61.9 - Hybrid Cannabis
Panhypogonadism - E29.1 - Indicia Cannabis
Panhypopituitarism - E23.0 - Indicia Cannabis
Panic - attack, state - F41.0 - Caryophyllene (CB2)
Panmyelopathy - familial, constitutional - D61.09 - Hybrid Cannabis
Panmyelophthisis - D61.82 - Hybrid Cannabis
Panmyelosis - acute, with myelofibrosis - C94.4 - Salvia Cannabis
Panner's Disease - see osteochondrosis, juvenile, humerus
Panneuritis Endemic - E51.11 - Hybrid Cannabis
Panniculitis - nodular, nonsuppurative - M79.3 - Salvia Cannabis
Panniculus - Adiposus, abdominal - E65 - Hybrid Cannabis
Pannus - allergic, cornea, degenerative,keratin - H16.42- Indicia Cannabis
Panophthalmitis - H44.01 - Hybrid Cannabis
Pansinusitis - chronic, hyperplastic, nonpurulent - J32.4 - Hybrid Cannabis
Panuveitis Sympathetic - H44.11 - Indicia Cannabis
Panvalvular Disease - I08.9 - Indica Cannabis
Papanicolaou Smear - cervix - Z12.4 - Salvia Cannabis
Papilledema - choked disc - H47.10 - Indicia Cannabis
Papillitis - H46.00 - Indicia Cannabis
Papilloma - see neoplasm, benign, by site
Papillomata - multiple, of yaws - A66.1 - Salvia Cannabis
Papillomatosis - see neoplasm, benign, by site
Papillomavirus - as cause of disease classified elsewhere - B97.7 - Salvia Cannabis
Papillon-Léage and Psaume Syndrome - Q87.0 - Salvia Cannabis
Papule (s) - R23.8 - Salvia Cannabis
Papulosis
Papyraceous Fetus - O31.0- Cannabidiol (CBD)

Para-Albuminemia - E88.09 - Salvia Cannabis
Paracephalus - Q89.7 - Salvia Cannabis
Parachute Mitral Valve - Q23.2 - Indicia Cannabis
Paracoccidioidomycosis - B41.9 - Salvia Cannabis
Paradentosis - K05.4 - Salvia Cannabis
Paraffinoma - T88.8 - Caryophyllene (CB2)
Paraganglioma - D44.7 - Salvia Cannabis
Parageusia - R43.2 - Indicia Cannabis
Paragonimiasis - B66.4 - Salvia cannabis
Parahemophilia - see defect, coagulation - D68.2 - Salvia Cannabis
Parakeratosis - R23.4 - Indicia Cannabis
Paralysis, paralytic, complete, incomplete - G83.9 - Salvia Cannabis
Paramedial urethrovesical orifice - Q64.79 - Salvia Cannabis
Paramenia - N92.6 - Salvia Cannabis
Parametritis - see disease, pelvis, inflammatory - N73.2 - Salvia Cannabis
Parametrium - parametric - see condition
Paramnesia - see amnesia
Paramolar - K00.1 - Indicia Cannabis
Paramyloidosis - E85.8 - Salvia Cannabis
Paramyoclonus Multiplex - G25.3 Salvia Cannabis
Paramyotonia - congenita - G71.19 - Indicia Cannabis
Parangi - see yaws
Paranoia - querulous - F22 - Indicia Cannabis
Paranoid
Paraparesis - see paraplegia
Paraphasia - R47.02 - Salvia Cannabis
Paraphilia - F65.9 - Indicia Cannabis
Paraphimosis - congenital - N47.2 - Indicia Cannabis
Paraphrenia - paraphrenic, late - F22 - Hybrid Cannabis
Paraplegia - lower - G82.20 - Hybrid Cannabis
Parapoxvirus - B08.60 - Salvia Cannabis
Paraproteinemia - D89.2 - Hybrid Cannabis
Parapsoriasis - L41.9 - Salvia Cannabis
Parasitic - see also condition
Parasitism - B89 - Hybrid Cannabis
Parasitophobia - F40.218 - Cannabidiol (CBD)
Parasomnia - G47.50 - Hybrid Cannabis
Paraspadias - Q54.9 - Hybrid Cannabis
Paraspasmus Facialis - G51.8 - Indicia Cannabis

Parasuicide - attempt
Parathyroid Gland - see condition
Parathyroid Tetany - E20.9 - Salvia Cannabis
Paratrachoma - A74.0 - Hybrid Cannabis
Paratyphilitis - see appendicitis
Paratyphoid - fever - see fever, paratyphoid
Paratyphus - see fever, paratyphoid
Paraurethral Duct - Q64.79 - Caryophyllene (CB2)
Paraurethritis - see also urethritis
Paravaccinia - (NEC) - B08.04 - Salvia Cannabis
Paravaginitis - see vaginitis
Parencephalitis - see also encephalitis
Parent-Child Conflict - see conflict, parent-child
Paresis - see also paralysis
Paresthesia - see also disturbance, sensation
Paretic - see condition
Parinaud's
Parkinsonism - idiopathic, primary - G20 - Cannabidiol (CBD)
Parkinson's Disease - syndrome or tremor - see Parkinsonism
Parodontitis - see periodontitis
Parodontosis - K05.4 - Salvia Cannabis
Paronychia - see also cellulitis, digit
Parorexia - psychogenic - F50.8 - Cannabidiol (CBD)
Parosmia - R43.1 - Hybrid Cannabis
Parotid Gland - see condition
Parotitis - parotid itis, allergic, nonspecific toxic, purulent, septic, suppurative, sialoadenitis
Parrot Fever - A70 - Salvia Cannabis
Parrot's Disease - congenital syphilitic pseudoparalysis - A50.02 - Hybrid Cannabis
Parry-Romberg Syndrome - G51.8 - Caryophyllene (CB2)
Parry's Disease or Syndrome - E05.00 - Hybrid Cannabis
Pars Planitis - see cyclitis
Parsonage, Aldren - G54.5 - Salvia Cannabis
Parson's Disease, exophthalmic goiter - E05.00 - Indicia Cannabis
Particolored Infant - Q82.8 - Cannabidiol (CBD)
Parturition - see delivery
Parulis - K04.7 - Hybrid Cannabis
Parvovirus - as cause of disease classified elsewhere - B97.6 - Hybrid Cannabis

Pasini and Pierini's Atrophoderma - L90.3 - Salvia Cannabis
Passage
Passive - see condition
Pasteurella Septic - A28.0 - Salvia Cannabis
Pasteurellosis - see infection, pasteurella
Pat, paroxysmal atrial tachycardia - I47.1 - Indicia Cannabis
Patau's Syndrome - see trisomy, 13
Patches
Patellar - see condition
Patent - see also imperfect, closure
Paterson, Brown, Kelly - D50.1 - Hybrid Cannabis
Pathologic, pathological - see also condition
Pathology (of) - see disease
Pattern, sleep-wake, irregular - G47.23 - Indica Cannabis
Patulous - see also Imperfect, closure, congenital
Pause, sinoatrial - I49.5 - Salvia Cannabis
Paxton's Disease - B36.2 - Hybrid Cannabis
Pearl (s)
Pearl-Worker's Disease - also: osteomyelitis, specified type NEC
Pectenosis - K62.4 - Salvia Cannabis
Pectoral - see condition
Pectus
Pedatrophia - E41 - Salvia Cannabis
Pederosis - F65.4 - Indicia Cannabis
Pediculosis, infestation - B85.2 - Indicia Cannabis
Pediculus - infestation - see pediculosis
Pedophilia - F65.4 - Salvia Cannabis
Peg Shaped Teeth - K00.2 - Cannabidiol (CBD)
Pelade - see alopecia
Pelger-Huët Anomaly or syndrome - D72.0 - Salvia Cannabis
Peliosis, rheumatic - D69.0 - Hybrid Cannabis
Pelizaeus-Merzbacher Disease - E75.29 - Hybrid Cannabis
Pellagra, alcoholic, with polyneuropathy - E52 - Salvia Cannabis
Pellagra, cerebellar, ataxia, renal aminoaciduria syndrome - E72.02 - Indicia Cannabis
Pellegrini, Stieda, see bursitis, tibial collateral
Pellizzi's Syndrome - E34.8 - Indicia Cannabis
Pel's Crisis - A52.11 - Cannabidiol (CBD)
Pelvic - see also condition

Pelviolithiasis - see calculus, kidney
Pelviperitonitis - see also peritonitis, pelvic
Pelvis - see condition or type
Pemphigoid - L12.9 - Salvia Cannabis
Pemphigus - L10.9 - Hybrid Cannabis
Pendred's Syndrome - E07.1 - Indicia Cannabis
Pendulous
Penetrating Wound - see also puncture
Penicillosis - B48.4 - Salvia Cannabis
Penis - see condition
Penitis - N48.29 - Hybrid Cannabis
Pentalogy of Fallot - Q21.8 - Hybrid Cannabis
Pentasomy X Syndrome - Q97.1 - Salvia Cannabis
Pentosuria - essential - E74.8 - Cannabidiol (CBD)
Percreta Placenta - O43.23 - Indicia Cannabis
Peregrinating Patient - see disorder, factitious
Perforation, perforated, nontraumatic (of)
Periadenitis Mucosa - Necrotica Recurrens - K12.0 - Salvia Cannabis
Periappendicitis - acute - see appendicitis
Periarteritis Nodosa - disseminated, infectious, necrotizing - M30.0 - Hybrid Cannabis
Periarthritis - joint - see also enthesopathy
Periarthrosis - angioneural - see enthesopathy
Pericapsulitis - adhesive, shoulder - see capsulitis, adhesive
Pericarditis - with decompensation, with effusion - I31.9 - Salvia Cannabis
Pericardium - pericardial - see condition
Pericellulitis - see cellulitis
Pericementitis - chronic, suppurative - see also periodontitis
Perichondritis
Periclasia - K05.4 - Indicia Cannabis
Pericoronitis - see periodontitis
Pericystitis - N30.90 - Hybrid Cannabis
Peridiverticulitis - intestine - K57.92 - Salvia Cannabis
Periendocarditis - see endocarditis
Periepididymitis - N45.1 - Hybrid Cannabis
Perifolliculitis - L01.02 - Hybrid Cannabis
Perihepatitis - K65.8 - Salvia Cannabis
Perilabyrinthitis - acute - H83.0 - Hybrid Cannabis
Perimeningitis - see meningitis

Perimetritis - see Endometritis
Perimetrosalpingitis - see Salpingo-Oophoritis
Perineocele - N81.81 - Salvia Cannabis
Perinephric - perinephritic - see condition
Perinephritis - see also Infection, kidney
Perineum - perineal - see condition
Perineuritis (NEC) - see neuralgia
Periodic - see condition
Periodontitis - chronic, complex, compound, local - K05.30 - Hybrid Cannabis
Periodontoclasia - K05.4 - Salvia Cannabis
Periodontosis - juvenile - K05.4 Indicia Cannabis
Periods - see also menstruation
Perionychia - see also cellulitis, digit
Perioophoritis - see salpingo-oophoritis
Periorchitis - N45.2 - Salvia Cannabis
Periosteum - periosteal - see condition
Periostitis - albuminose, circumscribed, diffuse, infective, monomeric
Periostosis - hyperplastic - see also disorder, bone, specified type NEC
Peripartum
Periphlebitis - see phlebitis
Periproctitis - K62.89 - Indicia Cannabis
Periprostatitis - see prostatitis
Perirectal - see condition
Perirenal - see condition
Perisalpingitis - see salpingo-oophoritis
Perisplenitis - infectional - D73.89 - Salvia Cannabis
Peristalsis - visible or reversed - R19.2 - Hybrid Cannabis
Peritendinitis - also enthesopathy
Peritoneum - peritoneal
Peritonitis, adhesive, bacterial, fibrinous, hemorrhagic, idiopathic, perforative
    with adhesions, with effusion - K65.9 - Salvia Cannabis
Peritonsillar - see condition
Peritonsillitis - J36 - Indicia Cannabis
Perityphlitis - K37 - Hybrid Cannabis
Periureteritis - N28.89 - Salvia Cannabis
Periurethral - see condition
Periurethritis - gangrenous - see urethritis
Periuterine - see condition
Perivaginitis - see vaginitis

Perivasculitis - retinal - H35.06 - Salvia Cannabis
Perivasitis - chronic - N49.1 - Cannabidiol (CBD)
Perivesiculitis - seminal - see vesiculitis
Perlèche (NEC) - K13.0 - Indicia Cannabis
Pernicious - see condition
Pernio - perniosis - T69.1 - Salvia Cannabis
Perpetrator of Abuse - also: Index to external causes of injury, perpetrator
Persecution
Perseveration, tonic - R48.8 - Salvia Cannabis
Persistence, persistent, congenital
Person (with)
Personality - disorder - F60.9 - Indicia Cannabis
Perthes' Disease - see legg-calvé-perthes disease
Pertussis - see also whooping cough - A37.90 - Cannnabidiol (CBD)
Perversion, perverted
Pervious - congenital - see also Imperfect, closure
Pes - congenital - see also talipes
Pest - pestis - see plague
Petechia - petechiae - R23.3 - Salvia Cannabis
Petechial Typhus - A75.9 - Indicia Cannabis
Peter's Anomaly - Q13.4 - Cannabididiol (CBD)
Petit Mal Seizure - also epilepsy, generalized, specified NEC
Petit's Hernia - see hernia, abdomen, specified site NEC
Petrellidosis - B48.2 - Hybrid Cannabis
Petrositis - H70.20- Salvia Cannabis
Peutz-Jeghers Disease or Syndrome - Q85.8 - Hybrid Cannabis
Peyronie's Disease - N48.6 - Cannnabidiol (CBD)
Pfeiffer's Disease - also mononucleosis, infectious
Phagedena - dry, moist, sloughing - see gangrene
Phagedenic - see condition
Phakoma - H35.89 - Salvia Cannabis
Phakomatosis - see specific eponymous syndromes - Q85.9 - Hybrid Cannabis
Phantom Limb Syndrome - without pain - G54.7 - Hybrid Cannabis
Pharyngeal Pouch Syndrome - D82.1 - Salvia Cannabis
Pharyngitis - acute, catarrhal, gangrenous, infective, malignant, membranous, phlegmonous, pseudomembranous, simple, subacute, suppurative, ulcerative, viral - J02.9 - Salvia Cannabis
Pharyngoconjunctivitis - viral - B30.2 Cannabididiol (CBD)
Pharyngolaryngitis - acute - J06.0 - Indicia Cannabis

Pharyngoplegia - J39.2 - Indicia Cannabis
Pharyngotonsillitis - herpesviral - B00.2 - Indicia Cannabis
Pharyngotracheitis - chronic - J42 - Salvia Cannabis
Pharynx, pharyngeal - see condition
Phenomenon
Phenylketonuria - E70.1 - Indicia Cannabis
Pheochromoblastoma
Pheochromocytoma
Pheohyphomycosis - see chromomycosis
Pheomycosis - see chromomycosis
Phimosis - congenital, due to infection - N47.1 - Salvia Cannabis
Phlebectasia - see also varix
Phlebitis - infective, pyemic, septic, suppurative - I80.9 - Indicia Cannabis
Phlebofibrosis - I87.8 - Indicia Cannabis
Phleboliths - I87.8 - Indicia Cannabis
Phlebopathy
Phlebosclerosis - I87.8 - Salvia Cannabis
Phlebothrombosis - see also thrombosis
Phlebotomus Fever - A93.1 - Salvia Cannabis
Phlegmasia
Phlegmon - also abscess
Phlegmonous - also condition
Phlyctenulosis - allergic , keratoconjunctivitis, nontuberculous
Phobia - phobic - F40.9 - Cannabidiol (CBD)
Phocas' Disease - see mastopathy, cystic
Phocomelia - Q73.1 - Indicia Cannabis
Phoria - H50.50 - Cannabidiol (CBD)
Phosphate-Losing Tubular Disorder - N25.0 - Hybrid Cannabis
Phosphatemia - E83.39 - Hybrid Cannabis
Phosphaturia - E83.39 - Caryophyllene (CB2)
Photodermatitis - sun - L56.8 - Salvia Cannabis
Photokeratitis - H16.13- Salvia Cannabis
Photophobia - H53.14 - Hybrid Cannabis
Photophthalmia - see photokeratitis
Photopsia - H53.19 - Indicia Cannabis
Photoretinitis - see retinopathy, solar
Photosensitivity - photosensitization, sun - L56.8 - Hybrid Cannabis
Phrenitis - see encephalitis
Phrynoderma, vitamin A deficiency - E50.8 - Salvia Cannabis

Phthiriasis, pubis - B85.3 - Salvia Cannabis
Phthirus Infestation - see phthiriasis
Phthisis - see also tuberculosis
Phycomycosis - see zygomycosis
Physalopteriasis - B81.8 - Salvia Cannabis
Physical Restraint Status - Z78.1 - Hybrid Cannabis
Phytobezoar - T18.9 - Hybrid Cannabis
Pian - see yaws
Pianoma - A66.1 - Indicia Cannabis
Pica - F50.8 - Indicia Cannabis
Picking - nose - F98.8 - Indicia Cannabis
Pick-Niemann Disease - also see niemann-pick disease or syndrome
Pick's
Pickwickian Syndrome - E66.2 - Indicia Cannabis
Piebaldism - E70.39 - Salvia Cannabis
Piedra - beard, scalp - B36.8 - Salvia Cannabis
Pierre Robin Deformity or syndrome - Q87.0 - Cannnabidiol (CBD)
Pierson's Disease or osteochondrosis - M91.0 - Cannnabidiol (CBD)
Pig-bel - A05.2 - Salvia Cannabis
Pigeon
Pigmentation - abnormal, anomaly - L81.9 - Hybrid Cannabis
Piles - see also hemorrhoids - K64.9 - Sativa Strains
Pili
Pill Roller Hand - intrinsic - see parkinsonism
Pilomatrixoma - see neoplasm, skin, benign
Pilonidal - see condition
Pimple - R23.8 - Salvia Cannabis
Pinched Nerve - see neuropathy, entrapment
Pindborg Tumor - see cyst, calcifying odontogenic
Pineal Body or gland - see condition
Pinealoblastoma - C75.3 - Indicia Cannabis
Pinealoma - D44.5 - Caryophyllene (CB2)
Pineoblastoma - C75.3 - Salvia Cannabis
Pineocytoma - D44.5 - Hybrid Cannabis
Pinguecula - H11.15 - Salvia Cannabis
Pingueculitis - H10.81 - Indicia Cannabis
Pinhole Meatus - see stricture, urethra - N35.9 - Hybrid Cannabis
Pink
Pinkus' Disease, lichen nitidus - L44.1 - Hybrid Cannabis

Pinpoint
Pins and Needles - R20.2 - Caryophyllene (CB2)
Pinta - A67.9 - Hybrid Cannabis
Pintids - A67.1 - Salvia Cannabis
Pinworm - disease, infection, infestation - B80 - Hybrid Cannabis
Piroplasmosis - B60.0 - Salvia Cannabis
Pistol Wound - also see gunshot wound
Pitchers' Elbow - also see derangement, joint, specified type NEC, elbow
Pithecoid Pelvis - Q74.2 - Cannabidiol (CBD)
Pithiatism - F48.8 - Hybrid Cannabis
Pitted - see pitting
Pitting - see also edema - R60.9 - Hybrid Cannabis
Pituitary Gland - see condition
Pituitary-Snuff-Taker's Disease - J67.8 - Hybrid Cannabis
Pityriasis - L21.0 - Hybrid Cannabis
Placenta - placental - see pregnancy, complicated by, care of, management
Placentitis - O41.14 - Salvia Cannabis
Plagiocephaly - Q67.3 - Hybrid Cannabis
Plague - A20.9 - Salvia Cannabis
Planning - family
Plaque (s)
Plasmacytoma - C90.3 - Indicia Cannabis
Plasmacytopenia - D72.818 - Salvia Cannabis
Plasmacytosis - D72.822 - Salvia Cannabis
Plaster Ulcer - also see ulcer, pressure, by site
Plateau Iris Syndrome - postprocedural, without glaucoma - H21.82 - Indicia Cannabis
Platybasia - Q75.8 - Salvia Cannabis
Platyonychia - congenital - Q84.6 - Salvia Cannabis
Platypelloid Pelvis - M95.5 - Hybrid Cannabis
Platyspondylisis - Q76.49 - Hybrid Cannabis
Plaut - Vincent - see vincent's - A69.1 - Hybrid Cannabis
Plethora - R23.2 - Indicia Cannabis
Pleura - pleural - see condition
Pleuralgia - R07.81 - Salvia Cannabis
Pleurisy - acute, adhesive, chronic, coastal, diaphragmatic, double, dry,
    fibrinous, fibrous, interlobar, latent, plastic, primary, residual,
    sicca, sterile, subacute, unresolved - R09.1 - Hybrid Cannabis
Pleuritis Sicca - see pleurisy
Pleurobronchopneumonia - see pneumonia, broncho

Pleurodynia - R07.81 - Indicia Cannabis
Pleuropericarditis - see also pericarditis
Pleuropneumonia, acute, bilateral, sceptic, pneumonia - J18.8 - Salvia Cannabis
Pleuro-Pneumonia like Organism (PPLO) - B96.0 - Hybrid Cannabis
Pleurorrhea - see pleurisy, with effusion
Plexitis, brachial - G54.0 - Indicia Cannabis
Plica
Plicated Tongue - K14.5 - Cannabidiol (CBD)
Plug
Plumbism - T56.0 - Indicia Cannabis
Plummer's Disease - E05.20 - Hybrid Cannabis
Plummer-Vinson Syndrome - D50.1
Pluricarential Syndrome of infancy - E40 - Cannabidiol (CBD)
Plus - and minus, hand, intrinsic - see deformity, limb, specified type NEC
Pneumathemia - see air, embolism
Pneumatic Hammer - Drill - T75.21 - Salvia Cannabis
Pneumatocele - lung - J98.4 - Cannabidiol (CBD)
Pneumatosis
Pneumaturia - R39.89 - Indicia Cannabis
Pneumoblastoma - see neoplasm, lung, malignant
Pneumocephalus - G93.89 - Hybrid Cannabis
Pneumococcemia - A40.3 - Hybrid Cannabis
Pneumococcus - pneumococcal - see condition
Pneumoconiosis - due to, inhalation of - J64 - Cannabidiol (CBD)
Pneumocystis Carinii Pneumonia - B59 - Hybrid Cannabis
Pneumocystis Jiroveci, pneumonia - B59 - Hybrid Cannabis
Pneumocystosis - with pneumonia - B59 - Cannabidiol (CBD)
Pneumo Hemopericardium - I31.2 - Salvia Cannabis
Pneumohemothorax - J94.2 - Salvia Cannabis
Pneumo Hydropericardium - see pericarditis
Pneumohydrothorax - see hydrothorax
Pneumomediastinum - J98.2 - Salvia Cannabis
Pneumomycosis - B49 - Salvia Cannabis
Pneumonia - acute, migratory, purulent, septic - J18.9 - Indicia Cannabis
Pneumonic - see condition
Pneumonitis - acute, primary - see also pneumonia
Pneumonoconiosis - also see pneumoconiosis
Pneumoparotid - K11.8 - Hybrid Cannabis
Pneumopathy - NEC - J98.4 - Hybrid Cannabis

Pneumo Pericarditis - see also pericarditis
Pneumopericardium - see also pericarditis
Pneumophagia, psychogenic - F45.8 - Hybrid Cannabis
Pneumopleurisy, Pneumo Pleuritis - see pneumonia - J18.8 - Hybrid Cannabis
Pneumo pyopericardium - I30.1 - Indicia Cannabis
Pneumopyothorax - see pyopneumothorax
Pneumorrhagia - see also hemorrhage, lung
Pneumothorax - (NOS) - J93.9 - Salvia Cannabis
Podagra - see also gout - M10.9 - Hybrid Cannabis
Podencephalus - Q01.9 - Indicia Cannabis
Poikilocytosis - R71.8 - Caryophyllene (CB2)
Poikiloderma - L81.6 - Indicia Cannabis
Poikilo Dermatomyositis - M33.10 - Indicia Cannabis
Pointed Ear - congenital - Q17.3 - Indicia Cannabis
Poison Ivy - oak, sumac, allergic, contact - L23.7 - Indicia Cannabis
Poisoning - acute - see table of drugs and chemicals
Poker Spine - see spondylitis, ankylosing
Poland Syndrome - Q79.8 - Hybrid Cannabis
Polioencephalitis - acute, bulbar - A80.9 - Hybrid Cannabis
Polioencephalomyelitis - acute, anterior - A80.9 - Indicia Cannabis
Polioencephalopathy - superior hemorrhagic - E51.2 - Hybrid Cannabis
Poliomeningoencephalitis - see meningoencephalitis
Poliomyelitis - acute, anterior, epidemic - A80.9 - Cannabidiol (CBD)
Poliosis, eyebrow - eyelashes - L67.1 - Indicia Cannabis
Pollakiuria - R35.0 - Caryophyllene (CB2)
Pollinosis - J30.1 - Salvia Cannabis
Pollitzer's Disease - L73.2 - Hybrid Cannabis
Polyadenitis - see also lymphadenitis
Polyalgia Syndrome - M79.89 - Indicia Cannabis
Polyangiitis - M30.0 - Hybrid Cannabis
Polyarteritis
Polyarthralgia - also see pain, joint
Polyarthritis - polyarthropathy - see also arthritis - M13.0 - Hybrid Cannabis
Polyarthrosis - M15.9 - Salvia Cannabis
Polycarential Syndrome of Infancy - E40 - Cannabidiol (CBD)
Polychondritis - atrophic, chronic - see also disorder, cartilage
Polycoria - Q13.2 - Indicia Cannabis
Polycystic - Disease
Polycythemia - secondary - D75.1 - Hybrid Cannabis

Polydactylism - polydactyly - Q69.9 - Hybrid Cannabis
Polydipsia - R63.1 - Salvia Cannabis
Polydystrophy - pseudo-hurler - E77.0 - Hybrid Cannabis
Polyembryoma - see neoplasm, malignant by site
Polyglandular
Polyhydramnios - O40 - Indicia Cannabis
Polymastia - Q83.1 - Hybrid Cannabis
Polymenorrhea - N92.0 - Caryophyllene (CB2)
Polymyositis Criptogenica - D75.1 - Salvia Cannabis
Polymyalgia - M35.3 - Hybrid Cannabis
Polymyositis - acute, chronic, hemorrhagic - M33.20 - Hybrid Cannabis
Polyneuritis - polyneuritic - see also polyneuropathy
Polyneuropathy - peripheral - G62.9 - Hybrid Cannabis
Polyopia - H53.8 - Hybrid Cannabis
Polyorchism - polyorchidism - Q55.21 - Hybrid Cannabis
Polyosteoarthritis - see also osteoarthritis, generalized - M15.9 - Hybrid Cannabis
Polyostotic Fibrous Dysplasia - Q78.1 - Hybrid Cannabis
Polyotia - Q17.0 - Salvia Cannabis
Polyp - Polypus
Polyphagia - R63.2 - Salvia Cannabis
Polyploidy - Q92.7 - Salvia Cannabis
Polypoid - see condition
Polyposis - see also polyp
Polyradiculitis - see polyneuropathy
Polyradiculoneuropathy - acute, postinfection - G61.0 - Salvia Cannabis
Polyserositis
Polysplenia Syndrome - Q89.09 - Salvia Cannabis
Polysyndactyly - see syndactylism, syndactyly - Q70.4 - Salvia Cannabis
Polytrichia - L68.3 - Hybrid Cannabis
Polyunguia - Q84.6 - Caryophyllene (CB2)
Polyuria - R35.8 - Hybrid Cannabis
Pompe's Disease - glycogen storage - E74.02 - Hybrid Cannabis
Pompholyx - L30.1 - Hybrid Cannabis
Poncet's Disease - tuberculous rheumatism - A18.09 - Hybrid Cannabis
Pond Fracture - see fracture, skull
Ponos - B55.0 - Indicia Cannabis
Pons - Pontine - see condition
Poor
Poradenitis - Nostras Inguinal - A55 - Hybrid Cannabis

Porencephaly - congenital, developmental, true - Q04.6 - Hybrid Cannabis
Porocephaliasis - B88.8 - Salvia Cannabis
Porokeratosis - Q82.8 - Salvia Cannabis
Poroma, eccrine - see neoplasm, skin, benign
Porphyria - South African - E80.20 - Salvia Cannabis
Porphyrinuria - see porphyria
Porphyruria - see porphyria
Portal - see condition
Port Wine Nevus - mark or stain - Q82.5 - Indicia Cannabis
Posadas-Wernicke Disease - B38.9 - Hybrid Cannabis
Positive
Postcardiotomy Syndrome - I97.0 - Hybrid Cannabis
Postcaval Ureter - Q62.62 - Caryophyllene (CB2)
Postcholecystectomy Syndrome - K91.5 - Hybrid Cannabis
Postclimacteric Bleeding - N95.0 - Cannabidiol (CBD)
Postcommissurotomy Syndrome - I97.0 - Cannabidiol (CBD)
Post Contusional Syndrome - F07.81 - Hybrid Cannabis
Post Contusional Syndrome - F07.81 - Hybrid Cannabis
Postcricoid Region - see condition
Post Dates (40-42 weeks) - pregnancy, mother - O48.0 - Cannabidiol (CBD)
Postencephalitic Syndrome - F07.89 - Salvia Cannabis
Posterior - see condition
Posterolateral Sclerosis - spinal cord - also see degeneration, combined
Postexanthematous - see condition
Postfebrile - see condition
Postgastrectomy Dumping Syndrome - K91.1 - Salvia Cannabis
Posthemiplegic Chorea - see monoplegia
Posthemorrhagic Anemia - chronic - D50.0 - Caryophyllene (CB2)
Postherpetic Neuralgia - zoster - B02.29 - Indicia Cannabis
Posthitis - N47.7
Postimmunization Complication or reaction - see complications, vaccination
Postinfectious - see condition
Postlaminectomy Syndrome NEC - M96.1 - Hybrid Cannabis
Postleukotomy Syndrome - F07.0 - Hybrid Cannabis
Postmastectomy Lymphedema - syndrome - I97.2 - Hybrid Cannabis
Postmaturity - postmature (over 42 weeks)
Postmeasles Complication (NEC) - see also condition
Postmenopausal
Postnasal Drip - R09.82 - Salvia Cannabis

Postnatal - see condition
Postoperative - postprocedural - see complication, postoperative
Postpancreatectomy Hyperglycemia - E89.1 - Salvia Cannabis
Postpartum - see puerperal
Postphlebitic Syndrome - see syndrome, postthrombotic
Postpoliomyelitic (PPS) - see also condition
Postpolio - myelitic - G14 - Indicia Cannabis
Postprocedural - see also postoperative
Postschizophrenic Depression - F32.8 - Salvia Cannabis
Postsurgery Status - see also status, post
Post Term (40-42 weeks) - pregnancy, mother - O48.0 - Cannabidiol (CBD)
Post Traumatic Brain Syndrome - nonpsychotic - F07.81 - Indicia Cannabis
Post-Typhoid Abscess - A01.09 - Indicia Cannabis
Postures - hysterical - F44.2 - Indicia Cannabis
Postvaccinal Reaction or complication - also see complications, vaccination
Postvalvulotomy Syndrome - I97.0 - Hybrid Cannabis
Potain's
Potter's
Pott's
Pouch
Pouchitis - K91.850 - Salvia Cannabis
Poultrymen's Itch - B88.0 - Indicia Cannabis
Poverty (NEC) - Z59.6 - Indicia Cannabis
Poxvirus (NEC) - B08.8 - Salvia Cannabis
Prader-Willi Syndrome - Q87.1 - Hybrid Cannabis
Preauricular Appendage or tag - Q17.0 - Hybrid Cannabis
Precipitate Labor or delivery - O62.3 - Indicia Cannabis
Preclimacteric Bleeding Menorrhagia - N92.4 - Hybrid Cannabis
Precocious
Precocity - sexual, constitutional, cryptogenic, female - E30.1 - Indicia Cannabis
Precordial Pain - R07.2 - Hybrid Cannabis
Predeciduous Teeth - K00.2 - Cannnabidiol (CBD)
Prediabetes - prediabetic - R73.09 - Indicia Cannabis
Predislocation Hip at Birth - Q65.6 - Cannabidiol (CBD)
Pre Eclampsia - O14.9- Indicia Cannabis
Pre Eruptive Color Change - teeth, tooth - K00.8 - Caryophyllene (CB2)
Pre Excitation Atrioventricular Conduction - I45.6 - Hybrid Cannabis
Preglaucoma - H40.00 - Salvia Cannabis
Pregnancy Single - uterine - also see delivery

Preiser's Disease - also see osteonecrosis, secondary, due to, trauma, metacarpus
Pre-Kwashiorkor - also see malnutrition, severe
Preleukemia Syndrome - D46.9 - Hybrid Cannabis
Preluxation - hip, congenital - Q65.6 - Indicia Cannabis
Premature - see also condition
Preterm - newborn
Premenstrual
Premolarization - cuspids - K00.2 - Hybrid Cannabis
Prenatal
Preparatory Care for Subsequent Treatment (NEC)
Prepartum - see condition
Preponderance - left or right ventricular - I51.7 - Hybrid Cannabis
Prepuce - see condition
Posterior Reversible Encephalopathy Syndrome (PRES) - I67.83 - Hybrid Cannabis
Presbycardia - R54 - Hybrid Cannabis
Presbycusis - H91.1- Caryophyllene (CB2)
Presbyesophagus - K22.8 - Salvia Cannabis
Presbyophrenia - F03 - Salvia Cannabis
Presbyopia - H52.4 - Salvia Cannabis
Prescription of Contraceptives - initial - Z30.019 - Cannabidiol (CBD)
Presence (of)
Presenile - see condition
Presentation - fetal - also delivery, complicated by, malposition
Prespondylolisthesis - congenital - Q76.2 - Hybrid Cannabis
Pressure
Pre-Syncope - R55 - Hybrid Cannabis
Preterm
Previa
Priapism - N48.30 - Indicia Cannabis
Prickling Sensation - skin - R20.2 - Indicia Cannabis
Prickly Heat - L74.0 - Indicia Cannabis
Primary - see condition
Primigravida
Primipara
Primus Varus - bilateral - Q66.2 - Salvia Cannabis
Prolonged Reversible Ischemic Neurologic Deficit (PRIND) - I63.9 - Hybrid Cannabis
Pringle's Disease - tuberous sclerosis - Q85.1 - Sativa Strains
Prinzmetal Angina - I20.1 - Hybrid Cannabis

Prizefighter Ear - see cauliflower
Problem (with) related to
Procedure - surgical
Procidentia - uteri - N81.3 - Hybrid Cannabis
Proctalgia - K62.89 - Hybrid Cannabis
Proctitis - K62.89 - Hybrid Cannabis
Proctocele
Proctocolitis, mucosal - see rectosigmoiditis, ulcerative
Proptosis - K62.3 - Caryophyllene (CB2)
Proctorrhagia - K62.5 - Indicia Cannabis
Proctosigmoiditis - K63.89 - Indicia Cannabis
Proctospasm - K59.4 - Indicia Cannabis
Profichet's Disease - also see disorder, soft tissue, specified type NEC
Progeria - E34.8 - Hybrid Cannabis
Prognathism - mandibular, maxillary - M26.19 - Salvia Cannabis
Progonoma - melanotic - see neoplasm, benign, by site
Progressive - see condition
Prolactinoma
Prolapse - prolapsed
Prolapsus - female - N81.9 - Cannabidiol (CBD)
Proliferation (s)
Proliferative - see condition
Prolonged - prolongation (of)
Prominence - prominent
Promiscuity - see high, risk, sexual behavior
Pronation
Prophylactic
Propionic Acidemia - E71.121 - Salvia Cannabis
Proptosis - ocular - see also exophthalmos
Prosecution - anxiety concerning - Z65.3 - Indicia Cannabis
Prosopagnosia - R48.3 - Hybrid Cannabis
Prostadynia - N42.81 - Hybrid Cannabis
Prostate, prostatic - see condition
Prostatism - see hyperplasia, prostate
Prostatitis - congestive, suppurative, with cystitis - N41.9 - Hybrid Cannabis
Prostatocystitis - N41.3 - Hybrid Cannabis
Prostatorrhea - N42.89 - Caryophyllene (CB2)
Prostatosis - N42.82 Indicia Cannabis
Prostration - R53.83 - Indicia Cannabis

Protanomaly - anomalous trichromat - H53.54 - Salvia Cannabis
Protanopia - complete, incomplete - H53.54 - Salvia Cannabis
Protection - against, from - see prophylactic
Protein
Proteinemia - R77.9 - Indicia Cannabis
Proteinosis
Proteinuria - R80.9 - Indicia Cannabis
Proteolysis - pathologic - D65 Indicia Cannabis
Proteus - mirabilis - B96.4 - Hybrid Cannabis
Prothrombin Gene Mutation - D68.52 - Caryophyllene (CB2)
Protoporphyria - erythropoietic - E80.0 - Hybrid Cannabis
Protozoal - see also condition
Protrusion
Prune Belly Syndrome - Q79.4 - Hybrid Cannabis
Prurigo - forex, gravies, simplex - L28.2 - Hybrid Cannabis
Pruritus - pruritic, essential - L29.9 - Indicia Cannabis
Pseudarthrosis - pseudoarthrosis, bone - see nonunion, fracture
Pseudoaneurysm - see aneurysm
Pseudoangiomatous Stromal - I81 - Salvia Cannabis
Pseudoangina - see angina
Pseudo Arteriosus - Q28.8 - Indicia Cannabis
Pseudoarthrosis - see pseudarthrosis
Pseudobulbar Affect - PBA - F48.2 - Salvia Cannabis
Pseudochromhidrosis - L67.8 - Indicia Cannabis
Pseudocirrhosis - liver, pericardial - I31.1 - Hybrid Cannabis
Pseudocowpox - B08.03 - Cannabidiol (CBD)
Pseudocoxalgia - M91.3- Indicia Cannabis
Pseudocroup - J38.5 - Hybrid Cannabis
Pseudo-Cushing's Syndrome - alcohol-induced - E24.4 - Salvia Cannabis
Pseudocyesis - F45.8 - Indicia Cannabis
Pseudocyst
Pseudoelephantiasis Neuroarthritica - Q82.0 - Caryophyllene (CB2)
Pseudoexfoliation - capsule, lens, also see cataract, specified NEC
Pseudofolliculitis Barbae - L73.1 - Salvia Cannabis
Pseudoglioma - H44.89 - Salvia Cannabis
Pseudohemophilia - Bernuth's, hereditary, type B - D68.0 - Salvia Cannabis
Pseudohermaphroditism - Q56.3 - Indicia Cannabis
Pseudo-Hurler's Polydystrophy - E77.0 - Salvia Cannabis
Pseudohydrocephalus - G93.2 - Salvia Cannabis

Pseudohypertrophic Muscular Dystrophy (Erb's) - G71.0 - Cannabidiol (CBD)
Pseudohypertrophy - muscle - G71.0 - Indicia Cannabis
Pseudo Hypoparathyroidism - E20.1 - Indicia Cannabis
Pseudoinsomnia - F51.03 - Indicia Cannabis
Pseudoleukemia - infantile - D64.89 - Caryophyllene (CB2)
Pseudomembranous - see condition
Pseudomonas - (newborn) - P54.6 - Cannabidiol (CBD)
Pseudomenstruation - (newborn) - P54.6 Cannabidiol (CBD)
Pseudomeningocele - cerebral, infective, posttraumatic - G96.19 - Cannabidiol (CBD)
Pseudomonas
Pseudomyotonia - G71.19 - Salvia Cannabis
Pseudomyxoma Peritonei - C78.6 - Salvia Cannabis
Pseudoneuritis - optic, nerve, disc, papilla - Q14.2 - Indicia Cannabis
Pseudo-Obstruction Intestine - acute, chronic, idiopathic - K59.8 - Hybrid Cannabis
Pseudopapilledema - H47.33- Indicia Cannabis
Pseudoparalysis
Pseudopelade - L66.0 - Hybrid Cannabis
Pseudophakia - Z96.1 - Salvia Cannabis
Pseudo-Polyarthritis - M35.3 - Hybrid Cannabis
Pseudopolycythemia - D75.1 - Hybrid Cannabis
Pseudopseudohypoparathyroidism - E20.1 - Hybrid Cannabis
Pseudopterygium - H11.81 - Indicia Cannabis
Pseudoptosis - eyelid - see blepharochalasis
Pseudopuberty - precocious
Pseudorickets - renal - N25.0 - Indicia Cannabis
Pseudorubella - B08.20 - Indicia Cannabis
Pseudosclerema - newborn - P83.8 - Cannabidiol (CBD)
Pseudosclerosis - brain
Pseudotetanus - see convulsions
Pseudotetany 29.0 - Salvia Cannabis
Pseudotruncus Arteriosus - Q25.4 - Hybrid Cannabis
Pseudotuberculosis - A28.2 - Hybrid Cannabis
Pseudotumor
Pseudoxanthoma Elasticum - Q82.8 - Hybrid Cannabis
Psilosis - sprue, tropical - K90.1 - Salvia Cannabis
Psittacosis - A70 - Caryophyllene (CB2)
Psoitis - M60.88 - Indicia Cannabis
Psoriasis - L40.9 - Cannabidiol (CBD)
Psychasthenia - F48.8 - Hybrid Cannabis

Psychiatric Disorder or problem - F99 - Hybrid Cannabis
Psychogenic - see also condition
Psychological and Behavioral Factors - F59 - Hybrid Cannabis
Psychoneurosis - psychoneurotic - see also neurosis
Psychopathy - psychopathic
Psychosexual Identity Disorder of Childhood - F64.2 - Cannabidiol (CBD)
Psychosis - psychotic - F29 - Cannabidiol (CBD)
Psychosomatic - see disorder, psychosomatic
Psychosyndrome - organic - F07.9 - Salvia Cannabis
Psychotic Episode - associated with physical condition - F06.8 - Hybrid Cannabis
Pterygium, eye - H11.00 - Cannabidiol (CBD)
Ptilosis - eyelid - see madarosis
Ptomaine - poisoning - see poisoning, food
Ptosis - see also blepharoptosis
PTP - D69.51 - Indicia Cannabis
Ptyalism - periodic - K11.7 - Hybrid Cannabis
Ptyalolithiasis - K11.5 - Hybrid Cannabis
Pubarche - precocious - E30.1 - Hybrid Cannabis
Pubertas Praecox - E30.1 - Caryophyllene (CB2)
Puberty - development state - Z00.3 - Salvia Cannabis
Puckering - macula - see degeneration, macula, puckering
Pudenda - pudendum- see condition
Puente's Disease - simple glandular cheilitis - K13.0 - Salvia Cannabis
Puerperal - puerperium, complicated by, complications
Puerperium - see puerperal
Pulmolithiasis - J98.4 - Salvia Cannabis
Pulmonary - see condition
Pulpitis - acute, anachoretic, chronic, hyperplastic, irreversible, putrescent, reversible, suppurative, ulcerative - K04.0 - Salvia Cannabis
Pulpless tooth - K04.99 - Cannabidiol (CBD)
Pulse
Pulsus Alternans or trigeminus - R00.8 - Indicia Cannabis
Punch Drunk - F07.81 - Indicia Cannabis
Punctum Lacrimale Occlusion - see obstruction, lacrimal
Puncture
Pyrexia of unknown origin (PUO) - R50.9 - Cannadidiol (CBD)
Pupillary Membrane - persistent - Q13.89 - Indicia Cannabis
Pupillotonia - also see anomaly, pupil, function, tonic pupil
Purpura - D69.2 - Indicia Cannabis

Purpuric Spots - R23.3 - Salvia Cannabis
Purulent - see condition
Pus
Pustular Rash - L08.0 - Indicia Cannabis
Pustule, nonmalignant - L08.9 - Hybrid Cannabis
Pustulosis Palmaris Et Plantaris - L40.3 - Hybrid Cannabis
Putnam - Dana - see degeneration, combined
Putrescent Pulp - dental - K04.1 - Indicia Cannabis
Pyarthritis - pyarthrosis - also see arthritis, pyogenic or pyemic
Pyelectasis - also see hydronephrosis
Pyelitis - Congenital, uremic - see pyelonephritis
Pyelocystitis - see pyelonephritis
Pyelonephritis - see also nephritis, tubulointerstital
Pyelonephrosis - obstructive - N11.1 - Hybrid Cannabis
Pyeloureteritis Cystic - N28.85 - Caryophyllene (CB2)
Pyemia - pyemic, fever, infection, purulent - see sepsis
Pygopagus - Q89.4 - Salvia Cannabis
Pyknoepilepsy - idiopathic - see pyknolepsy
Pyknolepsy - G40.A09 - Indicia Cannabis
Pylephlebitis - K75.1 - Indicia Cannabis
Pyle's Syndrome - Q78.5 - Hybrid Cannabis
Pylethrombophlebitis - K75.1 - Hybrid Cannabis
Pylethrombosis - K75.1 - Hybrid Cannabis
Pyloritis - K29.90 - Hybrid Cannabis
Pylorospasm - reflex - K31.3 - Indicia Cannabis
Pylorus, pyloric - see condition
Pyoarthrosis - see arthritis, pyogenic or pyemic
Pyocele
Pyocolpos - see vaginitis
Pyocystitis - N30.80 - Hybrid Cannabis
Pyoderma - L08.0 - Hybrid Cannabis
Pyodermatitis - L08.0 - Salvia Cannabis
Pyogenic - see condition
Pyohydronephrosis - N13.6 - Salvia Cannabis
Pyometra - see endometritis
Pyomyositis - tropical - see myositis, infective
Pyonephritis - N12 - Salvia Cannabis
Pyonephrosis - N13.6 - Salvia Cannabis
Pyo-oophoritis - see salpingo-oophoritis

Pyo-Ovarium - see salpingo-oophoritis
Pyopericarditis - I30.1 - Salvia Cannabis
Pyophlebitis - see phlebitis
Pyopneumopericardium - I30.1 - Hybrid Cannabis
Pyopneumothorax - infective - J86.9 - Hybrid Cannabis
Pyosalpinx - pyosalpingitis - see also salpingo-oophoritis
Pyothorax - J86.9 - Indicia Cannabis
Pyoureter - N28.89 - Caryophyllene (CB2)
Pyramidopallidonigral Syndrome - G20 - Hybrid Cannabis
Pyrexia - of unknown origin - R50.9 - Hybrid Cannabis
Pyroglobulinemia NEC - E88.09 - Hybrid Cannabis
Pyromania - F63.1 - Salvia Cannabis
Pyrosis - R12 - Indicia Cannabis
Pyuria - bacterial - N39.0 - Indicia Cannabis

Q

Q fever - A78 - Indicia Cannabis
Quadricuspid Aortic Valve - Q23.8 - Caryophyllene (CB2)
Quadrilateral Fever - A78 - Indicia Cannabis
Quadriparesis - see quadriplegia
Quadriplegia - G82.50 - Hybrid Cannabis
Quadruplet - pregnancy - see pregnancy, quadruplet
Quarrelsomeness - F60.3 - Cannabidiol (CBD)
Queensland Fever - A77.3 - Indicia Cannabis
Quervain's Disease - M65.4 - Hybrid Cannabis
Queyrat's Erythroplasia - D07.4 - Hybrid Cannabis
Quincke's Disease or edema - T78.3 - Hybrid Cannabis
Quinsy, gangrenous - J36 - Hybrid Cannabis
Quintan Fever - A79.0 - Indicia Cannabis
Quintuplet - pregnancy - see pregnancy, quintuplet

R

Rabbit fever - see tularemia
Rabies - A82.9 - Salvia Cannabis
Rachischisis - see spina bifida
Rachitic - see also condition
Rachitis - Rachitis, acute, trade - see also rickets
Radial Nerve - see condition

Radiation
Radiculitis - pressure, vertebra genic - see radiculopathy
Radiculomyelitis - see also encephalitis
Radiculopathy - M54.10 - Salvia Cannabis
Radiodermal Burns - acute, chronic, or occupational - see burn
Radiodermatitis - L58.9 - Indicia Cannabis
Radiotherapy Session - Z51.0 - Indicia Cannabis
Rage - meaning rabies - see rabies
Ragpicker's Disease - A22.1 - Hybrid Cannabis
Ragsorter's Disease - A22.1 - Hybrid Cannabis
Raillietiniasis - B71.8 - Caryophyllene (CB2)
Railroad Neurosis - F48.8 - Hybrid Cannabis
Railway Spine - F48.8 - Hybrid Cannabis
Raised - see also elevated
Rake Teeth - M26.39 - Cannabidiol (CBD)
Rales - R09.89 - Indicia Cannabis
Ramifying Renal Pelvis - Q63.8 - Hybrid Cannabis
Ramsay-Hunt Disease or Syndrome - see hunt's disease - B02.21 - Hybrid Cannabis
Ranula - K11.6 - Indicia Cannabis
Rarefaction, bone - also see disorder, bone, density and structure, specified (NEC)
Rash - toxic - R21 - Salvia Cannabis
Rasmussen an Aneurysm - see tuberculosis, pulmonary
Rasmussen Encephalitis - G04.81 - Indicia Cannabis
Rat Bite Fever - A25.9 - Caryophyllene (CB2)
Rathke's Pouch Tumor - D44.3 - Hybrid Cannabis
Raymond - Céstan - I65.8 - Salvia Cannabis
Raynaud's Disease - phenomenon or syndrome, secondary - I73.00 - Hybrid Cannabis
RDS - newborn, type I - P22.0 - Cannabidiol (CBD)
Reaction - see also disorder
Reactive Airway Disease
Reactive Depression - see reaction, depressive
Rearrangement
Recalcitrant Patient - see noncompliance
Recanalization - thrombus - see thrombosis
Recession - receding
Recklinghausen Disease - Q85.01 - Hybrid Cannabis
Reclus' Disease - cystic - see mastopathy, cystic
Recrudescent Typhus - fever - A75.1 - Hybrid Cannabis

Recruitment - auditory - H93.21- Hybrid Cannabis
Rectalgia - K62.89 - Indicia Cannabis
Rectitis - K62.89 - Hybrid Cannabis
Rectocele
Rectosigmoid Junction - see condition
Rectosigmoiditis - K63.89 - Salvia Cannabis
Rectourethral - see condition
Rectovaginal - see condition
Rectovesical - see condition
Rectum - rectal - see condition
Recurrent - see condition
Red Bugs - B88.0 - Indicia Cannabis
Red Cedar Lung or pneumonitis - J67.8 - Caryophyllene (CB2)
Red Tide - see also table of drugs and chemicals - T65.82 - Indicia Cannabis
Reduced
Redundant, redundancy
Reduplication - see duplication
Reflex - R29.2 - Indicia Cannabis
Reflux - K21.9 - Caryophyllene (CB2)
Reforming - artificial openings - also see attention to, artificial, opening
Refractive Error - also see disorder, refraction
Refsum's Disease or Syndrome - G60.1 - Hybrid Cannabis
Refusal of
Regional - see condition
Regurgitation - R11.10 - Hybrid Cannabis
Reifenstein Syndrome - E34.52 - Hybrid Cannabis
Reinsertion - contraceptive device - Z30.433 - Hybrid Cannabis
Reiter's Disease - Syndrome or urethritis - M02.30 - Hybrid Cannabis
Reichmann's Disease or Syndrome - K31.89 - Salvia Cannabis
Rejection
Relapsing Fever - A68.9 - Salvia Cannabis
Relationship
Relaxation
Release from Prison - anxiety concerning - Z65.2 - Indicia Cannabis
Remains
Remittent Fever - malaria - B54 - Hybrid Cannabis
Remnant
Removal - from (of)
Ren

Renal - see condition
Rendu-Osler-Weber Disease or Syndrome - I78.0 - Hybrid Cannabis
Reninoma - D41.0 - Hybrid Cannabis
Renon-Delille Syndrome - E23.3 - Hybrid Cannabis
Reovirus - as cause of disease classified elsewhere - B97.5 - Salvia Cannabis
Repeated Falls (NEC) - R29.6 - Caryophyllene (CB2)
Replaced Chromosome by dicentric ring - Q93.2 - Salvia Cannabis
Replacement of artificial or mechanical device or prosthesis of
Request for expert evidence - Z04.8 - Sativa Strains
Reserve - decreased or low
Residual - see also condition
Resistance - resistant (to)
Resorption
Respiration
Respiratory - see also condition
Respite Care - Z75.5 - Indicia Cannabis
Response (drug)
Restless Legs - Syndrome - G25.81 - Hybrid Cannabis
Restlessness - R45.1 - Indicia Cannabis
Restriction of housing space - Z59.1 - Salvia Cannabis
Restoration (of)
Restorative - Material, dental
Rests - ovarian, in fallopian tube - Q50.6 - Salvia Cannabis
Restzustand - schizophrenic - F20.5 - Cannabidiol (CBD)
Retained - see also retention
Retardation
Retching - see vomiting
Retention - see also retained
Reticular Erythematous Mucinosis - L98.5 - Hybrid Cannabis
Reticulation - dust - see pneumoconiosis
Reticulocytosis - R70.1 - Hybrid Cannabis
Reticuloendotheliosis
Reticulohistiocytoma - giant-cell - D76.3 - Hybrid Cannabis
Reticuloid, actinic - L57.1 - Hybrid Cannabis
Reticulosis (skin)
Retina - retinal - see also condition
Retinitis - see also Inflammation, chorioretinal
Retinoblastoma - C69.2 - Hybrid Cannabis
Retinochoroiditis - see also Inflammation, chorioretinal

Retinopathy (background) - H35.00 - Hybrid Cannabis
Retinoschisis - H33.10 - Indicia Cannabis
Retortamonads - A07.8 - Hybrid Cannabis
Retractile Testis - Q55.22 - Hybrid Cannabis
Retraction
Retrobulbar - see condition
Retrocecal - see condition
Retrocession - see retroversion
Retrodisplacement - see retroversion
Retroflection - retroflection - see retroversion
Retrognathia - retrognathism, mandibular, maxillary - M26.19 - Hybrid Cannabis
Retrograde Menstruation - N92.5 - Indicia Cannabis
Retroperitoneal - see condition
Retroperitoneal - see condition
Retroperitonitis - K68.9 - Hybrid Cannabis
Retropharyngeal - see condition
Retroplacental - see condition
Retroposition - see retroversion
Retro Prosthetic Membrane - T85.398 - Tetrahydrocannabinol (THC)
Retrosternal Thyroid - congenital - Q89.2 - Hybrid Cannabis
Retroversion - retroverted
Retrovirus - as cause of disease classified elsewhere - B97.30 - Salvia Cannabis
Retrusion - premaxilla, developmental - M26.09 - Hybrid Cannabis
Rett's Disease or Syndrome - F84.2 - Hybrid Cannabis
Reverse Peristalsis - R19.2 - Hybrid Cannabis
Reye's Syndrome - G93.7 - Hybrid Cannabis
Rh - Factor
Rhabdomyolysis - idiopathic - M62.82 - Indicia Cannabis
Rhabdomyoma - see neoplasm, connective tissue, benign
Rhabdomyosarcoma (any type)
Rhabdosarcoma - see rhabdomyosarcoma
Rhesus - factor - see (Rh), incompatibility
Rheumatic - acute, subacute, chronic
Rheumatism - particular, neuralgic, nonarticular - M79.0 - Indicia Cannabis
Rheumatoid - see also condition
Rhinitis - atrophic, catarrhal, chronic, croupous, fibrinous, granulomatous, hyperplastic, hypertrophic, membranous, obstructive, purulent, suppurative, ulcerative - J31.0 - Cannabidiol (CBD)
Rhinoantritis - chronic - see sinusitis, maxillary

Rhinodacryolith - see dacryolith
Rhinolith - nasal sinus - J34.89 - Indicia Cannabis
Rhinomegaly - J34.89 - Hybrid Cannabis
Rhinopharyngitis - acute, subacute - see also nasopharyngitis
Rhinophyma - L71.1 - Indicia Cannabis
Rhinorrhea - J34.89 - Hybrid Cannabis
Rhinosalpingitis - see salpingitis, eustachian
Rhinoscleroma - A48.8 - Hybrid Cannabis
Rhinosporidiosis - B48.1 - Cannabidiol (CBD)
Rhinovirus Infection NEC - B34.8 - Salvia Cannabis
Rhizomelic Chondrodysplasia Punctuate - E71.540 - Hybrid Cannabis
Rhythm
Rhytidosis Facials - L98.8 - Hybrid Cannabis
Rib - see also condition
Riboflavin Deficiency - E53.0 - Salvia Cannabis
Rice Bodies - see loose, body, joint
Richter Syndrome - also see leukemia, chronic lymphocytic, B-cell type
Richter's Hernia - also see abdomen, hernia, and obstruction
Ricinism - see also poisoning, food, noxious, plant
Rickets - active, acute, adolescent, chest wall, congenital - E55.0 - Indicia Cannabis
Rickettsial Disease - A79.9 - Hybrid Cannabis
Rickettsialpox - Rickettsia - A79.1 - Hybrid Cannabis
Rickettsiosis - A79.9 - Indicia Cannabis
Rider's Bone - also see ossification, muscle, specified NEC
Ridge - alveolus - see also condition
Ridged - ear, congenital - Q17.3 - Cannabidiol (CBD)
Riedel's
Rieger's Anomaly or Syndrome - Q13.81 - Hybrid Cannabis
Riehl's Melanosis - L81.4 - Hybrid Cannabis
Rietti-Greppi-Micheli Anemia - D56.9 - Indicia Cannabis
Rieux's Hernia - see also hernia, abdomen, specified site (NEC)
Riga - Fede - K14.0 - Hybrid Cannabis
Riggs' Disease - see periodontitis
Right Middle Lobe Syndrome - J98.11 - Hybrid Cannabis
Rigid - rigidity - see also condition
Rigors - R68.89 - Indicia Cannabis
Riley-Day Syndrome - G90.1 - Hybrid Cannabis
Reversible Ischemic Neurologic Deficit (RIND) - I63.9 - Indicia Cannabis
Ring (s)

Ringed Hair - congenital - Q84.1 - Indicia Cannabis
Ringworm - B35.9 - Indicia Cannabis
Rise - venous pressure - I87.8 - Salvia Cannabis
Risk - suicidal
Ritter's Disease - L00 - Hybrid Cannabis
Rivalry - sibling - Z62.891 - Caryophyllene (CB2)
Rivalta's Disease - A42.2 - Hybrid Cannabis
River Blindness - B73.01 - Caryophyllene (CB2)
Robert's Pelvis - Q74.2 - Hybrid Cannabis
Robin - Pierre - Q87.0 - Salvia Cannabis
Robinow-Silvermann-Smith Syndrome - Q87.1 - Hybrid Cannabis
Robinson's, hidrotic - Q82.4 - Indicia Cannabis
Robles' Disease - B73.01 - Hybrid Cannabis
Rocky Mountain - spotted - A77.0 - Hybrid Cannabis
Roethel - see rubella
Roger's Disease - Q21.0 - Hybrid Cannabis
Rokitansky-Aschoff Sinuses, gallbladder - K82.8 - Hybrid Cannabis
Rolando's Fracture - displaced - S62.22 - Indicia Cannabis
Romano-Ward - prolonged QT interval - I45.81 - Indicia Cannabis
Romberg's Disease or Syndrome - G51.8 - Hybrid Cannabis
Roof - mouth - see condition
Rosacea - L71.9 - Indicia Cannabis
Rosary - rachitic - E55.0 - Indicia Cannabis
Rose
Rosenbach's Erysipeloid - A26.0 - Hybrid Cannabis
Rosenthal's Disease or Syndrome - D68.1 - Hybrid Cannabis
Roseola - B09 - Hybrid Cannabis
Rossbach's Disease - K31.89 - Hybrid Cannabis
Ross River Disease or fever - B33.1 - Hybrid Cannabis
Rostan's Asthma - cardiac - see failure, ventricular, left
Rotation
Rotes Quérol Disease or Syndrome - see hyperostosis, ankylosing
Roth, Bernhardt - see meralgia paraesthetica
Rothmund - Thomson - Q82.8 - Indicia Cannabis
Rotor's Disease or Syndrome - E80.6 - Hybrid Cannabis
Round
Roussy-Lévy Syndrome - G60.0 - Salvia Cannabis
Rubella - German Measles - B06.9 - Cannabidiol (CBD)
Rubeola - meaning measles - see measles

Rubeosis - Iris - see disorder, iris, vascular
Rubinstein-Taybi Syndrome - Q87.2 - Indicia Cannabis
Rudimentary - congenital - see also agenesis
Ruled Out Condition - see observation, suspected
Rumination - R11.10 - Salvia Cannabis
Runeberg's Disease - D51.0 - Hybrid Cannabis
Runny Nose - R09.89 - Caryophyllene (CB2)
Rupia, syphilitic - A51.39 - Salvia Cannabis
Rupture Ruptured
Russell-Silver Syndrome - Q87.1 - Indicia Cannabis
Russian Spring - Summer type encephalitis - A84.0 - Salvia Cannabis
Rust's Disease - tuberculous cervical spondylitis - A18.01 - Hybrid Cannabis
Ruvalcaba-Myhre-Smith Syndrome - E71.440 - Hybrid Cannabis
Rytand-Lipsitch Syndrome - I44.2 - Hybrid Cannabis

S

Saber Shin Ortibia - syphilitic - A50.56 - Salvia Cannabis
Sac Lacrimal - see condition
Saccharomyces Infection - B37.9 - Indicia Cannabis
Saccharopinuria - E72.3 - Salvia Cannabis
Saccular - see condition
Sacculation
Sachs' Amaurotic Familial Idiocy or disease - E75.02 - Hybrid Cannabis
Sachs-Tay Disease - E75.02 - Hybrid Cannabis
Sacks-Libman Disease - M32.11 - Hybrid Cannabis
Sacralgia - M53.3 - Indicia Cannabis
Sacralization - Q76.49 - Hybrid Cannabis
Sacroiliac Joint - see condition
Sacroiliitis (NEC) - M46.1 - Hybrid Cannabis
Sacrum - see condition
Saddle Sadism (sexual) - F65.52 - Hybrid Cannabis
Sadness - Postpartum - O90.6
Sadomasochism - F65.50 - Sativa Strains
Saemisch's Ulcer - cornea - see also ulcer, cornea, central
Sahib Disease - B55.0 - Hybrid Cannabis
Sailors' Skin - L57.8 - Cannabidiol (CBD)
Saint
Salaam
Salicylism

Salivary Duct or gland - see condition
Salivation - excessive - K11.7 - Hybrid Cannabis
Salmonella - see infection, salmonella
Salmonellosis - A02.0 - Caryophyllene (CB2)
Salpingitis - catarrhal, fallopian tube, modular - N70.91 - Indicia Cannabis
Salpingocele - N83.4 - Indicia Cannabis
Salpingo-Oophoritis - catarrhal, purulent, ruptured - N70.93 - Indicia Cannabis
Salpingo-Ovaritis - see salpingo-oophoritis
Salpingoperitonitis - see salpingo-oophoritis
Salzmann's Nodular Dystrophy - see degeneration, cornea, modular
Sampson's Cyst or tumor - N80.1 - Hybrid Cannabis
San Joaquin - Valley - B38.0 - Indicia Cannabis
Sandblaster's Asthma - lung or pneumoconiosis - J62.8 - Cannabidiol (CBD)
Sander's Disease - paranoia - F22 - Hybrid Cannabis
Sandfly Fever - A93.1 - Salvia Cannabis
Sandhoff's Disease - E75.01 - Hybrid Cannabis
Sanfilippo - Type B, Type C, Type D - E76.22 - Hybrid Cannabis
Sanger-Brown Ataxia - G11.2 - Hybrid Cannabis
Sao Paulo Fever or typhus - A77.0 - Hybrid Cannabis
Saponification - mesenteric - K65.8 - Salvia Cannabis
Sarcocele (benign)
Sarcocystosis - A07.8 - Hybrid Cannabis
Sarcoepiplocele - see hernia
Sarcoepiplomphalocele - Q79.2 - Hybrid Cannabis
Sarcoid - see also sarcoidosis
Sarcoidosis - D86.9 - Hybrid Cannabis
Sarcoma (of) - see neoplasm, connective tissue, malignant
Sarcomatous
Sarcosinemia - E72.59 - Caryophyllene (CB2)
Sarcosporidiosis - intestinal - A07.8 - Salvia Cannabis
Satiety - early - R68.81 - Indicia Cannabis
Saturnine - see condition
Saturnism
Satyriasis - F52.8 - Hybrid Cannabis
Sauriasis - see ichthyosis
subacute Bacterial Endocarditis (SBE) - I33.0 - Salvia Cannabis
Scabs - R23.4 - Salvia Cannabis
Scabies - any site - B86 - Cannabidiol (CBD)
Scaglietti-Dagnini Syndrome - E22.0 - Hybrid Cannabis

Scald - see burn
Scalenus Antics - anterior - G54.0 - Hybrid Cannabis
Scales - R23.4 - Cannabidiol (CBD)
Scaling - skin - R23.4 - Cannabidiol (CBD)
Scalp - see condition
Scapegoating Affecting Child - Z62.3 - Indicia Cannabis
Scaphocephaly - Q75.0 - Salvia Cannabis
Scapulalgia - M89.8X1 - Hybrid Cannabis
Scapulohumeral Myopathy - G71.0 - Hybrid Cannabis
Scar, scarring - see cicatrix - L90.5 - Hybrid Cannabis
Scarabiasis - B88.2 - Indicia Cannabis
Scarlatina - angina, malignant, ulcers - A38.9 - Salvia Cannabis
Scarlet Fever - albuminuria, angina dermatosis - A38.9 - Hybrid Cannabis
Schamberg's Disease - progressive pigmentary - L81.7 - Hybrid Cannabis
Schatzki's Ring - acquired, esophagus, lower - K22.2 - Salvia Cannabis
Schaufenster Krankheit - I20.8 - Indicia Cannabis
Schaumann's
Scheie's Syndrome - E76.03 - Hybrid Cannabis
Schenck's Disease - B42.1 - Hybrid Cannabis
Scheuermann's Disease or osteochondrosis - see osteochondrosis
Schilder - Flatau - G37.0 - Hybrid Cannabis
Schilling Type Monocytic Leukemia - C93.0- Indicia Cannabis
Schimmelbusch's Disease - cystic mastitis, or hyperplasia, mastopathy, cystic
Schistosoma Infestation - see Infestation, schistosoma
Schistosomiasis - B65.9 - Cannabidiol (CBD)
Schizencephaly - Q04.6 - Cannabidiol (CBD)
Schizoaffective Psychosis - F25.9 - Salvia Cannabis
Schizophonia - K00.2 - Salvia Cannabis
Schizoid Personality - F60.1 - Salvia Cannabis
Schizophrenia - schizophrenia - F20.9 - Cannabidiol (CBD)
Schizothymia - persistent - F60.1 - Hybrid Cannabis
Schlatter-Osgood Disease or osteochondrosis
Schlatter's Tibia - see osteochondrosis, minor, tibia
Schmidt's Syndrome - polyglandular, autoimmune - E31.0 - Hybrid Cannabis
Schmincke's Carcinoma or tumor - see neoplasm,
Schmitz - Stutzer - A03.0 - Hybrid Cannabis
Schmorl's Disease or nodes
Schneiderian
Scholte's Syndrome - malignant Carcinoid - E34.0 - Indicia Cannabis

Scholz - Bielchowsky-Henneberg - E75.25 - Indicia Cannabis
Schönlein - Henoch Disease or purpura, rheumatic - D69.0 - Indicia Cannabis
Schottmuller's Disease - A01.4 - Indicia Cannabis
Schroeder's Syndrome - endocrine hypertensive - E27.0 - Salvia Cannabis
Schüller-Christian Disease or Syndrome - C96.5 - Hybrid Cannabis
Schultze's Type Acroparesthesia, simple - I73.89 - Hybrid Cannabis
Schultz's Disease or Syndrome - see agranulocytosis
Schwalbe-Ziehen-Oppenheim Disease - G24.1 - Hybrid Cannabis
Schwannoma - see also neoplasm, nerve, benign
Schwannomatosis - Q85.03 - Indicia Cannabis
Schwartz - Jampel - G71.13 - Hybrid Cannabis
Schwartz-Bartter Syndrome - E22.2 - Indicia Cannabis
Schweiger-Buzzi Anetoderma - L90.1 - Salvia Cannabis
Sciatic - see condition
Sciatica - infective
Scimitar Syndrome - Q26.8 - Indicia Cannabis
Sclera - see condition
Sclerectasia - H15.84 - Caryophyllene (CB2)
Scleredema
Sclerema, adipose, oedematous, neonate rum, newborn - P83.0 - Indicia Cannabis
Scleriasis - see scleroderma
Scleritis - H15.00- Hybrid Cannabis
Sclerochoroiditis - H31.8 - Salvia Cannabis
Scleroconjunctivitis - see scleritis
Spherocytic Ovary Syndrome - E28.2 - Caryophyllene (CB2)
Sclerodactyly - sclerodactyly - L94.3 - Hybrid Cannabis
Scleroderma - sclerodermic, acro sclerotic, generalized - M34.9 - Indicia Cannabis
Sclerokeratitis - H16.8 - Hybrid Cannabis
Scleroma as - A48.8 - Indicia Cannabis
Scleromalacia - perforant - H15.05- Hybrid Cannabis
Scleromyxedema - L98.5 - Hybrid Cannabis
Sclérose En Plaques - G35 - Hybrid Cannabis
Sclerosis - sclerotic
Scoliosis - acquired, postural - M41.9 - Indicia Cannabis
Scoliotic Pelvis
Scorbutus - scorbutic - see also scurvy
Scotoma - arcuate, central, ring - see also defect
Scratch - see abrasion
Scratchy Throat - R09.89 - Salvia Cannabis

Screening (for) - Z13.9 - Indicia Cannabis
Scrofula - scrofulosis, tuberculosis of cervical lymph glands - A18.2 - Hybrid Cannabis
Scrofula - primary, tuberculous - A18.4 - Hybrid Cannabis
Scrofuloderma - scrofuloderma any site primary - A18.4 - Hybrid Cannabis
Scrofulous Lichen - primary, tuberculous - A18.4 - Hybrid Cannabis
Scrofulous - see condition
Scrotal Tongue - K14.5 - Cannabidiol (CBD)
Scrotum - see condition
Scurvy - scorbutic - E54 - Salvia Cannabis
Sealpox - B08.62 - Cannabidiol (CBD)
Seasickness - T75.3 - Indicia Cannabis
Seatworm - infection, infestation - B80 - Salvia Cannabis
Sebaceous - see also condition
Seborrhea - seborrheic - L21.9 - Hybrid Cannabis
Seckel's Syndrome - Q87.1 - Hybrid Cannabis
Seclusion - pupil - see membrane, pupillary
Second-Hand Tobacco Smoke Exposure, acute - Z77.22 - Cannabidiol (CBD)
Secondary
Secretion
Section
Segmentation - incomplete, congenital - see also fusion
Spielberger's Syndrome - infantile neuroaxonal dystrophy - G31.89 - Hybrid Cannabis
Seizure (s) see also convulsions - R56.9 - Cannabidiol (CBD)
Selenium Deficiency - dietary - E59 - Salvia Cannabis
Self Damaging Behavior - lifestyle - Z72.89 - Tetrahydrocannabinol (THC)
Self-harm - attempted
Self-mutilation - attempted
Self-poisoning
Semicoma - R40.1 - Hybrid Cannabis
Seminal Vesiculitis - N49.0 - Hybrid Cannabis
Seminoma - C62.9- Caryophyllene (CB2)
Senior-Usher Disease or syndrome - L10.4 - Hybrid Cannabis
Senectus - R54 - Hybrid Cannabis
Senescence - without mention of psychosis - R54 - Tetrahydrocannabinol (THC)
Senile - senility - see condition - R41.81 - Tetrahydrocannabinol (THC)
Sensation
Sense loss
Sensibility Disturbance - cortical, deep, vibratory - R20.9 - Hybrid Cannabis

Sensitive - sensitivity - see also allergy
Sensitive Beziehungswahn - F22 - Cannabidiol (CBD)
Sensitization - auto-erythrocytic - D69.2 - Hybrid Cannabis
Separation
Sepsis - generalized, unspecified organism - A41.9 - Indicia Cannabis
Septate - see septum
Septic - see condition
Septicemia - A41.9 - Indicia Cannabis
Septum - septate, congenital - see anomaly by site
Sequelae (of) - see also condition
Sequestration - see also sequestrum
Sequestrum
Sequoiosis Lung or Pneumonitis - J67.8 - Hybrid Cannabis
Serology for Syphilis
Seroma - see also hematoma
Seropurulent - see condition
Serositis, multiple - K65.8 - Hybrid Cannabis
Serious - see condition
Sertoli Cell
Sertoli-Leydig Cell Tumor - see also neoplasm, benign, by site
Serum
Sesamoiditis - M25.8 - Indicia Cannabis
Sever's Disease or Osteochondrosis - see juvenile, tarsus
Severe Sepsis - R65.20 - Hybrid Cannabis
Sex
Sextuplet Pregnancy - see pregnancy, sextuplet
Sexual
Sexuality - pathologic - see deviation, sexual
Sézary Disease - C84.1 - Salvia Cannabis
Shadow - lung - R91.8 - Cannabidiol (CBD)
Shaking Palsy or paralysis - see Parkinsonism
Shallowness - acetabulum - see derangement, joint, specified
Shaver's Disease - J63.1 - Hybrid Cannabis
Sheath - tendon - see condition
Sheathing - retinal vessels - H35.01- Indicia Cannabis
Shedding
Sheehan's Disease or Syndrome - E23.0 - Hybrid Cannabis
Shelf - rectal - K62.89 - Cannabidiol (CBD)
Shell Teeth - K00.5 - Hybrid Cannabis

Shellshock - current - F43.0 - Hybrid Cannabis
Shield Kidney - Q63.1 - Hybrid Cannabis
Shift
Shifting Sleep - work schedule, affecting sleep - G47.26 - Cannabidiol (CBD)
Shiga - Kruse - A03.0 - Hybrid Cannabis
Shiga's Bacillus - A03.0 - Cannabidiol (CBD)
Shigella - dysentery - see dysentery, bacillary
Shigellosis - A03.9 - Hybrid Cannabis
Shin Splints - S86.89 - Indicia Cannabis
Shingles - see herpes, zoster
Shipyard Disease or eye - B30.0 - Cannabidiol (CBD)
Shirodkar Suture - in pregnancy - see also pregnancy, complicated
Shock - R57.9 - Caryophyllene (CB2)
Shoemaker's Chest - M95.4 - Indicia Cannabis
Short - shortening, shortness
Shortsightedness - see myopia
Shoshin - acute fulminating beriberi - E51.11 - Salvia Cannabis
Shoulder - see condition
Shovel-Shaped Incisors - K00.2 - Salvia Cannabis
Shower - thromboembolic - see embolism
Shunt
Shutdown - renal - N28.9 - Cannabidiol (CBD)
Shy-Drager Syndrome - G90.3 - Hybrid Cannabis
Sialadenitis - sialadenosis, any gland, chronic, periodic
Sialectasia - K11.8 - Indicia Cannabis
Sialidosis - E77.1 - Indicia Cannabis
Sialitis - colitis, any gland, chronic, suppurative - see sialoadenitis
Sialoadenitis - any gland, periodic, suppurative - K11.20 - Cannabidiol (CBD)
Sialoadenopathy - K11.9 - Salvia Cannabis
Salpingitis - see Sialoadenitis
Sialodochitis - Fibrin - see sialoadenitis
Sialodocholithiasis - K11.5 - Hybrid Cannabis
Sialolithiasis - K11.5 - Hybrid Cannabis
Sialometaplasia - necrotizing - K11.8 - Hybrid Cannabis
Sialorrhea - see also ptyalism
Sialosis - K11.7 - Indicia Cannabis
Siamese Twin - Q89.4 - Cannabidiol (CBD)
Sibling Rivalry - Z62.891 - Hybrid Cannabis
Sicard's Syndrome - G52.7 - Hybrid Cannabis

Sicca Syndrome - M35.00 - Hybrid Cannabis
Sick - R69 - Indicia Cannabis
Sick Euthyroid Syndrome - E07.81 - Hybrid Cannabis
Sickle-cell
Sicklemia - see also disease, sickle-cell
Sickness
Sideropenia - see Anemia, iron deficiency
Siderosilicosis - J62.8 - Caryophyllene (CB2)
Siderosis (lung) - J63.4 - Hybrid Cannabis
Siemens' Syndrome, ectodermal dysplasia - Q82.8 - Hybrid Cannabis
Sighing - R06.89 - Cannabidiol (CBD)
Sigmoid - see also condition
Sigmoiditis - see also enteritis - K52.9 - Hybrid Cannabis
Silfversköld's Syndrome - Q78.9 - Hybrid Cannabis
Silicosiderosis - J62.8 - Hybrid Cannabis
Silicosis, silicotic, pure, complicated - J62.8 - Salvia Cannabis
Silicotuberculosis - J65 - Hybrid Cannabis
Silo-fillers' Disease - J68.8 Indicia Cannabis
Silver's Syndrome - Q87.1 - Caryophyllene (CB2)
Simian Malaria - B53.1 - Cannabidiol (CBD)
Simmonds' Cachexia or disease - E23.0 - Hybrid Cannabis
Simons' Disease, progressive lipodystrophy - E88.1 - Hybrid Cannabis
Simple, simplex - see condition
Simulation, conscious, of illness - Z76.5 - Cannabidiol (CBD)
Simultanagnosia, simultanagnosia - R48.3 - Hybrid Cannabis
Sin Nombre Virus Disease - hantavirus, cardio, pulmonary - B33.4 - Hybrid Cannabis
Sinding-Larsen Disease or osteochondrosis - see osteochondrosis
Singapore Hemorrhagic Fever - A91 - Hybrid Cannabis
Singer's Node or module - J38.2 - Caryophyllene (CB2)
Single
Singultus - R06.6 - Indicia Cannabis
Sinus - see also fistula
Sinusitis, accessory, hyperplastic, nasal, nonpurulent - J32.9 - Indicia Cannabis
Sinusitis Bronchiectasis-situs, syndrome, triad - Q89.3 - Hybrid Cannabis
Sipple's Syndrome - E31.22 - Hybrid Cannabis
Sirenomelia, syndrome - Q87.2 - Hybrid Cannabis
Siriasis - T67.0 - Hybrid Cannabis

Sarkari's Disease - B55.0 - Hybrid Cannabis
Siti - A65 - Hybrid Cannabis
Situation - Psychiatric - F99 - Caryophyllene (CB2)
Situational
Situs or Transverses - abdominal, thoracic - Q89.3 - Hybrid Cannabis
Sixth Disease - B08.20 - Hybrid Cannabis
Sjögren-Larsson Syndrome - Q87.1 - Hybrid Cannabis
Sjögren's Syndrome or disease - see sicca syndrome
Skeletal - see condition
Skene's Gland - see condition
Skenitis - see urethritis
Sarajevo - A65 - Indicia Cannabis
Skevas-Zerfus Disease - see also toxicity, venom, marine
Skin - see also condition
Slate Dressers' or slate-miners' lung - J62.8 - Hybrid Cannabis
Sleep
Sleep hygiene
Sleeping Sickness - see sickness, sleeping
Sleeplessness - see Insomnia
Sleep-Wake Schedule Disorder - G47.20 - Indicia Cannabis
Slim Disease - in (HIV) infection - B20 - Hybrid Cannabis
Slipped, moving
Slocumb's Syndrome - E27.0 - Hybrid Cannabis
Sloughing - multiple, phagedenas, skin - see also gangrene
Slow
Slowing - Urinary stream - R39.19 - Hybrid Cannabis
Sluder's Neuralgia Syndrome - G44.89 - Hybrid Cannabis
Slurred - slurring speech - R47.81 - Indicia Cannabis
Small (ness)
Small, light, for, dates see small for dates
Small-for, dates, infant - P05.10 - Salvia Cannabis
Smallpox - B03 - Salvia Cannabis
Smearing - fecal - R15.1 - Salvia Cannabis
Smith-Lemli-Opitz Syndrome - E78.72 - Hybrid Cannabis
Smith's Fracture - S52.54 - Cannabidiol (CBD)
Smoker - see dependence, drug, nicotine
Smoker's
Smoking
Smothering Spells - R06.81 - Indicia Cannabis

Snaggle Teeth - tooth - M26.39 - Cannabidiol (CBD)
Snapping
Sneddon-Wilkinson Disease or Syndrome, sub-corneal pustular
Sneezing - intractable - R06.7 - Indicia Cannabis
Sniffing
Sniffles
Snoring - R06.83 - Indicia Cannabis
Snow Blindness - see photokeratitis
Snuffles - non-syphilitic - R06.5 - Indicia Cannabis
Social
Sodoku - A25.0 - Indicia Cannabis
Soemmerring's Ring - see cataract, secondary
Soft - see also condition
Softening
Soldier's
Solitary
Solvent Abuse - see abuse, drug, inhalant
Somatization Reaction, somatic reaction - see disorder, somatoform
Somnambulism - F51.3 - Indicia Cannabis
Somnolence - R40.0 - Indicia Cannabis
Sonne Dysentery - A03.3 - Indicia Cannabis
Soor - B37.0 - Indicia Cannabis
Sore
Soto's Syndrome - Cerebral gigantism - Q87.3 - Indicia Cannabis
South African Cardiomyopathy Syndrome - I42.8 - Hybrid Cannabis
Southeast Asian hemorrhagic fever - A91 - Hybrid Cannabis
Spacing
Spade-like Hand - congenital - Q68.1 - Indicia Cannabis
Spading Nail - L60.8 - Cannabidiol (CBD)
Spanish Collar - N47.1 - Salvia Cannabis
Sparganosis - B70.1 - Indicia Cannabis
Spasm (s) - see condition - R25.2 - Indicia Cannabis
Spasmodic - see condition
Spasmophilia - see tetany
Spasmus Mutants - F98.4 - Hybrid Cannabis
Spastic - spasticity - see also spasm
Speaker's Throat - R49.8 - Cannabidiol (CBD)
Specific - specified - see condition
Speech

Spencer's Disease - A08.19 - Hybrid Cannabis
Spens' Syndrome - syncope with heart block - I45.9 - Hybrid Cannabis
Sperm Counts - fertility testing - Z31.41 - Cannabidiol (CBD)
Spermatic Cord - see condition
Spermatocele - N43.40 - Hybrid Cannabis
Spermatocytoma - C62.9- Indicia Cannabis
Spermatorrhea - N50.8 - Hybrid Cannabis
Sphacelus - see gangrene
Sphenoidal - see condition
Sphenopalatine Ganglion Neuralgia - G90.09 - Indicia Cannabis
Sphericity - increased, lens, congenital - Q12.4 - Cannabidiol (CBD)
Spherocytosis - congenital, familial, hereditary - D58.0 - Hybrid Cannabis
Spherophakia - Q12.4 - Indicia Cannabis
Sphincter - see condition
Sphincteritis - Sphincter of oddi - see cholangitis
Sphingolipidosis - E75.3 - Hybrid Cannabis
Sphingomyelinosis - E75.3 - Hybrid Cannabis
Spicule Tooth - K00.2 - Indicia Cannabis
Spider
Spiegler-Fendt
Spielmeyer-Vogt Disease - E75.4 - Hybrid Cannabis
Spina Bifida - apart - Q05.9 - Hybrid Cannabis
Spindle - Krukenberg's - see pigmentation, cornea, posterior
Spine - spinal - see condition
Spiradenoma - eccrine - see neoplasm, skin, benign
Spirillosis - A25.0 - Hybrid Cannabis
Spirillum
Spirochetal - see condition
Spirochetosis - A69.9 - Hybrid Cannabis
Spirometrosis - B70.1 - Indicia Cannabis
Spitting Blood - see hemoptysis
Splanchnoptosis - K63.4 - Cannabidiol (CBD)
Spleen - splenic - see condition
Splenectomies - see splenomegaly
Splenitis - interstitial, malignant, nonspecific - D73.89 - Hybrid Cannabis
Splenocyte - D73.89 Indicia Cannabis
Splenomegaly - splenomegalies, bengal, cryptogenic, idiopathic - R16.1 - Salvia Cannabis
Splenopathy - D73.9 - Salvia Cannabis

Splenoptosis - D73.89 - Salvia Cannabis
Splenosis - D73.89 - Salvia Cannabis
Splinter - see also foreign body, superficial, by site
Split, splitting
Spondylarthrosis -see spondylosis
Spondylitis - chronic - see also spondylopathy, inflammatory
Spondylolisthesis - acquired, degenerative - M43.10 - Hybrid Cannabis
Spondylolysis - acquired - M43.00 - Hybrid Cannabis
Spondylopathy - M48.9 - Caryophyllene (CB2)
Spondylosis - M47.9 - Hybrid Cannabis
Sponge
Sponge Divers Disease - see toxicity, venom, marine, animal, sea anemone
Spongioblastoma - any type - see neoplasm, malignant, by site
Spongioneuroblastoma - see neoplasm, malignant, by site
Spontaneous - see also condition
Spoon nail - L60.3 - Salvia Cannabis
Sporadic - see condition
Sporothrix Schenck-ii infection - see sporotrichosis
Sporotrichosis - B42.9 - Hybrid Cannabis
Spots - spotting (in) (of)
Spotted Fever - see also fever, spotted - N92.3 - Hybrid Cannabis
Sprain, joint, ligament
Sprengel's Deformity, congenital - Q74.0 - Hybrid Cannabis
Sprue - tropical - K90.1 - Salvia Cannabis
Spur - Bone - see also enthesopathy
Spurway's Syndrome - Q78.0 - Indicia Cannabis
Sputum
Squamous - see also condition
Squashed Nose - M95.0 - Indicia Cannabis
Squeeze, driver's - T70.3 Caryophyllene (CB2)
Squint - see also strabismus
St. Hubert's Disease - A82.9 - Indicia Cannabis
Stab - see also laceration
Stafne's Cyst or Cavity - M27.0 - Hybrid Cannabis
Staggering Gait - R26.0 - Salvia Cannabis
Staghorn Calculus - see calculus, kidney
Stähli's Line, cornea, pigment - see pigmentation, cornea, anterior
Stain - staining
Stammering - see Disorder, fluency - F80.81 - Hybrid Cannabis

Standstill
Stannosis - J63.5 - Hybrid Cannabis
Stanton's Disease - see melioidosis
Staphylinids - acute, catarrhal, chronic, gangrenous, membranous suppurative, ulcerative - K12.2 - Hybrid Cannabis
Staphylococcal scalded skin syndrome - L00 - Indicia Cannabis
Staphylococcemia - A41.2 - Cannabidiol (CBD)
Staphylococcus - staphylococcal - see also condition
Staphyloma - sclera
Stargardt's Disease - see dystrophy, retina
Starvation - inanition, due to lack of food - T73.0 - Salvia Cannabis
Stasis
State (of)
Status - post - see also presence (of)
Stealing
Steam Burn - see burn
Steatocystoma Multiplex - L72.2 - Hybrid Cannabis
Steatohepatitis - non-alcoholic, Nash - K75.81 - Hybrid Cannabis
Steatoma - L72.3 - Salvia Cannabis
Steatorrhea, chronic - K90.4 - Indicia Cannabis
Steatosis - E88.89 - Salvia Cannabis
Steele-Richardson-Olszewski Disease or syndrome - G23.1 - Hybrid Cannabis
Steinbrocker's syndrome - G90.8 - Hybrid Cannabis
Steinert's disease - G71.11 - Hybrid Cannabis
Stein-Leventhal Syndrome - E28.2 - Hybrid Cannabis
Stein's syndrome - E28.2 - Hybrid Cannabis
Stemi - also - Infarct, myocardium, ST elevation - I21.3 - Hybrid Cannabis
Stenocardia - I20.8 - Salvia Cannabis
Stenosis - stenotic, cicatricial - see also Stricture
Stent jail - T82.897 - Salvia Cannabis
Stercolith - impaction - K56.41 - Hybrid Cannabis
Stercoraceous - stem coral ulcer - K63.3 - Hybrid Cannabis
Stereotypies NEC - F98.4 - Salvia Cannabis
Sterility - see infertility
Sterilization - see encounter (for) sterilization
Sternalgia - see angina
Sternopagus - Q89.4 - Caryophyllene (CB2)
Sternum Bifid Um - Q76.7 - Hybrid Cannabis
Steroid

Stevens-Johnson Disease or Syndrome - L51.1 - Hybrid Cannabis
Stewart-Morel Syndrome - M85.2 - Hybrid Cannabis
Sticker's Disease - B08.3 - Indicia Cannabis
Sticky Eye - see conjunctivitis, acute, mucopurulent
Stieda's Disease - see bursitis, tibial collateral
Stiff Neck - see torticollis
Stiff Man Syndrome - G25.82 - Caryophyllene (CB2)
Stiffness - joint (NEC) - M25.60 - Cannabidiol (CBD)
Stigmata Congenital Syphilis - A50.59 - Salvia Cannabis
Stillbirth - P95 - Indicia Cannabis
Still-Felty Syndrome - see felty's syndrome
Still's Disease or Syndrome, juvenile - M08.20 - Indicia Cannabis
Stimulation - ovary - E28.1 - Cannabidiol (CBD)
Sting Venomous, with allergic or anaphylactic shock - also table of drugs and chemicals, by animal or substance, poisoning
Stippled Epiphyses - Q78.8 - Indicia Cannabis
Stitch
Stokes-Adams Disease or Syndrome - I45.9 - Hybrid Cannabis
Stokes' Disease - E05.00 - Cannabidiol (CBD)
Stokvis - Talma - D74.8 - Hybrid Cannabis
Stoma Malfunction
Stomach - see condition
Stomatitis - denture, ulcerative - K12.1 - Hybrid Cannabis
Stomatocytosis - D58.8 - Hybrid Cannabis
Dermatomycosis - B37.0 - Hybrid Cannabis
Stomatorrhagia - K13.79 - Indicia Cannabis
Stone (s) - see also calculus
Stonecutter's Lung - J62.8 - Hybrid Cannabis
Stonemason's Asthma - disease, lung - J62.8 - Hybrid Cannabis
Stoppage
Storm - thyroid - see thyrotoxicosis
Strabismus - congenital, nonparalytic - H50.9 - Hybrid Cannabis
Strain
Straining - on urination - R39.16 - Cannabidiol (CBD)
Strand - vitreous - see also opacity, vitreous, membranes and strands
Strangulation - strangulated - see also asphyxia, traumatic
Strangury - R30.0 - Salvia Cannabis
Straw Itch - B88.0 - Cannabidiol (CBD)
Strawberry

Streak (s)
Strephosymbolia - F81.0 - Salvia Cannabis
Streptobacillary Fever - A25.1 - Salvia Cannabis
Streptobacillus - A25.1 - Hybrid Cannabis
Streptobacillus Moniliformin - A25.1 - Hybrid Cannabis
Streptococcus - Streptococcal - see also condition
Streptomyces - B47.1 - Hybrid Cannabis
Streptotrichosis - A48.8 - Hybrid Cannabis
Stress - F43.9 - Cannabidiol (CBD)
Stretching Nerve - see injury, nerve
Striae Alicante - atrophic or distance (cutis) - L90.6 - Hybrid Cannabis
Stricture - see also stenosis
Stridor - R06.1 - Salvia Cannabis
Stridulous - see condition
Stroke - apoplectic, brain, embolic, ischemic, paralytic - I63.9 - Hybrid Cannabis
Stromatolites - endometrial - D39.0 - Cannabidiol (CBD)
Strongyloidiasis - strongyloidiasis - B78.9 - Hybrid Cannabis
Strophulus Pruriginous - L28.2 - Hybrid Cannabis
Struck by Lightning - see lightning
Struma - see also goiter
Strumipriva Cachexia - E03.4 - Indicia Cannabis
Strümpell-Marie Spine - see spondylitis, ankylosing
Strümpell-Westphal Pseudosclerosis - E83.01 - Hybrid Cannabis
Stuart Deficiency Disease - factor X - D68.2 - Hybrid Cannabis
Stuart-Prower Factor Deficiency, factor X - D68.2 - Hybrid Cannabis
Student's Elbow - see bursitis, elbow, olecranon
Stump - see amputation
Stunting, nutritional - E45 - Hybrid Cannabis
Stupor - catatonic - R40.1 - Indicia Cannabis
Sturge - Weber, Dimitri, Kalischer - Q85.8 - Indicia Cannabis
Stuttering - F80.81 - Cannabidiol (CBD)
Sty - style, external, internal, meibomian, persian - see hordeolum
Subacidity - gastric - K31.89 - Cannabidiol (CBD)
Subacute - see condition
Subarachnoid - see condition
Subcortical - see condition
Subcostal Syndrome - nerve compression - see also mononeuropathy
Subcutaneous - subcuticular - see condition
Subdural - see condition

Subendocardium - see condition
Subependymoma
Suberosis - J67.3 - Salvia Cannabis
Subglossitis - see glossitis
Subhemophilia - D66 - Cannabidiol (CBD)
Subinvolution
Sublingual - see condition
Sublinguitis - see sialoadenitis
Sublimatable Hip - Q65.6 - Hybrid Cannabis
Subluxation - see also dislocation
Submaxillary - see condition
Submersion - fatal, nonfatal - T75.1 - Hybrid Cannabis
Submucous - see condition
Subnormal - subnormality
Subphrenic - see condition
Subscapular Nerve - see condition
Subseptus Uterus - Q51.2 - Hybrid Cannabis
Subsiding Appendicitis - K36 - Cannabidiol (CBD)
Substernal Thyroid - E04.9 - Hybrid Cannabis
Substitution Disorder - F44.9 - Indicia Cannabis
Subtentorial - see condition
Succenturiate Placenta - O43.19- Hybrid Cannabis
Sucking - thumb, child, excessive - F98.8 - Cannabidiol (CBD)
Sudamen - Sudamina - L74.1 - Salvia Cannabis
Sudanese Kala Azar - B55.0 - Caryophyllene (CB2)
Sudden
Sudeck's Atrophy - Disease, or Syndrome - see also algoneurodystrophy
Suffocation - see asphyxia, traumatic
Sugar
Suicide - suicidal, attempted - T14.91 - Hybrid Cannabis
Suipestifer Infection - see Infection, salmonella
Sulfhemoglobinemia - scalp hemoglobinemia, acquired - D74.8 - Hybrid Cannabis
Sumatran Mite Fever - A75.3 - Hybrid Cannabis
Summer - see condition
Sunburn - L55.9 - Indicia Cannabis
Sunct - short-lasting unilateral neuralgiform headache with conjunctival injection and tearing - G44.059 - Salvia Cannabis
Sunken Acetabulum - see also derangement, joint, specified type (NEC), hip

Sunstroke - T67.0 - Cannabidiol (CBD)
Superfecundation - see also pregnancy, multiple
Superfetation - see pregnancy, multiple
Superinvolution - uterus - N85.8 - Indicia Cannabis
Supernumerary - congenital
Supervision (of)
Supplemental Teeth - K00.1 - Indicia Cannabis
Suppression
Suppuration - suppurative - see also condition
Supraeruption of Tooth, teeth - M26.34 - Cannabidiol (CBD)
Supraglottitis - J04.30 - Hybrid Cannabis
Suprarenal - Gland - see condition
Suprascapular Nerve - see condition
Suprasellar - see condition
Surfer's Knots or nodules - S89.8 - Indicia Cannabis
Surgical
Surveillance (of) (for) - see also observation
Susceptibility to Disease - genetic - Z15.89 - Hybrid Cannabis
Suspected Condition - ruled out - see also observation, suspected
Suspended Uterus
Sutton's Nevus - D22.9
Suture
Swab - inadvertently left in operation wound - see also foreign body - accidentally left during a procedure
Swallowed - swallowing
Swan-Neck Deformity - finger - see deformity, finger, swan-neck
Swearing - compulsive - F42 - Caryophyllene (CB2)
Sweat - sweats
Sweating - excessive - R61 - Hybrid Cannabis
Sweeley-Klionsky Disease - E75.21 - Hybrid Cannabis
Sweet's Disease or Dermatosis - L98.2 - Hybrid Cannabis
Swelling (of) - R60.9 - Hybrid Cannabis
Swift - Feer
Swimmer's
Swimming in the Head - R42 - Hybrid Cannabis
Swollen - see swelling
Swyer Syndrome - Q99.1 - Hybrid Cannabis
Sycosis - L73.8 - Hybrid Cannabis
Sydenham's Chorea - see chorea, sydenham's

Sylvatic Yellow Fever - A95.0 - Cannabidiol (CBD)
Sylvest's Disease - B33.0 - Hybrid Cannabis
Symblepharon - H11.23- Indicia Cannabis
Symond's Syndrome - G93.2 - Indicia Cannabis
Sympathetic - see condition
Sympatheticotonia - G90.8 - Salvia Cannabis
Sympathicoblastoma
Sympathogonioma - see sympathicoblastoma
Symphalangy - fingers, toes - Q70.9 - Cannabidiol (CBD)
Symptoms (NEC) - R68.89 - Hybrid Cannabis
Syncephalus - Q89.4 - Salvia Cannabis
Synchondrosis
Synchysis - scintillant, senile, vitreous body - H43.89 - Salvia Cannabis
Syncope - near, pre - R55 Hybrid Cannabis
Syndactylism - syndactyly - Q70.9 - Hybrid Cannabis
Syndrome - see also disease
Synechia - anterior, iris, posterior, pupil - see also adhesions, iris
Synesthesia - R20.8 - Cannabidiol (CBD)
Syngamiasis - Syndesmosis - B83.3 - Hybrid Cannabis
Synodontia - K00.2 - Hybrid Cannabis
Synarchism - Synarchism - Q55.1 - Indicia Cannabis
Synostosis - congenital - Q78.8 - Caryophyllene (CB2)
Synovial Sarcoma - see also connective tissue, malignant, neoplasm
Synovioma (fatal) - also neoplasm, connective tissue
Synoviosarcoma - see neoplasm, connective tissue, malignant
Synovitis - see also tenosynovitis
Syphilid - A51.39 - Indicia Cannabis
Syphilis - syphilitic, acquired - A53.9 - Hybrid Cannabis
Syphiloma - A52.79 - Indicia Cannabis
Syphilophobia - F45.29 - Indicia Cannabis
Syringadenoma - see also neoplasm, skin, benign
Syringobulbia - G95.0 - Hybrid Cannabis
Syringocystadenoma - see neoplasm, skin, benign
Syringoma - see also neoplasm, skin, benign
Syringomyelia - G95.0 - Caryophyllene (CB2)
Syringomyelitis - see encephalitis
Syringomyelocele - see spina bifida
Syringopontia - G95.0 - Hybrid Cannabis
System - systemic - see also condition

T

Tabac, tabacosis, tribalism - see also poisoning, tobacco
Tabardillo - A75.9 - Salvia Cannabis
Tabes, tabetic - A52.10 - Hybrid Cannabis
Taboparalysis - A52.17 - Hybrid Cannabis
Taboparesis, remission - A52.17 - Hybrid Cannabis
Trigeminal Autonomic Cephalgia (TAC) - G44.099 - Hybrid Cannabis
Tache Noir - S60.22- Indicia Cannabis
Tachyalimentation - K91.2 - Hybrid Cannabis
Tachyarrhythmia, tachyarrhythmia - see tachycardia
Tachycardia - R00.0 - Cannabidiol (CBD)
Tachygastria - K31.89 - Hybrid Cannabis
Tachypnea - R06.82 - Hybrid Cannabis
Taenia, infection, infestation - B68.9 - Hybrid Cannabis
Taeniasis, intestine - see taenia
Transfusion - Associated Circulatory Overload Taco - E87.71 - Indicia Cannabis
Tag, hypertrophied skin, infected - L91.8 - Cannabidiol (CBD)
Tahyna Fever - B33.8 - Indicia Cannabis
Takahara's Disease - E80.3 - Hybrid Cannabis
Takayasu's Illness or syndrome - M31.4 - Hybrid Cannabis
Talcosis, pulmonary - J62.0 - Caryophyllene (CB2)
Talipes, congenital - Q66.89 - Salvia Cannabis
Tall Stature, constitutional - E34.4 - Hybrid Cannabis
Talma's Disease - M62.89 - Hybrid Cannabis
Talon Noir - S90.3- Hybrid Cannabis
Tamponade, heart - I31.4 - Indicia Cannabis
Tanapox, Virus, disease
Tantrum, child problem - F91.8 - Cannabidiol (CBD)
Tapeworm, infection, infestation - see infestation, tapeworm
Tapia's Syndrome - G52.7 - Hybrid Cannabis
Thrombocytopenia with Absent Radius (TAR) - Q87.2 - Hybrid Cannabis
Tarral-Besnier Disease - L44.0 - Hybrid Cannabis
Tarsal Tunnel Syndrome - see syndrome, tarsal tunnel
Tartaglia - see pain, limb, lower
Tarsitis, eyelid - H01.8 - Indicia Cannabis
Tartar, teeth, dental calculus - K03.6 - Cannabidiol (CBD)
Tattoo (mark) - L81.8 Indicia Cannabis
Tauri's Disease - E74.09 - Indicia Cannabis

Taurodontism - K00.2 Indicia Cannabis

Taussig-Bing Syndrome - Q20.1 - Hybrid Cannabis

Taybi's Syndrome - Q87.2 - Hybrid Cannabis

Tay-Sachs Amaurotic Familial Idiocy or disease - E75.02 - Cannabidiol (CBD)

Traumatic Brain Injury (TBI)

Teacher's node or nodule - J38.2 - Caryophyllene (CB2)

Tear, torn, traumatic - see also laceration

Tear-Stone - see dacryolith

Teeth - see also condition

Teething, syndrome - K00.7 - Indicia Cannabis

Telangiectasia, telangiectasis, verrucous - I78.1 - Hybrid Cannabis

Telephone Scatological - F65.89 - Hybrid Cannabis

Telescoped Bowel or intestine - K56.1 - Cannabidiol (CBD)

Temperature

Temple - see condition

Temporal - see condition

Temporomandibular Joint Pain-Dysfunction Syndrome - M26.62 - Hybrid Cannabis

Temporosphenoidal - see condition

Tendency

Tenderness, abdominal - R10.819 - Indicia Cannabis

Tendinitis, tendonitis - see also enthesopathy

Tendon - see condition

Tendosynovitis - see tenosynovitis

Tenesmus, rectal - R19.8 - Salvia Cannabis

Tennis Elbow - see epicondylitis, lateral

Tenonitis - see also tenosynovitis

Tenosynovitis - see tenosynovitis

Tenontothecitis - see tenosynovitis

Tenosynovitis - see also synovitis - M65.9 - Caryophyllene (CB2)

Tenovaginitis - see tenosynovitis

Tension

Tentorium - see condition

Teratencephalus - Q89.8 - Hybrid Cannabis

Teratism - Q89.7 - Hybrid Cannabis

Teratoblastoma, malignant - see neoplasm, malignant, by site

Teratocarcinoma - see also neoplasm, malignant, by site

Teratoma, solid - see also neoplasm, uncertain behavior, by site

Termination

Ternidens Infestation - B81.8 - Salvia Cannabis
Ternidensiasis - B81.8 - Salvia Cannabis
Terror (s) night, child - F51.4 - Cannabidiol (CBD)
Terrorism, victim of - Z65.4 - Hybrid Cannabis
Terry's Syndrome - H44.2- Indicia Cannabis
Tertiary - see condition
Test - tests, testing (for) - Caryophyllene (CB2)
Testicle - testicular, testis - see also condition
Tetanus - tetanic, cephalic, convulsions - A35 - Hybrid Cannabis
Tetany (due to) - R29.0 - Hybrid Cannabis
Tetralogy of Fallot - Q21.3 - Cannabidiol (CBD)
Tetraplegia - chronic - see also quadriplegia - G82.50 - Hybrid Cannabis
Thailand Hemorrhagic Fever - A91 - Salvia Cannabis
Thalassanemia - see thalassemia
Thalassemia - anemia, disease - D56.9 - Caryophyllene (CB2)
Thanatophoric Dwarfism or short stature - Q77.1 - Cannabidiol (CBD)
Thermoplegia - T67.0 - Hybrid Cannabis
Thaysen-Gee Disease, nontropical sprue
Thermoplegia - T67.0 - Hybrid Cannabis
Thaysen's Disease - K90.0 - Indicia Cannabis
Thecoma - D27- Indicia Cannabis
Thelarche - premature - E30.8 - Indicia Cannabis
Thelaziasis - B83.8 - Indicia Cannabis
Thelitis - N61 - Cannabidiol (CBD)
Therapeutic - see condition
Therapy
Thermic - see condition
Thermography - abnormal - see also abnormal, diagnostic imaging - R93.8 - Indicia Cannabis
Thermoplegia - T67.0 - Hybrid Cannabis
Thesaurismosis - glycogen - see disease, glycogen storage
Thiamin Deficiency - E51.9 - Hybrid Cannabis
Triaminic Deficiency with Beriberi - E51.11 - Cannabidiol (CBD)
Thibierge-Weissenbach Syndrome - see sclerosis, systemic
Thickening
Thigh - see condition
Thinning vertebra - see spondylopathy, specified NEC - Hybrid Cannabis
Thirst - excessive - R63.1 - Sativa Cannabis
Thomsen Disease - G71.12 - Hybrid Cannabis

Thoracic - see also condition - Hybrid Cannabis
Thoracogastroschisis, congenital - Q79.8 - Hybrid Cannabis
Thoracopagus - Q89.4 - Hybrid Cannabis
Thorax - see condition - Caryophyllene (CB2)
Thorn's Syndrome - N28.89 - Hybrid Cannabis
Thorson-Björck Syndrome - E34.0 - Hybrid Cannabis
Threadworm - infection, infestation - B80 - Hybrid Cannabis
Threatened
Three-Day Fever - A93.1 - Hybrid Cannabis
Threshers' Lung - J67.0 - Cannabidiol (CBD)
Thrix - congenital - Q84.1 - Salvia Cannabis
Throat - see condition
Thrombasthenia - Glanzmann, hemorrhagic, hereditary - D69.1 - Hybrid Cannabis
Thromboangiitis - I73.1 - Salvia Cannabis
Thromboarteritis - see arteritis
Thrombocytasthenia - D69.1 - Salvia Cannabis
Thrombocythemia - essential, hemorrhagic, idiopathic, primary - D47.3 - Indicia Cannabis
Thrombocytopathy - dystrophic, granulopenia - D69.1 - Hybrid Cannabis
Thrombocytopenia - thrombocytopenic - D69.6 - Hybrid Cannabis
Thrombocytosis, essential - D47.3 - Hybrid Cannabis
Thromboembolism - see embolism
Thrombopathy - Bernard-Soulier - D69.1 - Indicia Cannabis
Thrombopenia - see thrombocytopenia
Thrombophilia - D68.59 - Caryophyllene (CB2)
Thrombophlebitis - I80.9 - Hybrid Cannabis
Thrombosis - thrombotic, bland, multiple, progressive, silent, vessel - I82.90 - Hybrid Cannabis
Thrombus - see thrombosis
Thrush - see also candidiasis
Thumb - see also condition
Thymitis - E32.8 - Hybrid Cannabis
Thymoma - benign - D15.0 - Indicia Cannabis
Thymus - thymic, gland - see condition
Thyrocele - see goiter
Thyroglossal - see also condition
Thyroid - gland, body - see also condition
Thyroiditis - E06.9 - Cannabidiol (CBD)

Thyrolingual Duct, persistent - Q89.2 - Caryophyllene (CB2)
Thyromegaly - E01.0 - Indicia Cannabis
Thyrotoxic
Thyrotoxicosis, recurrent - E05.90 - Hybrid Cannabis
Tibia Vara - see osteochondrosis, juvenile, tibia
Tic, disorder - F95.9 - Hybrid Cannabis
Tick-Borne - see condition
Tietze's Disease or syndrome - M94.0 - Hybrid Cannabis
Tight, tightness
Tilting vertebra - see dorsopathy, deforming, specified NEC
Timidity, child - F93.8 - Cannabidiol (CBD)
Tin Miners Lung - J63.5 - Hybrid Cannabis
Tinea, intersect, tarsi - B35.9 - Salvia Cannabis
Tingling Sensation, skin - R20.2 - Salvia Cannabis
Tinnitus, audible, subjective - H93.1 - Hybrid Cannabis
Tipped Tooth, teeth - M26.33 - Caryophyllene (CB2)
Tipping
Tiredness - R53.83 - Hybrid Cannabis
Tissue - see condition
Tobacco, nicotine
Tocopherol Deficiency - E56.0 - Hybrid Cannabis
Todd's
Toe - see condition
Toilet, artificial opening - see attention to, artificial, opening
Tokelau, ringworm - B35.5 - Hybrid Cannabis
Tollwut - see Rabies
Tommaselli's Disease - R31.9 - Hybrid Cannabis
Tongue - see also condition
Tonic Pupil - see anomaly, pupil, function, tonic pupil
Toni-Fanconi Syndrome, cystinosis - E72.09 - Hybrid Cannabis
Tonsil - see condition
Tonsillitis, acute, catarrhal, croupous, follicular, gangrenous, infective, lacunar, lingual, malignant, membranous, parenchymatous, phlegmonous, pseudomembranous, purulent, septic, subacute, suppurative, toxic, ulcerative, vesicular, viral - J03.90 - Indicia Cannabis
Tooth, teeth - see condition
Toothache - K08.8 - Cannabidiol (CBD)
Topagnosis - R20.8 - Indicia Cannabis
Tophi - see gout, chronic

Torch Infection - see Infection, congenital
Torn - see tear
Tornwaldt's Cyst or Disease - J39.2 - Hybrid Cannabis
Torsion
Torticollis, intermittent, spastic - M43.6 - Indicia Cannabis
Tortipelvis - G24.1 - Salvia Cannabis
Tortuous
Torture, victim of - Z65.4 - Hybrid Cannabis
Torula, torula, infection - see cryptococcosis
Torulosis - see cryptococcosis
Torus, mandibular - M27.0 - Cannabidiol (CBD)
Touraine's Syndrome - Q79.8 - Hybrid Cannabis
Tourette's Syndrome - F95.2 - Cannabidiol (CBD)
Tourniquet Syndrome - external, by site
Tower Skull - Q75.0 - Caryophyllene (CB2)
Toxemia - R68.89 - Indicia Cannabis
Toxemia Cerebral Psychic, nonalcoholic - F04 - Indicia Cannabis
Toxic, poisoning - see also condition - T65.91 - Cannabidiol (CBD)
Toxemia - see toxemia
Toxicity - see drugs and chemicals, by substance, poisoning
Toxicosis - see also toxemia
To Infection, gastrointestinal - K52.1 - Salvia Cannabis
Toxocariasis - B83.0 - Hybrid Cannabis
Toxoplasma, toxoplasmosis, acquired - B58.9 - Hybrid Cannabis
Tpa (Rtpa) Z92.82 - Indicia Cannabis
Trabeculation, bladder - N32.89 - Hybrid Cannabis
Trachea - see condition
Tracheitis, catarrhal,infantile, membranous, plastic, septal suppurative, viral - J04.10 - Salvia Cannabis
Tracheitis, nonvenereal - see cervicitis
Tracheobronchial - see condition
Tracheobronchitis see also bronchitis
Tracheobronchomegaly - Q32.4 - Salvia Cannabis
Tracheobronchopneumonitis - see Pneumonia, broncho
Tracheocele, external, internal - J39.8 - Indicia Cannabis
Tracheomalacia - J39.8 - Hybrid Cannabis
Tracheopharyngitis, acute - J06.9 - Hybrid Cannabis
Tracheostenosis - J39.8 - Hybrid Cannabis
Tracheostomy

Trachoma - trachomatous - A71.9 - Hybrid Cannabis
Traction, vitreomacular - H43.82- Salvia Cannabis
Train Sickness - T75.3 - Hybrid Cannabis
Trait (s)
Tramp - Z59.0 - Caryophyllene (CB2)
Trance - R41.89 - Salvia Cannabis
Transaction
Transaminasemia - R74.0 - Indicia Cannabis
Transfusion
Transient - meaning homeless - see also condition - Z59.0 - Indicia Cannabis
Translocation
Translucency, iris - see degeneration
Transmission of chemical substances through the placenta - see absorption, chemical, through placenta
Transparency - lung, unilateral - J43.0 - Indicia Cannabis
Transplant (ed), status - Z94.9 - Salvia Cannabis
Transplants - ovarian, endometrial - N80.1 - Cannabidiol (CBD)
Transposed - see transposition
Transposition - congenital - see also malposition, congenital
Transsexualism - F64.1 - Hybrid Cannabis
Transverse - see also condition
Transvestism - transvestitism, dual-role - F64.1 Hybrid cannabis
Trapped Placenta, with hemorrhage - O72.0 - Cannabidiol (CBD)
Trauma - traumatism - see also Injury
Traumatic - see also condition
Treacher Collins Syndrome - Q75.4 - Indicia Cannabis
Treitz's Hernia - see hernia, abdomen, specified site NEC
Trematode Infestation - see infestation
Trematodiasis - see infestation, fluke
Trembling Paralysis - see parkinsonism
Tremor (s) - R25.1 - Hybrid Cannabis
Trench
Treponema Pallidum Infection - see Syphilis
Treponematosis
Triad
Trichiasis - eyelid - H02.059 - Hybrid Cannabis
Trichinella Spiralis, infection, infestation - B75 - Hybrid Cannabis
Trichinellosis - trichiniasis, trichinosis - B75 - Hybrid Cannabis
Trichobezoar - T18.9 - Caryophyllene (CB2)

Trichocephaliasis - B79 - Hybrid Cannabis
Trichocephalus Infestation - B79 - Hybrid Cannabis
Trichoclasis - L67.8 - Indicia Cannabis
Trichoepithelioma - see also neoplasm, skin, benign
Trichofolliculoma - see neoplasm, skin, benign
Tricholemmoma - see neoplasm, skin, benign
Trichomoniasis - A59.9 - Salvia Cannabis
Trichomycosis
Trichonodosis - L67.8 - Hybrid Cannabis
Trichophytic - Trichophyton infection - see dermatophytosis
Trichophytobezoar - T18.9 - Salvia Cannabis
Trichophytosis - see Dermatophytosis
Trichoptilosis - L67.8 - Indicia Cannabis
Trichorrhexis - L67.0 - Salvia Cannabis
Trichinosis - A48.8 - Hybrid Cannabis
Trichosporosis nodose - B36.2 - Salvia Cannabis
Trichostasis spinulose - congenital - Q84.1 - Hybrid Cannabis
Trichostrongyliasis - trichostrongyliasis, small intestine - B81.2 - Salvia Cannabis
Trichostrongylus Infection - B81.2 - Cannabidiol (CBD)
Trichotillomania - F63.3 - Indicia Cannabis
Trichromat - achromatopsia, anomalous, congenital - H53.55 - Hybrid Cannabis
Trichuriasis - B79 - Indicia Cannabis
Trichuris Trichiurid - infection, infestation, any site - B79 - Hybrid Cannabis
Tricuspid - valve - see condition
Trifid - see also accessory
Trigeminal Neuralgia - see neuralgia, trigeminal
Trigeminy - R00.8 - Indicia Cannabis
Trigger Finger (acquired) - M65.30 - Hybrid Cannabis
Trigonitis - bladder, chronic, pseudomembranous - N30.30 - Hybrid Cannabis
Trigonocephaly - Q75.0 - Hybrid Cannabis
Trilocular Heart - see cor trilocular
Trimethylaminuria - E72.52 - Indicia Cannabis
Tripartite Placenta - O43.19- - Caryophyllene (CB2)
Triphalangeal Thumb - Q74.0 - Indicia Cannabis
Triple - see also accessory
Triplegia - G83.89 - Hybrid Cannabis
Triplet, newborn - see also newborn, triplet
Triplication - see accessory

Triploidy - Q92.7 - Hybrid Cannabis
Trismus - R25.2 - Hybrid Cannabis
Trisomy Syndrome - Q92.9- Hybrid Cannabis
Tritanomaly, tritanopia - H53.55 Hybrid Cannabis
Trombiculosis - trombiculiasis, trombiculosis - B88.0 - Hybrid Cannabis
Trophedema - congenital, hereditary - Q82.0 - Salvia Cannabis
Trophoblastic Disease - see also mole, hydatidiform - O01.9 - Hybrid Cannabis
Tropholymphedema - Q82.0 - Indicia Cannabis
Trophoneurosis (NEC) - G96.8 - Cannabidiol (CBD)
Tropical - see condition
Trouble - see also disease
Trousseau's Syndrome, thrombophlebitis migrants - I82.1 - Hybrid Cannabis
Truancy, childhood
Truncus
Trunk - see condition
Trypanosomiasis
T-shaped Incisors - K00.2 - Salvia Cannabis
Tsutsugamushi Disease, fever - A75.3 - Cannabidiol (CBD)
Tube - tubal, tubular - see condition
Tubercle - see also Tuberculosis
Tuberculid - tuberculate, indurating, subcutaneous, lichenoid, military papule necrotic, primary, skin - A18.4 - Indicia Cannabis
Tuberculoma - see also tuberculosis
Tuberculosis - tubercular, tuberculous, calcification, calcified, caseous chromogenic acid-fast bacilli, degeneration, fibrocaseous, fistula interstitial, isolated circumscribed lesions, necrosis
Tuberculum
Tuberosity - entire maxillary - M26.07 - Salvia Cannabis
Tuberous sclerosis, brain - Q85.1
Tubo-ovarian - see condition
Tuboplasty - after previous sterilization - Z31.0 - Hybrid Cannabis
Tubotympanitis, catarrhal, chronic - see otitis, media, nonsuppurative, chronic, serious
Tularemia - A21.9 - Indicia Cannabis
Tularensis Conjunctivitis - A21.1 - Hybrid cannabis
Tumefaction - see also swelling
Tumor - see also neoplasm, unspecified behavior, by site
Tumor Lysis Syndrome - following antineoplastic chemotherapy spontaneous - E88.3 - Hybrid Cannabis

Tumorlet - see neoplasm, uncertain behavior, by site
Tungiasis - B88.1 - Hybrid Cannabis
Tunica Vascular Lentils - Q12.2 - Hybrid Cannabis
Turban Tumor - D23.4 - Indicia Cannabis
Türck's Trachoma - J37.0 - Cannabidiol (CBD)
Turner-Kieser Syndrome - Q79.8 - Hybrid Cannabis
Turner-Like Syndrome - Q87.1 - Hybrid Cannabis
Turner's
Turner-Ullrich Syndrome - Q96.9 - Hybrid Cannabis
Tussis Convulsive - see whooping cough
Twiddler's Syndrome, due to
Twilight State
Twin - newborn - see also newborn, twin
Twinning, teeth - K00.2 - Indicia Cannabis
Twist - twisted
Twitching - R25.3 - Indicia Cannabis
Tylosis (acquired) - L84 - Hybrid Cannabis
Tympanic - R14.0 - Indicia Cannabis
Tympanites - abdominal, intestinal - R14.0 - Hybrid Cannabis
Tympanitis - see myringitis
Tympanosclerosis - H74.0 - Hybrid Cannabis
Tympanum - see condition
Tympany
Type A Behavior Pattern - Z73.1 - Hybrid Cannabis
Typhlitis - see appendicitis
Typhoenteritis - see typhoid
Typhoid - abortive, ambulant, any site, clinical, fever hemorrhagic, infection, intermittent, malignant rheumatic, Widal negative - A01.00 - Indicia Cannabis
Typhomalarial - fever - see malaria
Typhomania - A01.00 - Hybrid Cannabis
Typhoperitonitis - A01.09 - Cannabidiol (CBD)
Typhus - fever - A75.9 - Indicia Cannabis
Tyrosinemia - E70.21 - Hybrid Cannabis
Tyrosinosis - E70.21 - Hybrid Cannabis
Tyrosinemia - E70.29 - Hybrid Cannabis

U

Uhl's Anomaly or disease - Q24.8 - Hybrid Cannabis

Ulcer - ulcerated, ulcerating, ulceration, ulcerative
Ulcerosa Scarlatina - A38.8 - Indicia Cannabis
Ulcus - see also ulcer - Hybrid Cannabis
Ulegyria - Q04.8 - Hybrid Cannabis
Ulerythema
Ullrich - Bonnevie, Turner - Q87.1 - Salvia Cannabis
Ullrich-Feichtiger Syndrome
Ulnar - see condition
Umbilicus - umbilical - see condition
Unacceptable
Unavailability (of)
Uncinaria Americana Infestation - B76.1 Hybrid Cannabis
Uncinariasis - B76.9 - Hybrid Cannabis
Uncongenial Work - Z56.5 - Salvia Cannabis
Unconscious (ness) - see coma
Under Observation - see observation
Underachievement in school - Z55.3 - Hybrid Cannabis
Underdevelopment - see also undeveloped
Underdosing - see also Table of Drugs and Chemicals, categories - T36- Hybrid Cannabis
Underfeeding - newborn - P92.3 - Cannabidiol (CBD)
Underfill - endodontic - M27.53 - Hybrid Cannabis
Underimmunization Status - Z28.3 - Salvia Cannabis
Undernourishment - see malnutrition
Undernutrition - see malnutrition
Underweight - R63.6 - Indicia Cannabis
Underwood's Disease - P83.0 - Indicia Cannabis
Undescended - see also malposition, congenital
Undeveloped - undeveloped - see also hypoplasia
Undiagnosed Disease - R69 - Indicia Cannabis
Undulant Fever - see brucellosis
Unemployment - anxiety concerning - Z56.0 - Salvia Cannabis
Unequal Length - acquired, limb - see also deformity, leg, unequal length
Unextracted Dental Root - K08.3 - Hybrid Cannabis
Unguis Incarnate - L60.0 - Hybrid Cannabis
Unhappiness - R45.2 - Indicia Cannabis
Unicornate Uterus - Q51.4 - Indicia Cannabis
Unilateral - see also condition
Unilocular Heart - Q20.8 - Cannabidiol (CBD)

Union - abnormal - see also fusion
Universal Mesentery - Q43.3 - Hybrid Cannabis
Unrepairable Overhanging of dental restorative materials - K08.52 - Cannabidiol (CBD)
Unsatisfactory
Unsoundness of Mind - see psychosis
Unstable
Unsteadiness on Feet - R26.81 - Salvia Cannabis
Untruthfulness - Child Problem - F91.8 Cannabidiol (CBD)
Unverricht - Lundborg - see epilepsy, generalized, idiopathic
Unwanted Pregnancy - Z64.0 - Hybrid Cannabis
Upbringing - institutional - Z62.22 - Cannabidiol (CBD)
Upper Respiratory - see condition
Upset
Urachus - see also condition
Urbach-Oppenheim Disease - necrobiosis lipoidica diabeticorum - see E08 - E13 with -620 - Hybrid Cannabis
Urbach's Lipoid Proteinases - E78.89 - Salvia Cannabis
Urbach-Wiethe Disease - E78.89 - Hybrid Cannabis
Urban Yellow Fever - A95.1 - Hybrid Cannabis
Urea
Uremia - uremic - N19 - Hybrid Cannabis
Ureter - ureteral - see condition
Ureteralgia - N23 - Cannabidiol (CBD)
Ureterectasis
Ureteritis
Ureterocele - N28.89 - Indicia Cannabis
Ureterolith - ureterolithiasis - see calculus, ureter
Ureterostomy
Urethra - urethral - see condition
Urethralgia - R39.89 - Hybrid Cannabis
Urethritis - anterior, posterior - N34.2 - Hybrid Cannabis
Urethrocele - N81.0 - Cannabidiol (CBD)
Ureterolithiasis - with colic or infection - N21.1 - Hybrid Cannabis
Urethrorectal - see condition
Urethrorrhagia - N36.8 - Hybrid Cannabis
Urethrorrhea - R36.9 - Salvia Cannabis
Urethrostomy
Urethrotrigonitis - see trigonitis

Urethrovaginal - see condition
Urgency
Uric Acid in blood, increased - E79.0 - Indicia Cannabis
Uricacidemia - asymptomatic - E79.0 - Cannabidiol (CBD)
Uricemia, asymptomatic - E79.0 - Salvia Cannabis
Uricosuria - R82.99 - Indicia Cannabis
Urinary - see condition
Urination
Urine
Urinemia - see uremia
Urinoma - urethra - N36.8 - Hybrid Cannabis
Uroarthritis, infectious, Reiter's - see reiter's disease
Urolithiasis - see calculus, urinary
Uronephrosis - see hydronephrosis
Uropathy - N39.9 - Salvia Cannabis
Urosepsis - code to condition
Urticaria - L50.9 - Hybrid Cannabis
Usher-Senear Disease or Syndrome - L10.4 - Hybrid Cannabis
Uta - B55.1 - Hybrid Cannabis
Uterovaginal - see condition
Ureterovesical - see condition
Uveal - see condition
Uveitis - anterior - see also Iridocyclitis
Uveoencephalitis - see Inflammation, chorioretinal
Uveokeratitis - see Iridocyclitis
Uveoparotitis - D86.89 - Hybrid Cannabis
Uvula - see condition
Uvulitis - acute, catarrhal, chronic, membranous, suppurative, ulcerative - K12.2 - Cannabidiol (CBD)

V

Vaccination - prophylactic
Vaccinia - generalized, localized - T88.1 - Hybrid Cannabis
Vacuum - in sinus, accessory, nasal - J34.89 - Indicia Cannabis
Vagabond - vagabondage - Z59.0 - Hybrid Cannabis
Vagabond's Disease - B85.1 - Hybrid Cannabis
Vagina - vagina - see condition
Vaginalitis - tunica, testis - N49.1 - Hybrid Cannabis
Vaginismus - reflex - N94.2 - Hybrid Cannabis

Vaginitis, acute, circumscribed, diffuse, emphysematous, nonvenereal, ulcerative - N76.0 - Hybrid Cannabis
Vaginosis - see vaginitis
Vagotonia - G52.2 - Salvia Cannabis
Vagrancy - Z59.0 - Indicia Cannabis
Vain - see neoplasia, intraepithelial, vagina
Vallecula - see condition
Valley Fever - B38.0 - Indicia Cannabis
Valsuani's Disease - see anemia, obstetric
Valve - valvular, formation - see also condition
Valvulitis - chronic - see endocarditis
Valvulopathy - see endocarditis
Van Bogaert's Leukoencephalopathy, sclerosing, subacute - A81.1 - Hybrid Cannabis
Van Bogaert-Scherer-Epstein Disease or Syndrome - E75.5 - Hybrid Cannabis
Van Buchem's Syndrome - M85.2 - Hybrid Cannabis
Van Creveld-Von Gierke Disease - E74.01 - Hybrid Cannabis
Van Der Hoeve - -de Kleyn - Q78.0 - Caryophyllene (CB2)
Van Der Woude's Syndrome - Q38.0 - Hybrid Cannabis
Van Neck's Disease or osteochondrosis - M91.0 - Hybrid Cannabis
Vanishing Lung - J44.9 - Indicia Cannabis
Vapor Asphyxia or suffocation - T59.9 - Hybrid Cannabis
Variance - lethal ball, prosthetic heart valve - T82.09 - Caryophyllene (CB2)
Variants - Thalassemia - D56.8 - Hybrid Cannabis
Variations in hair color - L67.1 - Cannabidiol (CBD)
Varicella - B01.9 - Indicia Cannabis
Varies-see varix
Varicocele - scrotum, thrombosed - I86.1 - Hybrid Cannabis
Varicose
Varicosis - varicosities, varicosity - see varix
Variola - larger, minor - B03 - Hybrid Cannabis
Varioloid - B03 - Indicia Cannabis
Varix - lower limb, ruptured - I83.90 - Salvia Cannabis
Vas Deferens - see condition
Vas Deferment - N49.1 - Hybrid Cannabis
Vasa Previa - O69.4 - Indicia Cannabis
Vascular - see also condition
Vascularization, cornea - see neovascularization, cornea
Vasculitis - I77.6 - Hybrid Cannabis

Vasculopathy - necrotizing - M31.9 - Hybrid Cannabis
Vasitis and Nodose - N49.1 - Hybrid Cannabis
Vasodilation - I73.9 - Hybrid Cannabis
Vasomotor - see condition
Vaginoplasty - after previous sterilization - Z31.0 - Cannabidiol (CBD)
Vasospasm - vasoconstriction - I73.9 - Hybrid Cannabis
Vasospastic - see condition
Vasovagal Attack, paroxysmal - R55 - Salvia Cannabis
Vater Syndrome - Q87.2 - Caryophyllene (CB2)
Vater's Ampulla - see condition
Vegetation - vegetative
Veil
Vein, venous - see condition
Veldt Sore - see ulcer, skin
Velpeau's Hernia - see hernia, femoral
Venereal
Venofibrosis - I87.8 - Hybrid Cannabis
Venom - venomous - see Table of Drugs and Chemicals, by animal or substance, poisoning
Venous - see condition
Ventilator lung - newborn - P27.8 - Cannabidiol (CBD)
Ventral - see condition
Ventricle - ventricular - see also condition
Ventriculitis - cerebral - see also encephalitis G04.90 - Hybrid Cannabis
Ventriculostomy Status - Z98.2 - Hybrid Cannabis
Vernet's Syndrome - G52.7 - Hybrid Cannabis
Verneuil's Disease - syphilitic bursitis - A52.78 - Cannabidiol (CBD)
Verruca - due to (HPV), filiform, simplex, viral, Vulgaris - B07.9 - Hybrid Cannabis
Varicosities - see verruca
Verruga Peruana - Peruvian - A44.1 - Salvia Cannabis
Version
Vertebra - vertebral - see condition
Vertical Talus - congenital - Q66.80 - Hybrid Cannabis
Vertigo - R42 - Indicia Cannabis
Very Low-Density-Lipoprotein-Type (VLDL) - E78.1 - Salvia Cannabis
Vesania - see psychosis
Vesical - see condition
Vesicle
Vesicocolic - see condition

Vesicoperineal - see condition
Vesicorectal - see condition
Vesicourethrorectal - see condition
Vesicovaginal - see condition
Vesiculiti - seminal - N49.0 - Hybrid Cannabis
Vestibulitis - ear - see also subcategory - H83.0 - Hybrid Cannabis
Vestibulopathy - acute peripheral, recurrent - see neuronitis, vestibular
Vestige - vestigial - see also persistence
Vibration
Vibriosis - A28.9 - Cannabidiol (CBD)
Victim (of)
Vidal's Disease - L28.0 - Salvia Cannabis
Villaret's Syndrome - G52.7 - Hybrid Cannabis
Villous - see condition
Vin - see neoplasia, intraepithelial, vulva
Vincent's Infection - angina, gingivitis - A69.1 - Hybrid Cannabis
Vinson Plummer Syndrome - D50.1 - Salvia Cannabis
Violence - physical - R45.6 - Indicia Cannabis
Viosterol Deficiency - see deficiency, calciferol
Vipoma - see neoplasm, malignant, by site
Viremia - B34.9 - Indicia Cannabis
Virilism - adrenal - E25.9 - Salvia Cannabis
Virilization - female, suprarenal - E25.9 - Hybrid Cannabis
Virulent Bubo - A57 - Hybrid Cannabis
Virus Viral - see also condition
Viscera - visceral - see condition
Visceroptosis - K63.4 - Cannabidiol (CBD)
Visible Peristalsis - R19.2 - Hybrid Cannabis
Vision - visual
Vitality - lack or want of - R53.83 - Hybrid Cannabis
Vitamin Deficiency - see deficiency, vitamin
Vitelline Duct - persistent - Q43.0 - Indicia Cannabis
Vitiligo - L80 - Hybrid Cannabis
Vitreal Corneal Syndrome - H59.01 - Caryophyllene (CB2)
Vitreoretinopathy - proliferative - see also retinopathy, proliferative
Vitreous - see also condition
Vocal Cord - see condition
Vogt-Koyanagi Syndrome - H20.82 - Hybrid Cannabis
Vogt's Disease or Syndrome - G80.3 - Salvia Cannabis

Vogt-Spielmeyer Amaurotic Idiocy or illness - E75.4 - Hybrid Cannabis
Voice
Volhynian Fever - A79.0 - Hybrid Cannabis
Volkmann's Ischemic Contracture or paralysis - complicating trauma - T79.6 - Hybrid Cannabis
Volvulus - bowel, colon, duodenum, intestine - K56.2 - Salvia Cannabis
Vomiting - R11.10 - Indicia Cannabis
Vomito - see fever, yellow
Von Bezold's Abscess - see mastoiditis, acute
Von Economo-Cruchet Disease - A85.8 - Hybrid Cannabis
Von Eulenburg's Disease - G71.19 - Hybrid Cannabis
Von Gierke's Disease - E74.01 - Indicia Cannabis
Von Hippel - Lindau - Q85.8 - Hybrid Cannabis
Von Jaksch's Anemia or Disease - D64.89 - Hybrid Cannabis
Von Recklinghausen
Von Schroetter's Syndrome - I82.890 - Salvia Cannabis
Von Willebrand - Jurgens, Minot - D68.0 - Cannabidiol (CBD)
Von Zumbusch's Disease - L40.1 - Hybrid Cannabis
Voyeurism - F65.3 - Indicia Cannabis
Vrolik's Disease - Q78.0 - Hybrid Cannabis
Vulva - see condition
Vulvitis - N94.2 - Hybrid Cannabis
Vulvitis - acute, allergic, atrophic, hypertrophic, intertriginous, senile - N76.2 - Hybrid Cannabis
Vulvodynia - N94.819 - Cannabidiol (CBD)
Vulvovaginitis - acute - see vaginitis

W

Waiting List - person on - Z75.1 - Indicia Cannabis
Waldenström-Kjellberg Syndrome - D50.1 - Salvia Cannabis
Waldenström
Walking
Wall - abdominal - see condition
Wallenberg's Disease or syndrome - G46.3 - Hybrid Cannabis
Wallgren's Disease - I87.8 - Hybrid Cannabis
Wandering
War Neurosis - F48.8 - Caryophyllene (CB2)
Wart due to (HPV), filiform, infectious, viral - B07.9 - Hybrid Cannabis

Warthin's Tumor - also see neoplasm, salivary gland, benign
Vassiliev's Disease - A27.0 Hybrid Cannabis
Wasting
Water
Waterbrash - R12 - Hybrid Cannabis
Waterhouse - Friderichsen, syndrome or illness, meningococcal - A39.1 - Hybrid Cannabis
Water Losing Nephritis - N25.89 - Hybrid Cannabis
Watermelon Stomach - K31.819 - Hybrid Cannabis
Watsoniasis - B66.8 - Indicia Cannabis
Wax in Ear - see Impaction, cerumen
Weak - weakening, weakness, generalized - R53.1 - Salvia Cannabis
Wear - worn, with regular or routine use
Whether Weathered
Weaver's Syndrome - Q87.3 - Hybrid Cannabis
Web - webbed, congenital
Weber-Christian Disease - M35.6 - Hybrid Cannabis
Weber-Cockayne Syndrome Epidermolysis Bullosa - Q81.8 - Hybrid Cannabis
Weber-Gubler Syndrome - G46.3 - Salvia Cannabis
Weber-Leyden Syndrome - G46.3 - Indicia Cannabis
Weber-Osler Syndrome - I78.0 - Hybrid Cannabis
Weber's Paralysis or Syndrome - G46.3 - Cannabidiol (CBD)
Wedge Shaped or wedging vertebra - also see collapse, vertebra (NEC)
Wegener's Granulomatosis or Syndrome - M31.30 - Hybrid Cannabis
Wegner's Disease - A50.02 - Hybrid Cannabis
Weight
Weightlessness - effect of - T75.82 - Indicia Cannabis
Weil (I) - Q87.1 - Hybrid Cannabis
Weil's Disease - A27.0 - Hybrid Cannabis
Weingarten's Syndrome - J82 - Hybrid Cannabis
Weir Mitchell's Condition - I73.81 - Caryophyllene (CB2)
Weiss-Baker Syndrome - G90.09 - Hybrid Cannabis
Wells' Disease - L98.3 - Hybrid Cannabis
Wen - see cyst, sebaceous
Wenckebach's Block or phenomenon - I44.1 - Hybrid Cannabis
Werdnig Hoffmann Syndrome - muscular atrophy - G12.0 - Salvia Cannabis
Werlhof's Disease - D69.3 - Indicia Cannabis
Wermer's Illness or syndrome - E31.21 - Hybrid Cannabis

Werner His Disease - A79.0 - Hybrid Cannabis
Werner's Disease or Syndrome - E34.8 - Hybrid Cannabis
Wernicke-Korsakoff's Syndrome or psychosis alcoholic - F10.96 - Hybrid Cannabis
Wernicke-Posadas Disease - B38.9 - Caryophyllene (CB2)
Wernicke's
West African Fever - B50.8 - Hybrid Cannabis
Westphal-Strümpell Syndrome - E83.01 - Hybrid Cannabis
West's Syndrome - see epilepsy, spasms
Wet
Wharton's Duct - see condition
Wheel - see urticaria
Wheezing - R06.2 - Indicia Cannabis
Whiplash Injury - S13.4 - Indicia Cannabis
Whipple's Disease - see also subcategory - M14.8- K90.81 - Salvia Cannabis
Whipworm - disease, infection, infestation - B79 - Cannabidiol (CBD)
Whistling Face - Q87.0 Indicia Cannabis
White - see also condition
Whitehead - L70.0 - Hybrid Cannabis
Whitlow - see also cellulitis, digit
Whitmore's Disease or fever - see melioidosis
Whooping Cough - A37.90 - Cannabidiol (CBD)
Wichman's Asthma - J38.5 - Hybrid Cannabis
Wide Cranial Sutures - newborn - P96.3 - Indicia Cannabis
Widening Aorta - see ectasia, aorta
Wilkie's Disease or Syndrome - K55.1 - Hybrid Cannabis
Wilkinson Sneddon Disease or Syndrome - L13.1 - Hybrid Cannabis
Willebrand, Jürgens - D68.0 - Hybrid Cannabis
Willige-Hunt Disease or Syndrome - G23.1 - Hybrid Cannabis
Wilms' Tumor - C64- Hybrid Cannabis
Wilson-Mikity Syndrome - P27.0 - Salvia Cannabis
Wilson's
Window - see also imperfect, closure
Winter - see condition
Wiskott-Aldrich Syndrome - D82.0 - Hybrid Cannabis
Withdrawal State - see also dependence, drug by type, with withdrawal
Witts' Anemia - D50.8 Indicia Cannabis
Witzelsucht - F07.0 - Hybrid Cannabis

Woakes' Ethmoiditis or syndrome - J33.1 - Cannabidiol (CBD)
Wolff-Hirschhorn Syndrome - Q93.3 - Hybrid Cannabis
Wolff-Parkinson-White Syndrome - I45.6 - Hybrid Cannabis
Wolhynian Fever - A79.0 - Salvia Cannabis
Wolman's Disease - E75.5 - Hybrid Cannabis
Wood Lung or Pneumonitis - J67.8 - Hybrid Cannabis
Wooly - wooly hair, congenital, nevus - Q84.1 - Hybrid Cannabis
Woolsorter's Disease - A22.1 - Hybrid Cannabis
Word
Worm (s) - infection, infestation - see also Infestation, helminth
Worm - Eaten Soles - A66.3 - Hybrid Cannabis
Worn Out - see exhaustion
Worried Well - Z71.1 - Hybrid Cannabis
Worries - R45.82 - Hybrid Cannabis
Wound - open
Wound - superficial - see Injury - see also specified injury type
Wright's Syndrome - G54.0 - Hybrid Cannabis
Wrist - see condition
Wrong Drug - by accident, given in error - see table of drugs and chemicals, by drug, poisoning
Wryneck - see torticollis
Wuchereria - Bancroft - B74.0 - Hybrid Cannabis
Wuchereriasis - B74.0 - Indicia Cannabis
Wuchernde Struma Langhans - C73 - Salvia Cannabis

X

Xanthelasma - eyelid, palpebra rum - H02.60 - Cannabidiol (CBD)
Xanthelasmatosis - essential - E78.2 - Hybrid Cannabis
Xanthinuria - hereditary - E79.8 - Salvia Cannabis
Xanthoastrocytoma
Xanthofibroma - see neoplasm, connective tissue, benign
Xanthogranuloma - D76.3 - Hybrid Cannabis
Xanthoma (s) - primary, hereditary - E75.5 - Cannabidiol (CBD)
Xenophobia - F40.10 - Hybrid Cannabis
Xeroderma - see also Ichthyosis
Xerophthalmia, vitamin deficiency - E50.7 - Hybrid Cannabis
Xerosis
Xerostomia - K11.7 - Salvia Cannabis

Xiphopagus - Q89.4 - Hybrid Cannabis
XO syndrome - Q96.9 - Cannabidiol (CBD)

X

X-Ray (of)
XXXXY Syndrome - Q98.1 - Hybrid Cannabis
XXY Syndrome - Q98.0 - Cannabidiol (CBD)

Y

Yaba Pox, virus disease - B08.72 - Hybrid Cannabis
Yatapoxvirus - B08.70 - Cannabidiol (CBD)
Yawning - R06.89 - Salvia Cannabis
Yaws - A66.9 - Indicia Cannabis
Yeast Infection - B37.9 - also see candidiasis
Yellow
Yersiniosis - see also Infection, Yersinia

Z

Zahorsky's Syndrome, her angina - B08.5- Hybrid Cannabis
Zellweger's Syndrome, - Q87.89 - Cannabidiol (CBD)
Zenker's Diverticulum, esophagus - K22.5 - Caryophyllene (CB2)
Ziehen-Oppenheim Disease - G24.1 - Salvia
Zieve's Syndrome - K70.0 - Hybrid Cannabis
Zinc
Zollinger-Ellison Syndrome - E16.4 - Cannabidiol (CBD)
F40.218 - Zona - see herpes, zoster
Zoophobia
Zoster (herpes) - see herpes, zoster
Zygomycosis - B46.9 - Hybrid Cannabis

INDEX

A

Abdominal pain, 8, 11–12, 14–15, 21, 25, 40, 43, 47, 52, 55, 64, 69, 71–72, 74–76, 79
Abnormal muscles, 17, 49, 80
Acquired hypothyroidism, xiv, 2, 34, 64, 97
Acquired Immune Deficiency Syndrome (AIDS), xiv, 29, 34, 46, 59, 65, 77, 94, 97, 122
Acute Gastritis, xiv, 2, 34, 64
acute myelogenous leukemia (AML), 18, 50, 82
Agoraphobia, xiv, 2, 34, 64, 97, 121
Alcohol, 2, 11–12, 34–35, 45, 65, 105
Alcohol Abuse, xiv, 2, 34, 65
Alcoholism, xiv, 47, 65
alcohol use disorder (AUD), xiv, 2, 35, 65, 97
alcohol withdrawal delirium (AWD), 9, 42, 73, 103
Alzheimer's disease (AD), xiv, 2, 65
Amyloidosis, xiv, 3, 35, 65
Amyloids, xiv, 3, 35, 65, 98
Amyotrophic Lateral Sclerosis (ALS), xv, 15, 21, 48, 66, 79, 84, 98
Anandamide, viii
Angina Pectoris, xv, 3–4, 9, 14, 42, 66, 73, 85, 89, 98, 109

Ankylosis, xv
Anorexia, xv, 3, 35
Anorexia Nervosa, xv, 3, 36, 66, 98
Anxiety, viii, xii, 5, 8, 14, 16, 19, 21, 24, 27–28, 34, 36, 38, 40, 42, 44, 47, 50–51, 55, 58–59, 64, 69, 71, 73, 78–79, 82–84, 88, 91–93, 110, 135, 214, 227
Appetite, xii, 12, 16, 24, 41–42, 44–45, 55, 64, 76, 85, 87, 129
Arteriosclerotic Health Disease, xv, 4, 36, 66, 98
Arthritis, xv, 4, 36–37, 51, 67, 83, 87, 98–99, 113, 130
Arthropathy, xv, 4, 37, 67, 140, 200, 218
Asthma, xvi, 10, 36–37, 67, 74, 99, 132, 234
Ataxia, 12, 44, 76–77, 132
Atrophic scarring, 75
Attention-Deficit Hyperactivity Disorder (ADHD), xvi, 37, 67, 99
Autism, 4, 37, 68, 133
autism spectrum disorder (ASD), 68
Autoimmune diseases, ix, xvi, 5, 13, 37, 45, 68, 76, 99, 105
Autonomic neuropathy, 43

B

B-caryophyllene, ix
Bell's Palsy, xvi, 38
Bipolar Disorder, 5, 38, 69, 108
Birthmark, 26, 57, 90, 138
Blisters, 11, 25, 43, 55, 75, 89, 104
Bloating, 22, 52, 69, 85, 139
Blood Pressure, 21, 24, 52, 55
  High, 14, 35, 47, 65, 78, 106
  Low, 69
Body Mass Index (BMI), 19, 50, 82, 139
Bowel movements, 8, 10–11, 40–41, 43–44, 71, 73, 75
Bradykinesia, 20, 51, 83, 141
Brainstem, 15, 48, 79
Brain Tumor, xvi, 5, 38, 69, 101
Breathlessness, 41, 72, 141
Bruxism, 5, 38, 69, 101
Bulimia Nervosa, 6, 25, 38, 69, 99
butane hash oil, x

C

Cachexia, 6, 38, 70, 100, 144
Cancer
  Adrenal cortical, xiv, 2, 34, 64, 97
  Brain tumor, 5
  Endometrial, 11, 43, 74, 104
  Ovarian, 6, 38, 70, 100
  Prostate, 22, 52, 85, 112
  Testicular, 27, 58, 92
  Uterine, 28, 59, 94, 104, 117
Cannabis, viii–ix, xi, 121–22, 125, 135, 140, 145, 150, 156, 159, 161, 164, 168–69, 178, 180–81, 189, 194–96, 205, 209–10, 213, 215, 217–22, 225, 229, 234
Cannabis indica, xii

Cannabis ruderalis, ix
Cannabis sativa, ix–x
Carpal Tunnel Syndrome, 6, 17, 39, 49, 70
Caryophyllene, viii–ix, 164, 176–77, 213–14, 216, 219–20, 222–24, 226–29, 232–34
CB2, viii–ix, 164, 176–77, 213–14, 216, 219–20, 222–24, 226–29, 232–34
Cerebral Cortex, 15, 48, 79
Cerebral Palsy, 6, 39, 53, 70
Cervical Disc Disease, 6, 70, 103
Cervical Disc Disease Degeneration, 6, 70
Charcot Disease. *See* Amyotrophic Lateral Sclerosis (ALS)
Chemotherapy, 7, 39, 70, 101, 150
Chest pain. *See* angina pectoris
Chronic Fatigue Syndrome, 7, 39, 70
Chronic Obstructive Pulmonary Disease (COPD), 10, 74, 104
Chronic Renal Failure (CRF), 7, 40, 71
Clamminess, 14, 47, 78
Clonus, 25, 90
Cocaine, 8, 40, 71, 155
Cocaine Dependence, 8, 40, 71
Colitis Inflammation, 40, 71
Conjunctivitis, 8, 23, 40, 53, 72
Constipation, 2, 8, 17, 21, 24, 28, 34, 41, 52, 54, 59, 64, 69, 72, 81, 93, 158–59
Coordination, 12, 14, 18, 20, 34, 42, 46, 49, 51, 65, 84, 214
Costochondritis, 28, 58, 93, 159
Crohn Disease, 72, 102, 112
Crohn's Disease, 41, 72, 102, 112
Cystic Fibrosis (CF), 8, 41, 72, 102

D

Darier's Disease, 9, 72, 102
Delirium Tremens, 9, 42, 73, 103
Delusions, 9, 23, 42, 54, 73, 87, 165
Depression, viii–x, 3, 10, 14,
    16–17, 20–23, 29, 36, 43–44,
    47–48, 51–52, 54, 59, 66,
    74, 76, 78, 81, 83–84, 87,
    94, 104, 108, 112–13, 166
  Clinical, 16, 36, 48, 108
Dermatomyositis, 9, 42, 73, 103, 167
Diabetes, 9, 23, 42, 47, 54, 73,
    79, 87, 103, 168, 220
Diabetes Mellitus, 9, 12
Diarrhea, 10, 13–14, 25, 28–29, 43,
    45, 47, 55, 59, 72–73, 76–77,
    79, 88, 93–94, 103, 168, 173
Digestive Tract, 3, 7, 39, 70, 72, 107
Disorder
  Behavioral, 15, 47, 79
  Life-troublesome, 23, 54
  Mental, 21, 24, 54, 69, 87
  Metabolic, 9, 17, 42, 49,
    73, 81, 103, 109
  Movement, 20, 88
  Neurological, 26, 29, 44, 57,
    60, 91, 94, 104, 117
  Psychiatric, 14, 46, 78, 99, 106
  Schizoaffective, 23, 54, 87, 113
  Skin, 90, 115
  Temporomandibular Joint,
    12, 26, 57, 91, 101, 116
Diverticulitis, 10, 74, 103
Dizziness, 3, 5, 14, 17–18, 24–26, 38,
    47, 49, 55, 57, 69, 78, 81, 88, 171
Drowsiness, 12–14, 47, 71, 76, 78, 172
Dysmenorrhea, 11, 43, 74–75, 173
Dysthymic Disorder, 10, 43, 74, 104

E

Eczema, 10, 74, 104
Ejaculation, 11, 14, 44, 75, 176
Emphysema, 10, 74, 104, 177
  Primary Symptom of, 10, 74
Endometriosis, 11, 43, 69, 75, 104
Epidermolysis Bullosa,
    11, 43, 75, 104
Epididymitis, 11, 44, 75, 104, 180
Erection, 14, 47, 79, 107, 181
Esophagus, 18, 50, 81, 109,
    128, 146, 182
Euphoria, 2–3, 16–17, 24, 26,
    28, 34–35, 55, 57, 59,
    64, 80–81, 88, 91, 93

F

Fear, xiv–xv, 3, 14, 19, 24, 35,
    44, 47, 50, 55, 66, 82,
    88, 97–98, 110, 185
Felty's Syndrome, 11, 44,
    75, 105, 185
Fever, 4, 11, 13–14, 16, 18, 25, 29, 34,
    36, 41, 46–48, 50, 55, 59, 65,
    67, 72, 77–79, 82, 87, 89, 94,
    135, 140, 142, 147, 166, 173,
    182, 185–86, 199, 219, 231
Fibromyalgia, xii, 12, 44, 76, 105
Flajani-Basedow-Graves disease.
    See Graves' disease
Friedreich's Ataxia (FRDA),
    12, 44, 76, 105

G

Gastritis, 12, 25, 45, 55,
    76, 105, 192–93
Genital Herpes, 12, 45, 76, 105

Glaucoma, 12, 19, 45, 76, 82, 90, 105, 194
Glioblastoma Multiforme (GBM), 12, 45, 76, 105
Graves' Disease, 13, 76, 105

H

Hallucinations, 23, 54, 78, 87, 198
Headache, 5, 7, 12–13, 22, 24–27, 38–39, 41, 45–46, 52, 55, 57, 69–70, 72, 76–77, 81, 88–89, 92, 148, 199
   Cluster, 7, 40, 71
   Migraine, 12, 17, 81
   Tension, 27, 57, 92
Heart Attack, 20, 28, 50–51, 58, 83, 111
Hemophilia, 77
Hemophilia A, 13, 77
Henoch-Schonlein Purpura, 13, 46, 77, 106
Hepatitis C, 13, 16, 29, 46, 59, 77, 94, 106, 204
hepatitis C virus (HCV), 29, 46, 59, 94, 106
herpes simplex virus (HSV), 12, 25, 45, 55, 76, 89, 114
herpes simplex virus (HSV-1) type 1, 12, 89
Hood syndrome. *See* nail-patella syndrome
Hormones, 2, 103–4
Hospice, 13, 27, 58, 78, 92, 106
Human Immunodeficiency Virus (HIV), 13, 46, 77, 106, 204
Huntington's Disease, 14, 46, 78, 106, 205
Hyperkinetic disorder. *See* Attention-Deficit Hyperactivity Disorder (ADHD)
Hypertension, 14, 47, 78, 106, 130, 146, 175, 209–10
Hyperventilation, 14, 47, 209–10, 221
Hypoglycemia, 14, 47, 78, 107

I

Immune System, xv, 5, 18, 37, 48–49, 68, 80–81, 98–99, 108
Impairment, 37, 67, 86, 94, 213
Impotence, 14, 47, 79, 107, 214
Infection, xiv, 5, 8, 12–14, 21, 23, 25, 29, 37, 40–42, 44–47, 53, 56, 59, 65, 72, 76–77, 79, 86, 89, 94, 105–6, 115, 117, 119, 126, 131, 134, 143, 160–61, 167–69, 171, 175, 179, 181–82, 195–97, 204, 207, 215, 223
   Frequent, 9, 18, 50, 82
   Opportunistic, xiv, 29, 34, 59, 65, 94, 97
   Viral, 8, 72
Inflammation, xiv–xv, 2, 4, 8, 12–13, 21–23, 25, 28–29, 34, 36–37, 44–46, 53, 55, 58–59, 64, 67, 72, 76–77, 85, 89, 94, 97, 99, 102, 104–6, 147, 153, 163, 181, 218, 226
Inflammatory Bowel Disease (IBD), 14, 41, 47, 72, 79, 107
Insomnia, viii–ix, xii, 16, 20–21, 24, 27–28, 51, 55, 58–59, 83–84, 93, 111, 216
Insulin, 9, 12, 42, 73, 103
Insulin Dependent Mellitus (IDDM), 42, 73, 103

Intermittent Explosive Disorder (IED), 15, 47, 79, 107
Irritability, 8, 10, 14, 27-28, 40, 43, 47, 58-59, 71, 74, 78, 85, 93, 108, 217

L

Leri Disease. *See* melorheostosis
Lou Gehrig's disease. *See* Amyotrophic Lateral Sclerosis (ALS)
Lyme Disease, xvi, 16, 48, 80, 108
Lymphocytes, 16, 48, 80
Lymphoma, 16, 108, 112, 204, 224, 229-30

M

Malignant Melanoma, 16, 49, 80, 108
Malnutrition, 3, 36, 66, 72, 145, 176, 232
Melanocytes, 16, 49, 80, 108
Melanomas, 16, 49, 80, 108
Melorheostosis, 17, 49, 80
Meniere's Disease, 17, 81
Morphine, 20, 50, 83
Motion Sickness, 17, 81, 89
Mucopolysaccharidosis (MPS), 17, 49, 81, 109
Mucoviscidosis. *See* Cystic Fibrosis (CF)
Multiple Sclerosis (MS), xii, 18, 49, 81, 109
Muscle Spasm, xii, 109
Muscular Dystrophy, 18, 82, 110
Myelin, 18, 49, 81, 109

N

Nail-Patella Syndrome, 19, 82, 110
Nausea, viii, xii, 2-3, 12, 15-16, 25, 29, 34, 45-46, 48, 55, 59, 64-65, 71, 76-77, 86, 94
Nerves
  Peripheral, 20-21, 51, 84, 111
  Trigeminal, 27, 58, 90, 92
Nervous System, 9, 12, 24, 28, 42, 51, 59, 73, 83, 93, 103, 108, 110-11, 117
  Central, 20, 24, 44, 50, 55, 88, 104, 110
  Peripheral, 25, 89, 110
  Somatic, 25, 89, 115
Nicotine Dependence. *See* tobacco dependence
Nightmares, 19, 22, 24, 50, 52, 55, 82, 84, 110

O

Obesity, 2, 14, 19, 50, 82, 107, 120, 159, 185
Obsession, 19, 50, 66, 69, 83
OCD (Obsessive-Compulsive Disorder), 19, 50, 83
Opiate dependence, 20, 50, 83
Osteoarthritis, 20-21, 51-52, 72, 83-84, 112, 130

P

PAD (peripheral arterial disease), 9, 73
Palpitations, 13, 20, 27, 45, 51, 58, 76, 83
Panic disorder, 20, 51, 83, 111
Paralysis, 4, 20, 26, 51, 53, 57, 84, 86, 143, 150, 171, 181, 220, 222

Parkinson's disease, 20, 51, 83, 111
Penis, 11, 27, 44, 58, 75, 92, 148–49
Peripheral neuropathy, 20, 51, 84, 111
Peritoneal dialysis, 21, 84, 111
Peritoneal Pain, 21, 84, 111
Persistent insomnia. *See* insomnia
Phobia, 2, 14, 34, 47, 64
Pink eye. *See* conjunctivitis
PMS (Premenstrual Syndrome), 22, 52, 85, 112
Porphyria, 21, 52, 111, 201
Porphyrin, 111
PPS (Post-polio Syndrome), 21, 52, 84, 112
Prostate gland, 22–23, 52–53
Prostatitis, 22, 53, 85
Proteins, 3, 13, 19, 45, 82, 110–11
Psoriasis, 22, 53, 85, 112
PTSD (Post-Traumatic Stress Disorder), 22, 52, 84, 112
Pulmonary fibrosis, 22, 53, 85, 112

R

Radiation Therapy, 23, 53, 86
Raynaud's disease, 23, 86
Reflexes, 25, 39, 42, 56, 70, 115, 130, 146, 193, 217
Reiter Syndrome, 23, 86
RLS (Restless Legs Syndrome), 23, 29, 54, 60, 87, 94, 117
Rosacea, 23, 54, 87, 113

S

Saliva, viii
Sativa, viii–ix, xii, 61, 63–64, 168
Schizophrenia, 23–24, 54, 87, 200, 221
Scoliosis, 21, 24, 52, 54, 84, 88, 114, 221
Scrotum, 27, 43, 58, 92
Seizures, 5, 12, 21, 24, 26, 34, 38–39, 44–45, 52, 55, 57, 65, 69–70, 75, 88, 90, 104, 114, 158
Senile dementia, 24, 55, 88, 114
Sensations, 8, 12, 17, 20–21, 29, 44, 49, 52, 60, 69, 81, 83, 86–87, 92, 94, 101, 105
Sensitivity, 20, 84
Shingles, 25, 55, 89, 114
Sinusitis inflammation, 25, 56
Sleep apnea, 17, 36, 49, 56, 81, 89, 115
Spasticity, 25, 56, 90, 115
Spinal cord, 8, 15, 41, 48, 72, 79, 90, 102, 110, 201
Spinal Stenosis, 25, 56, 90, 115
Sputum, 41, 72, 102
Stress, 11, 14, 21–23, 47, 51–53, 69, 84, 86, 112
Stuttering, 26, 56, 91, 115
SWS (Surge-Weber Syndrome), 26, 57, 90, 115

T

TD (Tardive Dyskinesia), 26, 57, 91, 115
THC (tetrahydrocannabinol), viii–ix, xi–xii, 176, 179–80, 187, 190, 192–93, 195, 198–200, 202, 204, 206–14, 216–22, 224–27, 229–30
Thyroiditis, 27, 58, 199
Tic douloureux. *See* trigeminal neuralgia
Tietze syndrome. *See* costochondritis

Tinnitus, 17, 26, 28, 49, 57–58, 81, 93, 117
Tobacco Dependence, 28, 93, 117
Tourette Syndrome, 28, 93, 117
Trauma, xv, 4, 36, 47, 67, 79, 98, 112, 117
Trichotillomania, 28, 59, 94, 117
Trigeminal neuralgia, 27, 58, 92

U

Ulcers, 25, 42, 55
Uterus, 11, 28, 43, 59, 74–75, 94, 104, 137, 160, 167, 170

V

Virus, 29, 40, 46, 59, 72, 77, 89, 94, 106, 117, 160

W

Weakness, 5, 9, 12, 14–15, 18, 20–21, 25–26, 38, 41–42, 45, 47–49, 51, 56–57, 66, 69, 72–73, 76, 78, 84–85, 90, 111, 223
Weight gain, 2–3, 34–35, 52, 64, 66
Weight loss, 4, 6, 9, 13, 15, 34, 36, 38, 41–42, 46, 48, 65–67, 70, 72–73, 77, 79, 107
Whiplash, 29, 60, 94, 117
Willis-Ekbom disease. *See* RLS restless legs syndrome
Wittmaack-Ekbom syndrome. *See* RLS restless legs syndrome
Writer's cramp, 29, 60, 118

www.ingramcontent.com/pod-product-compliance
Lightning Source LLC
Chambersburg PA
CBHW020626220526
45464CB00001B/44